METHODS AND DESIGNS FOR OUTCOMES RESEARCH

METHODS AND DESIGNS FOR OUTCOMES RESEARCH

2nd Edition

ELINOR G. BORGERT, PhD, MSc

Associate Professor
Department of Healthcare Leadership & Management
College of Health Professions
Medical University of South Carolina
Charleston, South Carolina

KIT N. SIMPSON, DrPH, MPH

Distinguished University Professor
Department of Healthcare Leadership & Management
College of Health Professions
Assistant Director for Pilot Studies
CEDAR Core (Comparative Effectiveness Data Analytics Resources)
Medical University of South Carolina
Charleston, South Carolina

ashp

Any correspondence regarding this publication should be sent to the publisher, American Society of Health-System Pharmacists, 4500 East-West Highway, Suite 900, Bethesda, MD 20814, attention: Special Publishing.

Senior Vice President, Professional Development and Publishing Office: Daniel J. Cobaugh, PharmD, DABAT, FAACT

Senior Editorial Director, Special Publishing: Ryan E. Owens, PharmD, BCPS

Editorial Coordinator, Special Publishing: Güneş Turhanlı, MA

Director, Production and Platform Services, Special Publishing: Johnna M. Hershey, BA

Cover Layout: DeVall Advertising

Cover Art: Mehau Kulyk/Shutterstock.com

Library of Congress Cataloging-in-Publication Data

Names: Bogert, Elinor G. editor | Simpson, Kit N. editor

Title: Methods and designs for outcomes research / [edited by] Elinor G. Bogert, PhD, MSc, Kit N. Simpson, DrPH.

Description: 2nd edition. | Bethesda, MD : ASHP, [2026] | Includes bibliographical references and index. | Summary: "Methods and Designs for Outcomes Research provides a comprehensive overview of the common research designs and statistical methods currently used in epidemiology and outcomes research. The book is organized into four integrated sections, offering comprehensive exploration of key domains in outcomes research. The first section introduces foundational study designs used in health services and clinical research. The second section focuses on statistical analysis. The third section explores the role of real-world evidence (RWE) in healthcare research. The fourth section introduces the principles and practices of pharmacoeconomic evaluations. The sections offer a cohesive and practical framework for assessing outcomes research and balancing theoretical rigor with real-world relevance. The second edition builds upon the foundation from the first edition and showcases the latest developments in study design, statistical methodology, data science, and health economics"-- Provided by publisher.

Identifiers: LCCN 2025053293 (print) | LCCN 2025053294 (ebook) | ISBN 9781585287659 paperback | ISBN 9781585287666 pdf | ISBN 9781585287673 epub

Subjects: LCSH: Outcome assessment (Medical care)--United States

Classification: LCC R853.O87 M48 2026 (print) | LCC R853.O87 (ebook)

LC record available at https://lccn.loc.gov/2025053293

LC ebook record available at https://lccn.loc.gov/2025053294

The authorized representative in the EU for product safety and compliance is Mare Nostrum Group B.V., Mauritskade 21D, 1091 GC Amsterdam, The Netherlands; gpsr@mare-nostrum.co.uk

Print ISBN: 978-1-58528-765-9

PDF ISBN: 978-1-58528-766-6

ePub ISBN: 978-1-58528-767-3

DOI: 10.37573/9781585287666

10 9 8 7 6 5 4 3 2 1

DEDICATION

To Andy, Morgan, Mary, and Gray for their steadfast encouragement throughout.
– E.B.

To Annie and Chris for their patience and support.
– K.S.

Furthermore, we jointly dedicate this book to our colleagues and students from whom we continue to learn so much.

TABLE OF CONTENTS

DOI: 10.37573/9781585287666.FM

ACKNOWLEDGMENTS

We would like to first acknowledge the tremendous contributions of our coauthors who are all experts in their respective fields. Their thoughtful scholarship and commitment to clarity and rigor made this collaborative effort both rewarding and successful. We are also grateful to our colleague Dr. Daniel Brinton for his early encouragement to undertake a second edition.

Special thanks are extended to Dr. Ryan Owens, Senior Editorial Director, and Güneş Turhanlı, Editorial Coordinator of Special Publishing, for their steady guidance, encouragement, and patience throughout the development of this edition. Their attention to detail and commitment to excellence were evident in every phase of the project, and we are beyond grateful for their support. We would similarly like to acknowledge Johnna Hershey, Director of Production and Platform Services, whose behind-the-scenes leadership ensured a smooth and timely production process.

We also extend our heartfelt thanks to the authors of the first edition of *Methods and Designs for Outcomes Research*. Their scholarly contributions provided a strong foundation for this second edition. In several chapters, their original work served as a valuable starting point for updates and revisions. We are grateful for their commitment to advancing the field and for the enduring relevance of their insights. Their work continues to inform and inspire the next generation of outcomes researchers.

DOI: 10.37573/9781585287666.FM

PREFACE TO THE SECOND EDITION

In today's complex and cost-conscious healthcare environment, the ability to generate, interpret, and apply health outcomes research is essential for informed decision-making. The past couple of decades have brought significant advances to the field. Our experiences teaching in colleges of pharmacy, health administration, and graduate studies convinced us of the pressing need for an updated edition of our textbook. As before, we approached leaders within each academic discipline and asked them to author chapters specific to their area of research. The result is a broad and updated overview of the field of outcomes research.

Whether evaluating clinical interventions, shaping policy, or allocating resources, outcomes research provides the methodological backbone for evidence-based practice. This second edition of *Methods and Designs for Outcomes Research* is primarily designed to support graduate students in health-related degree programs, including pharmacy, health administration, medicine, and nursing. It provides a comprehensive overview of the common research designs and statistical methods currently used in epidemiology and outcomes research. We were especially focused on conveying the relationship between study design and statistics and their combined role as tools for the appropriate interpretation of analysis results to guide practice decisions. We prioritized clear explanations over complex mathematical formulas, using healthcare databases and examples to illustrate important concepts.

The textbook is organized into four integrated sections, each offering a comprehensive exploration of key domains in outcomes research. The first section introduces foundational study designs used in health services and clinical research. From descriptive and analytic observational studies to quasi-experimental designs and randomized controlled trials, readers are guided through the strengths, limitations, and appropriate applications of each methodology. Chapters on performance metrics and systematic reviews emphasize the importance of aligning research design with real-world healthcare challenges and synthesizing evidence to inform practice and policy.

Building on this foundation, the second section focuses on statistical analysis, beginning with core concepts, such as data types, distributions, and hypothesis testing. Readers progress from descriptive statistics to multivariable modeling, gaining the analytical tools needed to critically evaluate published research and conduct their own investigations. Emphasis is placed on aligning statistical methods with study design and research questions, ensuring that students understand both the mechanics and strategic application of analysis.

The third section explores the expanding role of real-world evidence (RWE) in healthcare research. With the widespread availability of electronic health records, insurance claims, and patient registries, researchers now have unprecedented access to data generated in routine clinical practice. This section examines the regulatory frameworks, methodological innovations, and ethical considerations that shape the use of real-world data (RWD) in evaluating treatment effectiveness, informing policy, and supporting regulatory decisions. It highlights the growing importance of RWE in areas, such as rare disease research, postmarket surveillance, and health technology assessment.

The fourth section introduces the principles and practices of pharmacoeconomic evaluations, which are essential for assessing the value, affordability, and impact of healthcare interventions. Readers are guided through cost identification, cost-effectiveness analysis, budget-impact modeling, and cost-utility and cost-benefit frameworks. Special attention is given to decision analysis models and patient-centered outcomes, including quality-adjusted life-years

DOI: 10.37573/9781585287666.FM

(QALYs) and utility estimation techniques. These chapters provide a robust foundation for evaluating healthcare interventions in terms of both clinical benefit and economic sustainability, equipping students to contribute meaningfully to policy development, reimbursement decisions, and strategic planning.

Together, these sections offer a cohesive and practical framework for assessing outcomes research, balancing theoretical rigor with real-world relevance. This second edition reflects the latest developments in study design, statistical methodology, data science, and health economics, while maintaining a clear focus on the applications that matter most to students, clinicians, and decision-makers.

This edition also builds upon the strong foundation laid by the contributors to the first edition of *Methods and Designs for Outcomes Research*. We are deeply grateful for their original scholarship, which informed the structure and content of several chapters in this volume. Their insights and examples continue to shape the way outcomes research is taught and practiced, and we acknowledge their lasting impact on the field and on this text.

We hope our readers enjoy and learn from this second edition, and we wish them all the best in their pursuits related to outcomes research!

EDITORS AND CONTRIBUTORS

Editors

Elinor G. Borgert, PhD, MSc

Associate Professor
Department of Healthcare Leadership & Management
College of Health Professions
Medical University of South Carolina
Charleston, South Carolina

Kit N. Simpson, DrPH, MPH

Distinguished University Professor
Department of Healthcare Leadership & Management
College of Health Professions
Assistant Director for Pilot Studies
CEDAR Core (Comparative Effectiveness Data Analytics Resources)
Medical University of South Carolina
Charleston, South Carolina

Contributors

Heather Shaw Bonilha, PhD, CCC-SLP

Professor, Director of the Doctoral Program
Communication Sciences and Disorders
University of South Carolina
Columbia, South Carolina

Anita J. Brogan, PhD, MS

Vice President, Value Evidence, Modeling & Communication
AESARA
San Diego, California

Mary Dooley, PhD

Assistant Professor
Department of Clinical Sciences
College of Health Professions
Medical University of South Carolina
Charleston, South Carolina

Stephanie R. Earnshaw, PhD, MS

Senior Fellow
Medical Decision Modeling Inc.
Indianapolis, Indiana

Jada M. Johnson, MS

Senior Research Analyst
Medical University of South Carolina
Charleston, South Carolina

Jami Jones, PhD, MHA

Professor
Department of Healthcare Leadership & Management
Medical University of South Carolina
Charleston, South Carolina

Zahi Jurdi, DHA

MHA Program Director, Associate Professor
Health Services Policy and Management, Arnold School of Public Health
University of South Carolina
Columbia, South Carolina

DOI: 10.37573/9781585287666.FM

Caitlin Koob, PhD, MS, OTR/L
Research Associate
College of Health Professions
Department of Healthcare Leadership & Management
Medical University of South Carolina
Charleston, South Carolina

Sherry Livingston, PhD
Research Assistant Professor of Biostatistics
Department of Public Health Sciences
Medical University of South Carolina
Charleston, South Carolina

Patrick Mauldin, PhD
Professor (Ret.)
Department of Medicine
Division of General Internal Medicine, Geriatrics, and Palliative Care
Medical University of South Carolina
Charleston, South Carolina

Corey Morrow, PhD, MOT, OTR/L
Assistant Professor
Division of Occupational Therapy, College of Health Professions
Medical University of South Carolina
Charleston, South Carolina

Annie N. Simpson, PhD
Adjunct Professor
Division of Physician Assistant Studies
Medical University of South Carolina
Charleston, South Carolina

Caroline Vass, PhD
Senior Economist
Health Preference Assessments
RTI Health Solutions
Manchester, England

Todd L. Wandstrat, RPh, PharmD
President & Founder
Magnum Futurum Advisors, L.L.C.
Kissimmee, Florida

Ralph Ward, PhD
Research Associate Professor
Department of Public Health Sciences
Medical University of South Carolina
Charleston, South Carolina

Kevin Wiley, PhD, MPH
Assistant Professor
College of Health Professions
Department of Healthcare Leadership & Management
Medical University of South Carolina
Charleston, South Carolina

Dunc Williams, PhD
Associate Professor, Healthcare Financial Management
College of Health Professions, Department of Health Care Leadership & Management
Medical University of South Carolina
Charleston, South Carolina

Sorrel Wolowacz, PhD
Head
European Health Economics
RTI Health Solutions
Manchester, England

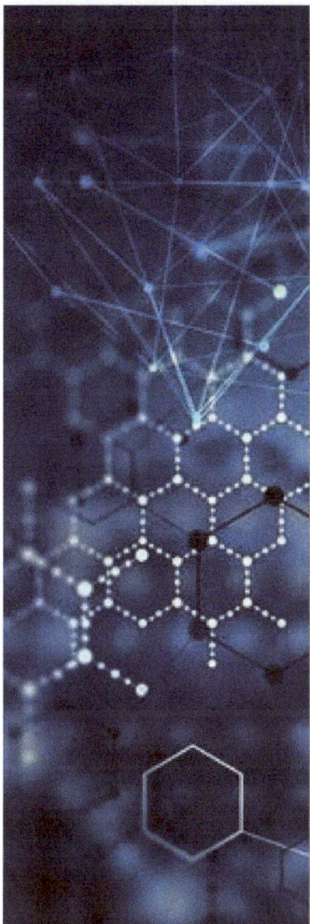

SECTION ONE
Study Design

DOI: 10.37573/9781585287666.TITLE

Introduction to Study Design

1

Elinor G. Borgert, PhD, MSc

Epidemiology is based on the fundamental assumption that bad outcomes (whether diseases or system failures) rarely occur at random, and that both causal and preventive factors can be identified through systematic investigations. Understanding epidemiologic study designs and outcome measures is essential for both interpreting and conducting high-quality research. This section introduces the key methodologies used in health sciences and clinical research, each with their own unique advantages and limitations. Taken as a whole, this provides readers with the tools to evaluate evidence critically and apply the findings to practice and policy.

In Chapter 2, Drs. Jami Jones and Zahi Jurdi introduce the foundational role of metrics in healthcare operations, tracing their evolution from traditional epidemiologic indicators, such as incidence, prevalence, and mortality rates, to more comprehensive performance measures that reflect the complexity of modern healthcare systems. In particular, key performance indicators (KPIs) play a major role in aligning operational goals with strategic objectives and improving patient care. Metrics, such as readmission rates, patient satisfaction scores, and hospital-acquired infection rates, can help to drive quality improvement, enhance accountability, and support strategic decision-making.

Chapter 3 provides a comprehensive overview of observational study designs, focusing on case-control, cohort, and ecologic studies. Whereas descriptive designs, such as case reports and cross-sectional studies, are useful for hypothesis generation, analytic designs that include control groups to assess associations between exposures and outcomes are a step above. A case-control study selects subjects based on whether they do (cases) or do not (controls) have the disease under investigation. The two groups are then compared based on their respective history of exposures. Because the outcome is known at the start of the study, case-control analyses are ideally suited for studying diseases that are rare and/or involve long latency periods.

In contrast, a cohort study enrolls disease-free subjects based on whether or not they were exposed to a suspected risk factor. Eligible participants are then followed for a period of time to determine the number of subjects in both groups who develop the disease. Because cohort studies often involve following a large number of subjects for long periods, they tend to be more time-consuming and expensive than case-control studies. However, by establishing a clear temporal relationship between exposure and disease, they also allow for the direct calculation of risk and by extension, the ubiquitous number needed to treat (NNT). Whereas other study designs under consideration focus on individual effects, ecologic analyses analyze group-level data to identify population-level trends and policy impacts.

Quasi-experimental designs (QEDs) are structured to infer causal relationships and to minimize bias when randomization is not feasible or ethical, essentially serving as a bridge between observational and experimental designs. In Chapter 4, Drs. Simpson and Simpson introduce interrupted time series, difference-in-differences, regression discontinuity, propensity score matching, inverse-probability weighting, and instrumental variable analysis. While most of these designs are not new, researchers have only recently begun to fully appreciate their applications to the large volumes of observational data

DOI: 10.37573/9781585287666.001

generated by electronic health records, billing data, and patient registries.

Chapter 5 covers randomized controlled trials (RCTs), which are widely considered the most rigorous study design in which patients are assigned to a particular therapy based on chance and then monitored for a period of time to determine health outcomes. Drs. Sherry Livingston and Patrick Mauldin integrate discussions of methodological rigor with practical insights, providing a thorough treatment of the design, conduct, and interpretation of RCTs. They outline the phases of clinical trials and include detailed descriptions of trial structures, types of analyses, and randomization methods.

Finally, we conclude this section with a chapter on systematic literature reviews and meta-analyses (Chapter 6). These study designs allow researchers to combine data from previously conducted studies to identify patterns, explain discrepancies, and inform clinical practice and policy. Dr. Heather Shaw Bonilha provides a step-by-step guide to conducting these, from topic selection and feasibility assessment to search strategy development, data extraction, and critical appraisal. She introduces meta-analysis as a powerful extension of systematic reviews, explaining how the statistical pooling of data can enhance precision and reveal treatment effects not evident in individual studies.

Taken together, these chapters provide a comprehensive foundation in study designs and outcome measures, equipping readers to critically evaluate and conduct research across a range of methodologies. Understanding these designs is essential for advancing evidence-based practice, improving healthcare outcomes, and contributing to the scientific community. This section serves as both a primer and a reference for researchers, clinicians, and students committed to rigorous and impactful inquiry.

Metrics in Healthcare Operations

2

Jami Jones, PhD, MHA, and Zahi Jurdi, DHA

INTRODUCTION

Healthcare metrics have evolved significantly over the years, transitioning from a primary focus on traditional epidemiologic measures, such as incidence, prevalence, and mortality rates, to a broader emphasis on population health, including organizational and system operational efficiency and performance outcomes. This shift, as highlighted by Donabedian,[1] reflects the growing complexity of healthcare systems and the need for metrics that capture not only health outcomes but also the effectiveness and quality of service delivery. In modern healthcare management and leadership, the integration of key performance indicators (KPIs) has emerged as a critical tool for improving efficiency, ensuring accountability, and promoting continuous improvement.[2] Key performance indicators enable organizations to assess performance across diverse domains, aligning operational goals with strategic objectives to deliver value-driven care.

This chapter provides a comprehensive exploration of healthcare metrics, beginning with a review of traditional epidemiologic measures and their relevance in contemporary contexts. It then examines the role of KPIs in healthcare management, emphasizing their importance in identifying critical success factors (CSFs) and enhancing both inpatient and outpatient operations. The discussion extends to innovation metrics and the integration of KPIs into performance dashboards, highlighting the practical challenges of developing and implementing effective metrics. The chapter concludes with real-world case studies demonstrating successful KPI implementation and its impact on improved healthcare outcomes, offering insights for healthcare leaders navigating the increasingly data-driven landscape of modern medicine.

TRADITIONAL EPIDEMIOLOGIC METRICS

In epidemiology and outcomes research, incidence and prevalence are the key measures used to understand how often diseases or events occur. Incidence refers specifically to the number of new cases of a disease or event that develop in a population at risk during a specified period of time. For a population to be "at risk," individuals must have the potential to develop the disease or experience the event being studied in a specified time period. For example, in a study examining the incidence of uterine cancer among women aged 50 to 59 in the year 2024, women who had undergone hysterectomies before this period would be excluded from the population at risk.

Incidence or cumulative incidence (CI) calculates the likelihood of new cases occurring in the at-risk population over a period of time. The denominator includes all individuals who are at risk of potentially developing the disease, whereas the numerator is just the new cases that develop during the study period. Incidence allows researchers to assess how frequently new cases arise and estimate the risk

DOI: 10.37573/9781585287666.002

within a given population over time using the following calculation:

$$\text{incidence} = \frac{\text{number of new cases that develop in a population at risk over a specified time}}{\text{number of persons at risk for developing the condition or disease over a specified time}}$$

In contrast, prevalence is defined as the number of people in a population who have a particular disease divided by the number of people in the population at a specific point in time.

$$\text{prevalence} = \frac{\text{number of cases of disease or outcome at a specified time}}{\text{number of people in the population at a specified time}}$$

The denominator in the prevalence formula includes both new cases and existing cases. Moreover, because it focuses on a particular point in time, prevalence is like a snapshot of the disease in a community, whereas incidence is a video of the development of disease or outcome over time.

Careful consideration must occur when interpretating incidence and prevalence values. For example, advances in pharmacotherapy have significantly reduced the number of acquired immunodeficiency syndrome (AIDS) deaths and slowed the transition from human immunodeficiency virus (HIV) to AIDS. The consequences of improved prevention and treatment led to a decrease in incidence and a commensurate increase in prevalence. Although increased prevalence may sound alarming, in this case it reflects the success of the intervention employed so that people are able to live longer after their diagnosis. Careful thought is essential to interpret both incidence and prevalence measures.

Mortality rates measure the likelihood of dying during a specific period. If the mortality rate includes all deaths regardless of cause or reason, the rate is called an all-cause mortality rate.

$$\text{mortality rate} = \frac{\text{number of deaths in a specified time period}}{\text{number of people in the population during the time period}}$$

Rates also can be restricted to a particular person or disease characteristic, or a combination of characteristics. For example, a researcher might be interested in the annual mortality rate for Reye's syndrome among children younger than 10 years. This formula is used to calculate that age- and disease-specific mortality rate:

$$\text{mortality rate} = \frac{\text{number of deaths from Reye's syndrome among children} < 10 \text{ years of age in 1 year}}{\text{number of children} < 10 \text{ years of age in population at midyear point}}$$

It is important to remember that the denominator is populated by individuals who satisfy the restriction criteria: in this case those younger than 10 years who had the potential to become cases during the time period.

Mortality information also can be presented as case fatality rates. Case fatality rates assess the rate at which people who have a particular disease or condition die. The difference between disease-specific mortality rates and case fatality rates exists in the denominator. The denominator of a mortality rate is the number of people in the population, typically measured at the midpoint of the time period studied. This can extend to the entire population or pertain to a particular age group. In contrast, the denominator of a case fatality rate is the number of people who have the disease or condition studied. Furthermore, case fatality rates typically omit any reference to a specified time period. They are used mostly in acute, short-term conditions when death is directly attributed to the condition. If death occurs, it will typically be close in time to the initial diagnosis. In effect, the case fatality rate is the rate at which people who have the disease die.

$$\text{case fatality rate} = \frac{\text{number of deaths from a specific condition}}{\text{number of people with the disease or condition}}$$

Proportionate mortality provides a different way to present mortality information. It is unique, because it does not require a measurement of the size of the population in which deaths occurred. Instead of the denominator as the number of people in the population, it is the total number of deaths in the population over a specified period of time. The numerator is the number of deaths attributed to a particular disease or event.

$$\text{proportionate mortality} = \frac{\text{number of deaths attributed to a disease within a time period}}{\text{total number of deaths in the population within a time period}}$$

The objective of proportionate mortality measures is to determine the percentage of deaths attributed to a particular disease, and it can also be restricted to groups. Proportionate mortality could demonstrate, for example, that accidents account for 40% of all deaths among migrant workers or that lung cancer accounts for 25% of all deaths from cancer in the United States during a particular time period.

CRITICAL SUCCESS FACTORS IN HEALTHCARE

Critical success factors are key activities and priorities that organizations need to address to reach their goals and stay relevant in a fast-changing and competitive world. In healthcare, these factors are especially important. They are the backbone of efforts to provide top-notch care, improve operations, and meet the expectations of patients, staff, and stakeholders. As the Institute for Healthcare Improvement explains, CSFs help organizations to align their work with their big-picture goals, ensuring that resources are used in the smartest way possible to support what truly matters.[3]

While every healthcare organization has its own unique challenges and priorities, some CSF areas may apply across the board. These include focusing on patient-centered care, improving clinical outcomes, achieving operational excellence, integrating technology, engaging with the community and market, fostering strong leadership and a positive culture, and maintaining effective governance and strategy.

The push toward patient-centered care has focused on measuring patient satisfaction to assess whether health systems and providers are understanding and addressing patients' needs effectively. One of the best ways to do this is by continuously gathering and acting on patient feedback. While many hospitals have long collected information on patient satisfaction for their own internal use, there were no common metrics/national standards for collecting and publicly reporting information about patient experiences. The Hospital Consumer Assessment of Healthcare Providers and Systems (HCAHPS) survey was designed to address this issue.[4] The HCAHPS survey data have been collected for the Hospital Inpatient Quality Reporting program since 2006, publicly reported since 2008 (allowing valid comparisons to be made across hospitals locally and nationally) and used in the Hospital Value-Based Purchasing (HVBP) program since 2012. The goal is to push towards consumer-driven healthcare.

The HCAHPS

- Produces comparable data for public reporting
- Creates incentives for organizations to improve
- Enhances public accountability and transparency

This survey, developed to measure patients' perspectives on their hospital stay, gives hospitals a standardized way to assess patient satisfaction and experiences. The HCAHPS survey offers a consistent framework to compare patient satisfaction across different healthcare organizations; thus, it plays a key role in the Centers for Medicare & Medicaid Services (CMS) Value-Based Purchasing Program. In other words, the hospitals' Medicare reimbursement is tied to how well they score on patient experience.[4] The survey itself is comprehensive; 29 questions cover various aspects of a patient's care experience. There has always been a moral imperative for hospitals and health systems to provide high-quality patient experiences, and now that CMS is tying reimbursements to HCAHPS scores, it is also a financial priority.

Research shows that hospitals following strong process measures often have more satisfied patients, indicating that the quality of care and how patients perceive it are closely linked.[5] Clear communication is a key driver of satisfaction. When hospitals prioritize clear and effective communication with patients and their families, it builds trust and creates a more comfortable experience.[6] Simple things, such as reducing wait times and making sure that patients feel at ease, can have a huge impact. Studies show that timely care leads to better outcomes and higher satisfaction levels.[7,8]

Optimizing clinical outcomes is one of the most important goals in healthcare. To achieve this, it is crucial to implement evidence-based care protocols and monitor hospital-acquired infections and readmissions.[9] Aligning care delivery with industry standards improves patient-centered care and boosts overall clinical effectiveness.[10-12]

A hospital's organizational culture can directly and indirectly impact patient outcomes. Research shows that hospitals with a positive, supportive culture tend to achieve better clinical results.[13] This highlights the importance of connecting clinical protocols with the cultural and organizational factors that shape the care environment. Fostering a culture that prioritizes quality care and patient safety is as essential as following clinical guidelines.

Indeed, creating a culture of safety is absolutely essential in healthcare organizations. It is about making sure that clinicians, staff, and leadership are on the same page when prioritizing patient safety. Rigorous training and open, transparent reporting systems are key to reducing medication errors and preventing adverse events.[14] Simple but critical practices, such as regular audits of hand hygiene and equipment sterilization, can make a huge difference in keeping patients safe.[15,16]

The overarching organizational culture also impacts patient safety. Research shows that when healthcare teams feel supported and empowered, they are more likely to follow safety protocols consistently,[17] which leads to better outcomes for patients.[18] Standardized processes, such as medication administration and patient monitoring, also play a big role in preventing adverse events and improving overall safety.[19,20] Promoting a culture of safety is not just about following rules—it is about creating an environment where every patient and team member feels valued and protected.

Operational excellence in hospitals is not just about running things efficiently—it is about caring for the people who make it happen. Staff efficiency and morale are at the heart of delivering high-quality patient care. Ensuring adequate staffing levels and workloads prevents burnout and keeps talented healthcare professionals on board.[21] When staff feel supported and valued, it directly impacts patient care. Offering opportunities for professional growth and taking the time to recognize great work can boost morale, which ultimately translates into better care for patients.[22] Additionally, using Lean management principles and improving procurement processes can help streamline workflows and reduce waste. When resources are used where they matter most, it improves both efficiency and patient outcomes.[23]

Integrating advanced technologies, such as electronic health records (EHRs) and telemedicine, is increasingly vital for healthcare organizations. These technologies enhance operational efficiency and improve the quality of patient care by facilitating better communication and data management.[24-26] Predictive analytics can aid decision-making and operational forecasting, allowing hospitals to anticipate patient needs and allocate resources effectively.[27] Additionally, innovations, such as artificial intelligence (AI) and robotic process automation, can further enhance efficiency. However, it is crucial to ensure that technology is well designed and implemented to avoid negative impacts on staff morale and patient safety.[28] Studies have shown that successful technology integration can lead to significant reductions in medication errors[29,30] and improved patient outcomes,[31] thus highlighting the importance of adopting advanced healthcare technologies.

Building a strong brand reputation through transparency in quality metrics and patient outcomes is essential for healthcare organizations.[32] Engaging with the community by addressing social determinants of health and partnering with local organizations can enhance the hospital's image and foster trust between patients and health providers.[33] Providing accessible care to underserved populations is critical to community engagement that can improve overall health outcomes.[34,35] Research indicates hospitals that actively engage with their communities and address health disparities contribute to better health outcomes for vulnerable populations and enhance the hospital's reputation.[36]

This engagement is particularly important for safety-net hospitals, which often serve high-risk populations and face unique challenges in delivering quality care.[37]

Effective leadership is a CSF in healthcare organizations.[38] Visionary leadership that inspires teams and promotes accountability is essential for achieving strategic goals. A culture of inclusivity and collaboration fosters innovation and adaptability, which are necessary for responding to evolving healthcare challenges, such as changing payment models, provider shortages, regulatory changes, and technological innovations.[39] Engaging staff in decision-making processes can enhance buy-in for new initiatives, improve overall morale, and reduce staff turnover.[40,41] Research also has shown that strong leadership and a positive organizational culture are linked to improved staff satisfaction and patient outcomes, demonstrating the importance of cultivating a supportive work environment.[42] Additionally, equipping leaders with the tools and training to manage organizational changes can lead to effective, smoother transitions that enhance overall organizational performance.[43,44]

Aligning an organization's governance and strategy with its goals is key to achieving long-term success. Hospitals thrive when they regularly evaluate their performance against clear, measurable objectives, keeping their focus on what matters most.[45,46] Staying on top of healthcare regulations and adopting proactive risk management strategies are also crucial for staying compliant and maintaining high standards of care.[47]

Sustainability is becoming increasingly important in healthcare. By adopting environmentally friendly practices, hospitals can improve operational efficiency and build a stronger reputation in their communities.[48] Research shows that prioritizing sustainability benefits the environment and improves a hospital's financial performance, making sustainability an essential part of modern healthcare governance.[49,50]

In conclusion, the interdependence of each CSF discussed above highlights the need for continuous assessment and adaptation in healthcare organizations. By focusing on these factors, hospitals can enhance patient care, streamline operations, and foster a resilient organizational culture driven by strong leadership.

KEY PERFORMANCE INDICATORS IN HEALTHCARE

The evaluation of healthcare-related KPIs is crucial for assessing the performance of healthcare systems and improving patient outcomes. This section will explore various KPIs, their definitions, importance, and the innovative metrics that have emerged in recent years, such as "days at home" and "days not in hospital." Additionally, KPIs and CSFs are differentiated to provide a comprehensive understanding of their roles in healthcare management.

In the context of healthcare, a KPI is defined as a quantifiable measure used to evaluate the success of an organization in achieving its objectives, particularly in delivering quality care and improving patient outcomes. KPIs serve as benchmarks that help healthcare organizations assess their performance across various dimensions, including clinical effectiveness, operational efficiency, patient satisfaction, and safety.[51] They are essential for guiding decision-making, informing policy development, and ensuring accountability within healthcare systems.[52]

The significance of KPIs in healthcare is multifaceted; KPIs provide a structured approach to performance measurement, enabling healthcare organizations to track their progress toward specific goals and objectives systematically. By utilizing KPIs, such as hospital readmission rates and patient satisfaction scores, healthcare providers can assess the quality of care they deliver and pinpoint areas that need improvement.[53] For example, a high readmission rate may indicate gaps in postdischarge care, prompting hospitals to implement targeted interventions, such as better discharge planning, patient education, and follow-up care. Similarly, patient satisfaction scores offer insights into patients' experiences, guiding efforts to enhance communication, reduce wait times, and improve overall service quality. By continuously monitoring these indicators, healthcare organizations can drive meaningful improvements in patient outcomes and operational efficiency.

Beyond performance measurement, KPIs also play a vital role in fostering accountability and transparency within healthcare organizations. Publicly reporting performance metrics demonstrates a commitment to quality care and patient safety and builds trust among patients, regulators, and other stakeholders.[54] When they are transparent about their outcomes, healthcare organizations create an environment of openness and continuous learning, thus motivating providers to maintain high standards of care. This level of accountability encourages data-driven decision-making and helps to identify best practices for sharing across institutions to elevate the overall standard of healthcare delivery.

Furthermore, KPIs are instrumental in supporting the transition toward value-based care. This model shifts the focus from the service volume to the quality and effectiveness of care. Traditional metrics, such as the number of hospital visits, are gradually being supplemented or replaced by value-based metrics, such as "days at home" and "days not in hospital." These innovative KPIs emphasize the importance of maintaining patients' independence, reducing unnecessary hospitalizations, and improving overall quality of life. By aligning performance measurements with value-based care principles, healthcare organizations can prioritize preventive care, enhance care coordination, and implement strategies that support a patient's recovery journey. Integrating these KPIs into healthcare decision-making ultimately promotes better outcomes, more efficient resource allocation, and a more sustainable healthcare system.

KPIs in the Inpatient Setting

In an inpatient hospital setting, KPIs are essential for measuring the quality, efficiency, and overall effectiveness of healthcare delivery. These metrics help hospitals to assess patient care outcomes, operational performance, and adherence to safety standards. The most commonly used KPIs include hospital readmission rates, which indicate the effectiveness of discharge planning and follow-up care, and average length of stay, which reflects hospital efficiency and resource utilization. Additionally, patient satisfaction scores provide insights into the overall patient experience. At the same time, hospital-acquired infection rates and medication error rates serve as critical indicators of patient safety and quality of care. By monitoring these KPIs, hospitals can identify areas for improvement, enhance patient outcomes, and optimize healthcare services in an increasingly value-driven environment. Below are definitions and brief descriptions of the most common KPIs in the inpatient setting.

30-Day Readmission Rate

This is the percentage of patients who are readmitted to the hospital within 30 days of discharge. This KPI is a critical measure of hospital performance and quality of care. High readmission rates can indicate inadequate discharge planning or poor postdischarge care.[55] The CMS uses this metric to adjust hospital reimbursements, emphasizing its significance in value-based care.[55]

30-Day Risk-Standardized Mortality Rate

This indicator adjusts mortality rates based on patient risk factors to compare hospital performance fairly. The risk-standardized mortality rate (RSMR) is essential for evaluating the quality-of-care hospitals provide, particularly for high-risk patients. The metric helps to identify hospitals that require quality improvement initiatives.[56]

Days at Home

This is the total number of days a patient spends at home after discharge from the hospital. This innovative metric emphasizes patient-centered care and quality of life. The KPI reflects the effectiveness of care transitions and postdischarge support, aligning with the goals of reducing hospitalizations and improving patient autonomy.[57]

Days Not in Hospital

This indicator measures the total number of days that patients remain out of the hospital during a specified period. This metric serves as an indicator of effective outpatient care and chronic disease management. The KPI highlights the ability of healthcare systems to manage patients' health in the community, thereby reducing unnecessary hospitalizations.[57]

90-Day Risk-Standardized Home Time

Like the 30-day home time metric, this KPI measures the number of days patients spend at home within 90 days postdischarge. This metric is particularly relevant for cardiac surgery patients, because it provides insights into longer-term recovery and the effectiveness of surgical interventions.[58]

Hospital-Acquired Infection Rates

This is the rate of infections acquired during hospital stays, often measured per 1,000 patient days. Monitoring these rates is crucial for infection control and quality improvement initiatives. High rates can indicate lapses in hygiene practices or inadequate infection prevention protocols.[59]

Average Length of Stay

This is the average duration of a patient's hospitalization. The average length of stay (ALOS) is a fundamental KPI that reflects operational efficiency and resource utilization. Shorter ALOS can indicate effective care delivery, but excessively short stays may compromise patient safety and care quality.[55]

Patient Satisfaction Scores

These metrics are derived from patient surveys assessing patient experiences and patient care satisfaction. Patient satisfaction is increasingly recognized as a vital component of healthcare quality. High satisfaction scores correlate with better patient outcomes and adherence to treatment.[55]

Emergency Department Utilization Rates

These rates are the frequency of patient visits to the emergency department (ED), often measured per 1,000 population. High ED utilization can indicate gaps in primary care access or inadequate management of chronic conditions. Monitoring this KPI helps healthcare systems identify areas for improvement in outpatient care.[60]

Days of Therapy Avoided

This metric quantifies the impact of antimicrobial stewardship programs by measuring the reduction in antibiotic use. This KPI is essential for assessing the effectiveness of interventions to reduce unnecessary antibiotic prescriptions, thereby combating antibiotic resistance.[61]

KPIs in the Outpatient Setting

Key performance indicators in the outpatient setting are quantifiable metrics that healthcare organizations use to evaluate the effectiveness, efficiency, and quality of care provided to patients who receive treatment without being admitted to a hospital. These indicators are essential for monitoring various aspects of outpatient care, including patient outcomes, service delivery efficiency, and overall patient satisfaction. The importance of KPIs in outpatient settings is highlighted by their role in enhancing care quality, optimizing resource utilization, and supporting continuous improvement initiatives. Below are definitions and brief descriptions of the most common KPIs in the outpatient setting.

Patient Satisfaction Scores

These metrics are derived from surveys assessing the experiences of patients and their satisfaction with outpatient services. High patient satisfaction scores indicate quality care, which can improve patient retention and treatment plan adherence.[62]

Appointment No-Show Rates

This is the percentage of scheduled outpatient appointments that patients fail to attend without prior notification. Monitoring no-show rates helps providers identify barriers to accessing care and implement strategies to improve patient engagement and attendance.[63]

Medication Reconciliation Rates

This is the percentage of patients who receive medication reconciliation during outpatient visits. Effective medication reconciliation is crucial for preventing medication errors and ensuring patient safety, particularly for patients with complex medication regimens.[64]

Follow-Up Appointment Compliance

This indicator is the percentage of patients who attend follow-up appointments as recommended by their healthcare providers. High compliance rates indicate effective care coordination and contribute to better health outcomes by ensuring ongoing management of chronic conditions.[65]

Time to First Appointment

This is the average time a patient receives the first outpatient appointment after a referral or request. Shorter appointment wait times are associated with improved patient satisfaction and timely access to necessary care.[66] This metric also relates to patient safety, because delayed treatment may exacerbate the patient's condition.

Clinical Outcomes

These metrics assess the effectiveness of treatments provided in outpatient settings, such as improvement in symptoms or disease management. Monitoring clinical outcomes helps healthcare providers evaluate the effectiveness of interventions and make data-driven decisions to enhance care quality.[67]

Cost per Patient Visit

This is the average cost incurred by the healthcare organization for each outpatient visit. Understanding the cost per visit is essential for financial management and resource allocation, allowing organizations to identify opportunities for cost reduction without compromising care quality.[68]

Implementing KPIs in outpatient care settings ensures high-quality, efficient, and patient-centered healthcare delivery. One of the primary benefits of KPIs is their role in quality improvement by providing a structured framework for continuous evaluation and enhancement of care delivery. For instance, tracking patient satisfaction scores can help healthcare organizations identify specific pain points in the patient experience, such as long wait times, communication gaps, or difficulties in accessing care, allowing for targeted interventions.[69]

Another critical advantage of KPIs in outpatient settings is resource optimization. By monitoring metrics, such as appointment no-show rates and time to the first appointment, healthcare organizations can improve their scheduling efficiency and resource allocation. High no-show rates, for example, can lead to wasted provider time and delayed care for other patients. Yet with effective KPI tracking, organizations can implement reminder systems, overbooking strategies, or telehealth options to minimize disruptions.[63] These measures help to ensure that providers maximize their capacity while maintaining timely access to care.

Key performance indicators also play a crucial role in enhancing patient safety, particularly through indicators related to medication reconciliation and follow-up compliance. Tracking these metrics helps to reduce the risk of medication errors, adverse drug interactions, and gaps in care continuity. For example, ensuring that patients adhere to follow-up appointments after a procedure or hospitalization can prevent complications and readmissions. By systematically monitoring these safety-related KPIs, outpatient clinics can implement best practices, such as automated reminders, pharmacist consultations, and streamlined prescription reconciliation to improve patient outcomes.[64]

Moreover, KPI data facilitate informed decision-making, enabling healthcare leaders to develop policies, refine care protocols, and allocate resources based on evidence rather than intuition. A data-driven approach fosters a culture of accountability and transparency, ensuring that healthcare providers continuously assess and improve their services to meet patient and organizational needs.[70]

Another significant benefit of KPIs in outpatient care is their impact on patient engagement. Metrics focused on patient satisfaction, treatment plan adherence, and preventive care encourage healthcare organizations to prioritize strategies that enhance the patient experience. Understanding patient needs and preferences allows providers to tailor their services by expanding telehealth options, improving communication, or offering more patient education resources, ultimately fostering a more patient-centered care model.[62]

Finally, KPIs serve as a tool for benchmarking and accountability, allowing outpatient clinics to compare their performance against industry standards or peer organizations. This external benchmarking provides insights into areas requiring improvement and motivates healthcare providers to adopt best practices and strive for excellence in care delivery. By establishing measurable goals and tracking progress over time, outpatient facilities can ensure that they remain competitive and continue to meet evolving healthcare demands.[71]

Key performance indicators in the outpatient setting are essential tools for measuring and improving patient care quality. By defining and monitoring relevant indicators, healthcare organizations can enhance patient outcomes, optimize resource utilization, and foster a culture of continuous improvement. As outpatient care continues to evolve, developing and refining KPIs will be crucial to ensure high-quality, patient-centered care.

DIFFERENTIATING KPIs FROM CSFs

While KPIs and CSFs are both essential for healthcare management, they serve different purposes. KPIs are specific, measurable indicators that reflect performance in various domains, such as clinical outcomes, operational efficiency, and patient satisfaction. In contrast, CSFs are broader elements that are critical for achieving organizational goals. For example, a CSF might be establishing a patient-centered care model, whereas a KPI could measure the percentage of patients who report satisfaction with their care experience. This distinction is crucial for healthcare leaders to prioritize the metrics that indicate performance and the broader strategic elements that drive success.[53]

The importance of healthcare-related KPIs in assessing and improving healthcare performance cannot be overstated. Metrics, such as 30-day readmission rates, RSMRs, and days at home, provide valuable insights into the quality of care delivered. Healthcare organizations can better align their performance measurement strategies with their overarching goals by differentiating KPIs from CSFs. As the healthcare field evolves, the ongoing development and refinement of KPIs will be essential for driving improvements and ensuring high-quality care.

CHALLENGES IN METRIC DEVELOPMENT AND IMPLEMENTATION

The development and implementation of metrics in the US healthcare system is a complex endeavor with numerous challenges that can hinder the effectiveness and reliability of these measures. These challenges are critical to address, because they directly impact the quality of patient care. Key areas of concern include data quality and interoperability, study power, staff training and engagement, and regulatory alignment.

Data quality and interoperability are fundamental to creating meaningful healthcare metrics. Good data quality does not just exist on paper; those data play a crucial role in supporting patient care, improving outcomes, boosting clinical efficiency, and advancing medical research. To achieve accurate metrics that truly reflect the quality of care, data must be collected, shared, and analyzed seamlessly across different healthcare systems.

The Healthcare Information and Management Systems Society (HIMSS), a global organization dedicated to advancing the transformation of the healthcare system, has outlined interoperability technology across four distinct levels: (1) Foundational, (2) Structural, (3) Semantic, and (4) Organizational.[72] The Foundational level establishes the basic requirements for connecting systems and securely exchanging data. The Structural level addresses the format, syntax, and data interpretation at the field level. The Semantic level enables the use of standardized terminologies, vocabularies, and publicly defined values to ensure a complete and accurate understanding of the exchanged information. The Organizational level includes governance, policy, legal, and organizational use of data within and between organizations.

Unfortunately, many healthcare organizations face ongoing challenges with fragmented data systems that do not communicate well with each other on multiple levels. This lack of interoperability often results in incomplete or even biased data.[73,74] Interoperability—the ability of different systems to exchange and use information—remains a persistent issue. Without interoperability, it becomes incredibly difficult to share critical information among providers and compare health metrics across populations.

Despite years of attention to this problem, interoperability holds healthcare organizations back, especially as they adopt more health information systems. These systems often introduce both internal and external challenges, further complicating data exchange.[75] Torab-Miandoab et al. highlight one of the key barriers: overly broad standards that are open to local interpretation.[76] This inconsistency creates confusion and undermines the goal of seamless data exchange.[76]

Data quality also depends heavily on how well data are exchanged. Accurate and reliable information is essential, yet studies show that inconsistencies in how EHRs are entered—and the lack of standardized protocols—often compromise data quality.[74] This inconsistency does not just impact the reliability of metrics; it makes it harder to implement quality improvement initiatives across different healthcare settings. Sometimes, it may completely fail to meet the demands of programs linking payment to quality measures.[77]

As de Mello et al. point out, well-established interoperability standards are key to improving data quality.[78] These standards ensure smoother data exchanges among departments in the same facility or across entirely different organizations.[78] The path forward may not be simple, but addressing interoperability and data quality issues head-on is essential to advancing healthcare as a whole.

Integrating emerging technologies, such as distributed ledger technologies (DLTs), blockchain, and AI, opens exciting possibilities to improve how data are shared and maintained in healthcare.[79-81] For example, Bundi's review explains how DLTs can tackle tough interoperability challenges by creating secure, unchangeable records that make it easier for different systems to share data.[79] Similarly, blockchain has the potential to help meet EHR standards, securely store and extract data, and enable the exchange of standardized information.[82]

Some big hurdles to overcome are scalability issues, privacy concerns, and regulatory requirements, such as the Health Insurance Portability and Accountability Act (HIPAA).[83] Artificial intelligence also shows promise in improving data quality, from enhancing quality control to streamlining data collection and cleaning processes.[81] However, integrating AI and big data analytics into healthcare has its challenges, notably, data privacy, security risks, algorithm bias, and the need for solid infrastructure.[84,85]

These technologies are advancing quickly, and to make the most of them, it is clear that healthcare professionals and organizations need to adapt continuously. The journey toward fully integrating these tools into clinical practice is both promising and complex; yet with the right effort, the potential benefits are enormous.

One of the biggest challenges in developing metrics is ensuring sufficient study power. Calculating study power is a critical step in research design because the calculation ensures that conclusions drawn from a study are reliable and valid. To obtain meaningful and applicable results, studies need sufficient sample sizes. Yet in reality, recruiting enough participants can be a real struggle, especially for specialized disease areas or in rural healthcare settings.[86] This often leads to metrics that do not accurately reflect the larger patient population, limiting their usefulness for drawing meaningful or accurate conclusions.[74] Moreover, the complexity of many healthcare interventions often requires layered, multifaceted approaches to data collection and analysis, which makes building robust metrics even more challenging.[87]

A power analysis helps address this issue by determining how likely a study is to detect an effect of a given size, assuming that effect truly exists. As discussed further in Chapter 8, this process considers key factors, such as effect size, sample size, significance level (alpha), and the statistical test used. Power is the probability of correctly rejecting the null hypothesis when it is false.[88] A common benchmark for adequate power is 0.8, meaning that there is an 80% chance of detecting an effect if one exists.[89]

Sample size plays a huge role here. Larger samples generally lead to higher power by reducing the standard error and making it easier to detect true effects.[90] In fact, Hedges and Pigott emphasize that determining the right sample size is critical to avoiding inconclusive results or misinterpretations in research.[90] Similarly, Topp et al. provides a detailed guide for conducting power analyses in health policy research, blending theory with practical strategies to design stronger studies.[91]

Adequate power is not just about sample size. The choice of statistical test also matters, because different tests vary in their ability to detect effects. Gelman and Carlin highlight the importance of tailoring power calculations to a study's specific design and context, even suggesting using external information to refine estimates of effect size.[88] The significance level (alpha) also plays a role. Lower alpha levels, such as 0.01 instead of 0.05, reduce the chance of Type I errors (rejecting a true null hypothesis); yet they also lower power by making it harder to reach statistical significance.[89] Striking the right balance between Type I and Type II errors is key.

Fortunately, power analysis has become much more accessible thanks to software tools that can calculate power for simple models and more complex ones, such as structural equation modeling.[92] Tools, such as R, SAS, SPSS, and Stata, are commonly used, although some require coding knowledge. Each option has pros and cons, so it is worth finding the software tool that best suits one's needs, comfort level, and budget.

Staff training and engagement are also critical to successful metric implementation.[93] Healthcare professionals must be adequately trained in the technical aspects of data collection and management as well as understanding the importance of metrics for improving patient care. For example, Stange et al. argue that engaging primary care providers in the metric development process can enhance metric relevance and usability, as well as improve the research team's ability to assess the performance of the primary care system.[94] However, time constraints and competing demands often limit interprofessional training opportunities, leading to knowledge gaps and potentially limited staff engagement.[95] Yet engaging healthcare workers in the metric development process and presentation is recommended, because it can increase the likelihood that the metrics will be accepted and utilized for quality improvement initiatives.[96] Without this engagement, there is a risk of resistance to new metrics and practices, making adoption challenging.

Regulatory alignment between healthcare metrics and clinical practice is important for several key reasons. When metrics align with clinical practice, care processes can be designed and monitored based on scientifically validated measures.[97] This alignment helps improve patient outcomes and reduces unnecessary variations in care. Programs, such as the HVBP and the Hospital Readmissions Reduction Program, go a step further by tying reimbursement to performance of these quality metrics.[98] This creates a strong financial incentive for providers to deliver high-quality, evidence-based, efficient care.

Moreover, aligning clinical practices with required reporting metrics also helps healthcare organizations stay compliant, avoid penalties, and maintain accreditation.[99] It is a way to ensure that hospitals and providers are held accountable for meeting quality standards. Also, having metrics that transparently evaluate performance builds trust among patients, regulators, and payers.[99]

The constantly evolving nature of healthcare regulations can create challenges for organizations as they work to align their practices with new regulatory requirements. Balancing compliance with practical, patient-centered care calls for ongoing collaboration and dialogue among healthcare providers and regulatory bodies.[100] It is an effort that requires flexibility, yet when done well, it ensures that metrics remain practical and meaningful for improving patient care.

CONCLUSION

The challenges associated with metric development and implementation in healthcare are complex and interconnected. Addressing data quality and interoperability issues, study power, staff training and engagement, and regulatory alignment is essential for successfully integrating metrics into healthcare systems. By overcoming these challenges, healthcare organizations can enhance the quality of care delivered to patients and improve overall health outcomes.

Integrating KPIs in healthcare has played a pivotal role in improving quality, efficiency, patient safety, and accountability in inpatient and outpatient settings. By systematically tracking metrics, such as hospital readmission rates, patient satisfaction scores, medication reconciliation, and follow-up compliance, healthcare organizations can identify areas for improvement and implement targeted interventions to enhance patient outcomes. Moreover, the shift toward value-based care has introduced innovative KPIs, such as "days at home" and "days not in hospital," emphasizing patient-centered outcomes and supporting care models that prioritize long-term health and well-being. Despite the benefits, challenges, such as data quality, interoperability, regulatory alignment, and staff engagement, must be addressed to ensure the effective development and implementation of healthcare metrics.

Future trends in healthcare metrics likely will be driven by advancements in AI, predictive analytics, and real-time data monitoring. Artificial intelligence-powered analytics will enable more precise risk stratification, allowing healthcare providers to intervene and prevent adverse outcomes proactively. Additionally, the growing adoption of wearable technology and remote monitoring devices will facilitate real-time patient data collection, expanding the scope of KPIs beyond traditional clinical settings. As value-based care models continue to evolve, new metrics will focus on health equity, social determinants of health, and personalized patient outcomes. To maximize the impact of these advancements, healthcare organizations must prioritize data integration, enhance interoperability among systems, and ensure that KPIs align with evolving healthcare policies and patient needs.

CASE STUDY EXAMPLES

The following case studies are included to stress the value of KPIs as essential tools in transforming healthcare delivery. In each instance, the application of carefully chosen, context-specific KPIs facilitated greater transparency, accountability, and continuous learning within healthcare systems. Whether improving access to specialized care, supporting critical care decision-making, or optimizing operational workflows, KPIs serve as a bridge between clinical excellence and strategic health-system management. The first case study centers on the development of KPIs, while the second and third illustrate how the use of KPIs resulted in improved quality outcomes. These examples demonstrate the practicality of KPIs and emphasize their capacity to shape organizational culture, empower healthcare professionals, and drive sustained improvements in patient care.

Adopting and utilizing KPIs in healthcare has emerged as an essential practice in quality improvement initiatives. These indicators facilitate the measurement and analysis of various dimensions of healthcare services, leading to enhanced patient care outcomes, operational efficiencies, and overall service quality. The following case studies explore real-world applications of KPIs across diverse clinical and organizational settings, offering rich insights into the practical and transformative potential of performance measurement tools in healthcare.

Case Study 1: Centralized Intake Systems for Rheumatology

A 2015 study in Alberta, Canada, explored KPIs to evaluate a centralized intake system for managing patients with osteoarthritis (OA) and rheumatoid arthritis (RA).[101] The study followed a three-phase process to develop and validate relevant KPIs. In the first phase, input was gathered from a wide range of stakeholders, including healthcare providers, managers, researchers, and patients who contributed to identifying candidate KPIs aligned with five dimensions of healthcare quality: appropriateness (services delivered based on best practices), accessibility (services delivered in timely manner), acceptability (services responsive to user expectations/preferences), efficiency (services optimally used), and effectiveness (services based on knowledge to achieve best outcomes). Perceived impact (identifiable health benefits), provider control over KPI performance (extent to which provider can influence outcomes), and measurement feasibility (available information to measure performance) were used to prioritize KPI development. The second phase involved comprehensive literature reviews to ensure that selected KPIs reflected best practices and were consistent with existing national standards. In the final phase, a three-round modified Delphi process was used to finalize the KPI set based on scientific validity (strength of scientific evidence or professional consensus), face validity (likelihood of better performance on an indicator reflects higher-quality outcomes), feasibility (likelihood of availability of information to report on an indicator), importance (importance of measuring and reporting an indicator when evaluating centralized intake in arthritis care), and likelihood to use (likelihood of use for quality improvement). A panel of 27 individuals participated in two rounds of rating using a 9-point Likert scale and a third round of online and in-person discussions. KPIs rated as valid and important (≥7) were retained. Consequently, 25 initial KPIs were submitted for review. After discussion, 3 were removed, and 6 new ones were suggested, yielding a final set of 28 KPIs. These included 9 focused on OA (ie, time from OA referral receipt to referral completion for initially incomplete referrals, percentage of OA referrals received with complete information), 10 on RA (ie, wait times for rheumatologist consultation for patients with new onset of RA, percentage of RA referrals categorized as early RA), and 9 applicable to the centralized intake process (ie, patient experience with centralized intake, referring clinician experience with centralized intake). All final KPIs were endorsed as valid and important. The study emphasized how a rigorous and collaborative process can produce meaningful, actionable

KPIs that reflect diverse stakeholder priorities and support continuous quality improvement. This study centered on creating a set of KPIs intended for feasibility testing. Upon validation, these indicators are intended to inform the design and assessment of an optimized centralized intake system for patients with OA and RA.[101]

Case Study 2: Process-Based Quality Improvement in Renal Care

A process improvement project was implemented in Cincinnati, Ohio, from 2012 to 2017 to assess continuous renal replacement therapy (CRRT) in critically ill patients.[102] The use of CRRT has increased significantly in acute kidney injury management; yet literature addressing the quality of its delivery remains limited. To address this gap, the authors developed a CRRT dashboard that captured performance metrics (KPIs) across three core categories: filter life/unplanned changes, dialysis prescription accuracy (eg, delivered vs. prescribed dose), and fluid balance (eg, attainment of targeted fluid removal goals). The dashboard was used for quarterly reviews from 2012 to 2017, covering 184 patients. The use of a dashboard to monitor these KPIs resulted in marked improvements. The mean filter life was 56 ± 28.4 hours; 62% of filters lasted at least 60 hours (targeted time). Unplanned filter changes were reduced from 40% to 15%. Regarding dosage, the average prescribed CRRT dose was 2,300 mL/1.73 m^2/hr, exceeding the institution's minimum standard of 2,000 mL/1.73 m^2/hr, resulting in at least 98% of patients receiving at least the minimum prescription. The proportion of patients receiving at least 90% of their prescribed dose rose from 87% in 2014 to 100% by 2017, maintaining 100% consistently in all following quarters. Fluid balance was also a key metric: 83% of CRRT patient-days met the desired target within a 10% deviation range. Achievement of fluid goals improved from 69% to 83% over eight quarters. The dashboard offers continuous performance monitoring and supports the analysis of variations and deviations from established standards of care. For instance, filter survival serves as an indicator of circuit functionality can be used to assess the quality and real-time maintenance of CRRT delivery.[103] These results demonstrate the value of real-time KPI dashboards to improve patient outcomes and treatment consistency, enable targeted provider education, and reinforce adherence to institutional standards in complex care settings.[102]

Case Study 3: Integrating Lean Models and KPIs

A comparative study was conducted in Sao Paulo, Brazil, in two private health institutions from 2012 to 2013 to examine the effectiveness of total quality (TQ) and Lean Production models in Brazilian hospitals.[104] One institution (Organization A), a large-scale medical diagnostics company, utilized a traditional TQ model. The second institution (Organization B), a mid-sized oncology hospital in São Paulo, implemented Lean Healthcare practices, which are commonly used in manufacturing. Organization A relied on a hierarchical, expert-driven TQ model where performance data were collected centrally, and corrective actions were proposed by unit coordinators. In this system, two primary KPIs were used: the service complaint index and the sample recollection index. The complaint index revealed that 28% of patient complaints stemmed from long wait times, whereas 15% were attributed to registration errors during patient intake. As a corrective measure, managers introduced a verification step whereby an additional staff member reviewed the patient's intake record before the procedure began. This intervention reduced registration errors, although precise postintervention metrics were not reported. The sample recollection index, another KPI, measured the frequency of lab specimens that required recollection due to preanalytical errors. The recollection rate in Organization A was reported to be 49% above the recommended threshold. Contributing factors included mislabeling, incorrect tube selection, and inadequate sample volume. In response, unit coordinators initiated individualized reviews of error causes and introduced additional cross-check procedures. However, as with the registration KPI, improvements were monitored internally, and quantified postintervention outcomes were not disclosed. In contrast, Organization B adopted a Lean Healthcare model characterized by its emphasis on team-based, systemic process evaluation and continuous improvement. A central part of the Lean approach was the use of Value Stream Mapping, Failure Mode and Effects Analysis (FMEA), and A3 problem-solving tools to track and address key quality indicators in real time. One of the critical KPIs used in Organization B was the prescription error rate during chemotherapy treatment preparation. Prior to Lean interventions, the hospital experienced frequent avoidable failures in the prescription process, including incorrect drug names, doses, and patient identifiers. To address these issues, a multidisciplinary team conducted regular assessments using FMEA and direct workflow observation (Gemba walks). Several specific quality controls were implemented, including double verification of patient weight, standardized drug-labeling protocols, and limits on prescription frequency to reduce confusion. As a result of these interventions, the hospital achieved a 30% reduction in risk associated with prescription errors. Another important KPI in Organization B measured workflow efficiency in the hospital pharmacy and nursing departments. Following the introduction of Lean tools such as Kanban labeling systems and streamlined medication-handling procedures, the pharmacy was able to eliminate 70 minutes of non-value-added work per day. At the same time, nurses gained an additional 9 minutes per day to spend in direct patient care, thanks to the reduction in redundant or inefficient tasks. The pharmacy also implemented additional KPIs to monitor accuracy in drug preparation and delivery, including checks for patient identification (name, birth date, and mother's name), sequential labeling of medications, and visual color-coding to prevent medication mix-ups. The Lean model enabled real-time adjustments and promoted collaboration between operational staff and management, significantly reducing errors without adding bureaucratic burden. This case study illustrates the tangible benefits of integrating KPIs into a Lean Healthcare framework. Unlike the TQ model, which often centralized decision-making and limited staff engagement to data collection, Lean empowered frontline workers to participate in root cause analysis, solution design, and implementation. Through collaborative, data-driven processes, Organization B not only improved clinical quality and safety but also enhanced workflow efficiency and staff satisfaction; the strategic use of KPIs in the Lean model resulted in measurable quality improvements. These outcomes highlight how KPIs, when aligned with Lean methodologies, can drive systemic improvements in healthcare delivery by enhancing both operational efficiency and patient-centered care. This case study offers valuable insights into how KPIs were employed to assess and improve the quality-of-care delivery, particularly within the Lean framework.[104]

REFERENCES

1. Donabedian A. Evaluating the quality of medical care. *Milbank Q*. 2005;83(4): 691-729. https://doi.org/10.1111/j.1468-0009.2005.00397.x
2. Porter ME, Teisberg EO. *Redefining Health Care: Creating Value-Based Competition on Results*. Brighton, MA: Harvard Business Review Press; 2006.
3. Institute for Healthcare Improvement. *Metrics for Value-Based Healthcare*. Published 2021. https://www.ihi.org/. Accessed April 6, 2026.
4. Centers for Medicare and Medicaid Services. *HCAHPS: Patients' Perspectives of Care Survey*. https://www.cms.gov/medicare/quality/initiatives/hospital-quality-initiative/hcahps-patients-perspectives-care-survey. Accessed March 4, 2026.
5. Girotra S, Cram P, Popescu I. Patient satisfaction at America's lowest performing hospitals. *Circ Cardiovasc Qual Outcomes*. 2012;5(3):365-372. https://doi.org/10.1161/circoutcomes.111.964361
6. Nabeel M, Prasad R, Kemnic T, Wang L. Structured, timely, and individualized patient feedback to residents and its effect on HCAHPS scores. *J Patient Exp*. 2022;9:1-8. https://doi.org/10.1177/23743735221112583
7. Jones S, Moulton C, Swift S, et al. Association between delays to patient admission from the emergency department and all-cause 30-day mortality. *Emerg Med J*. 2022;39(3):168-173. https://doi.org/10.1136/emermed-2021-211572
8. Glogovac G, Kennedy ME, Weisgerber MR, et al. Wait times in musculoskeletal patients: what contributes to patient satisfaction. *J Patient Exp*. 2020;7(4):549-553. https://doi.org/10.1177/2374373519864828
9. Trivedi KK, Schaffzin JK, Deloney VM, et al. Implementing strategies to prevent infections in acute-care settings. *Infect Control Hosp Epidemiol*. 2023;44(8):1232-1246. https://doi.org/10.1017/ice.2023.103
10. Jacobs D, Fowler E, Fleischer L, Sheshamani M. The Medicare value-based care strategy: alignment, growth, and equity. *Health Aff Forefront*. July 21, 2022. https://doi.org/10.1377/forefront.20220719.558038
11. Jarvik JG, Meier EN, James KT, et al. The effect of including benchmark prevalence data of common imaging findings in spine image reports on healthcare utilization among adults undergoing spine imaging: a stepped-wedge randomized clinical trial. *JAMA Netw Open*. 2020;3(9):e2015713. https://doi.org/10.1001/jamanetworkopen.2020.15713
12. Shittu AM, Hannon E, Kyriacou J, et al. Improving care for critical care patients by strategic alignment of quality goals with a physician financial incentive model. *Qual Manag Health Care*. 2021;30(1):21-26. https://doi.org/10.1097/QMH.0000000000000281
13. Braithwaite J, Herkes J, Ludlow K, et al. Association between organisational and workplace cultures, and patient outcomes: systematic review. *BMJ Open*. 2017;7:e017708. https://doi.org/10.1136/bmjopen-2017-017708
14. World Health Organization. *Medication Without Harm*. Geneva, Switzerland: WHO; 2017.
15. Smiddy MP, Murphy OM, Savage E, et al. Efficacy of observational hand hygiene audit with targeted feedback on doctors' hand hygiene compliance: a retrospective time series analysis. *J Infect Prev*. 2019;20(4):164-170. https://doi.org/10.1177/1757177419833165
16. Seavey R. Sterile processing accreditation surveys: risk reduction and process improvement. *AORN J*. 2015;102(4):358-368. https://doi.org/10.1016/j.aorn.2015.07.005
17. Arzahan I, Ismail Z, Yasin SM. Safety culture, safety climate, and safety performance in healthcare facilities: a systematic review. *Saf Sci*. 2022;147:105624. https://doi.org/10.1016/j.ssci.2021.105624
18. Labrague LJ. Nurses' adherence to patient safety protocols and its relationship with adverse patient events. *J Nurs Scholarsh*. 2024;56:282-290. https://doi.org/10.1111/jnu.12942
19. Leape LL, Kabcenell AI, Gandhi TK, et al. Reducing adverse drug events: lessons from a breakthrough series collaborative. *Jt Comm J Qual Improv*. 2000;26(6):321-331. https://doi.org/10.1016/S1070-3241(00)26026-4
20. McGrath SP, McGovern KM, Perreard IM, et al. Inpatient respiratory arrest associated with sedative and analgesic medications: impact of continuous monitoring on patient mortality and severe morbidity. *J Patient Saf*. 2021;17(8):557-561. https://doi.org/10.1097/PTS.0000000000000696
21. Humphries N, Morgan K, Conry MC, et al. Quality of care and health professional burnout: narrative literature review. *Int J Health Care Qual Assur*. 2014;27(4):293-307. https://doi.org/10.1108/IJHCQA-08-2012-0087
22. Shanafelt TD, Noseworthy JH. Executive leadership and physician well-being: nine organizational strategies to promote

engagement and reduce burnout. *Mayo Clin Proc*. 2017;92(1):129-146. https://doi.org/10.1016/j.mayocp.2016.10.004

23. Avinash B, Joseph G. Reimagining healthcare supply chains: a systematic review on digital transformation with specific focus on efficiency, transparency, and responsiveness. *J Health Organ Manag*. 2024;38(8):1255-1279. https://doi.org/10.1108/JHOM-03-2024-0076
24. Adapala V. Optimizing EHR data: a pathway to enhanced patient care and healthcare efficiency. *J Clin Eng*. 2024;49(4):140-142. https://doi.org/10.1097/JCE.0000000000000663
25. Hajjar L, Kragen B. Timely communication through telehealth: added value for a caregiver during COVID-19. *Front Public Health*. 2021;9:755391. https://doi.org/10.3389/fpubh.2021.755391
26. Zhao M, Hamadi H, Xu J, et al. Telehealth and hospital performance: does it matter? *J Telemed Telecare*. 2022;28(5):360-370. https://doi.org/10.1177/1357633X20932440
27. Bandi M, Masimukku AK, Vemula R, Vallu S. Predictive analytics in healthcare: enhancing patient outcomes through data-driven forecasting and decision-making. *Int J Mach Learn*. 2024;8(8):1-20.
28. Fihn SD, Saria S, Mendonça E, et al. Deploying AI in clinical settings. In: *Artificial Intelligence in Health Care: The Hope, the Hype, the Promise, the Peril*. Washington, DC: National Academies Press; 2019:145-165.
29. Bates DW, Cohen M, Leape LL, et al. Reducing the frequency of errors in medicine using information technology. *J Am Med Inform Assoc*. 2001;8(4):299-308. https://doi.org/10.1136/jamia.2001.0080299
30. Teich JM, Merchia PR, Schmiz JL, et al. Effects of computerized physician order entry on prescribing practices. *Arch Intern Med*. 2000;160(18):2741-2747. https://doi.org/10.1001/archinte.160.18.2741
31. Awad A, Trenfield SJ, Pollard TD, et al. Connected healthcare: improving patient care using digital health technologies. *Adv Drug Deliv Rev*. 2021;178:113958. https://doi.org/10.1016/j.addr.2021.113958
32. Hibbard JH, Stockard J, Tusler M. Hospital performance reports: impact on quality, market share, and reputation. *Health Aff (Millwood)*. 2005;24(4):1150-1160. https://doi.org/10.1377/hlthaff.24.4.1150
33. Hilts KE, Yeager VA, Gibson PJ, et al. Hospital partnerships for population health: a systematic review of the literature. *J Healthc Manag*. 2021;66(3):170-198. https://doi.org/10.1097/JHM-D-20-00172
34. Rhodes SD, Daniel-Ulloa J, Wright SS, et al. Critical elements of community engagement to address disparities and related social determinants of health: the Centers for Disease Control and Prevention Community Approaches to Reducing Sexually Transmitted Disease Initiative. *Sex Transm Dis*. 2021;48(1):49-55. https://doi.org/10.1097/OLQ.0000000000001267
35. Cyril S, Smith BJ, Possamai-Inesedy A, Renzaho AMN. Exploring the role of community engagement in improving the health of disadvantaged populations: a systematic review. *Glob Health Action*. 2015;18(8);29842. https://doi.org/10.3402/gha.v8.29842
36. Williams DR, Costa MV, Odunlami AO, Mohammed SA. Moving upstream: how interventions that address the social determinants of health can improve health and reduce disparities. *J Public Health Manag Pract*. 2008;14(6):S8-S17. https://doi.org/10.1097/01.PHH.0000338382.36695.42
37. Bachrach D, Braslow L, Karl A. Toward a high-performance healthcare system for vulnerable populations: funding for safety-net hospitals. *Commonwealth Fund*. 2012:1-56.
38. Bhati D, Deogade MS, Kanyal D. Improving patient outcomes through effective hospital administration: a comprehensive review. *Cureus*. 2023;15(10):e47731. https://doi.org/10.7759/cureus.47731
39. Fausett CM, Korentsides JM, Miller ZN, Keebler JR. Adaptive leadership in health care organizations: five insights to promote effective teamwork. *Psychol Lead Leaders*. 2024;27(1):6. https://psycnet.apa.org/doi/10.1037/mgr0000148
40. Applequist J, Miller-Day M, Cronholm PF, et al. "In principle we have agreement, but in practice it is a bit more difficult": obtaining organizational buy-in to patient-centered medical home transformation. *Qual Health Res*. 2017;27(6):909-922. https://doi.org/10.1177/1049732316680601
41. Weir R, Stewart L, Browne G, et al. The efficacy and effectiveness of process consultation in improving staff morale and absenteeism. *Med Care*. 1997;35(4):334-353. https://doi.org/10.1097/00005650-199704000-00005
42. Tsai Y. Relationship between organizational culture, leadership behavior, and job

satisfaction. *BMC Health Serv Res*. 2011;11:98. https://doi.org/10.1186/1472-6963-11-98

43. Tucker AL, Edmondson AC. Why hospitals don't learn from failures: organizational and psychological dynamics that inhibit system change. *Calif Manag Rev*. 2003;45(2):55-72.
44. McAlearney AS. Using leadership development programs to improve quality and efficiency in healthcare. *J Healthc Manag*. 2008;53(5):319-331. PMID: 18856137
45. Taylor N, Clay-Williams R, Hogden E, et al. High-performing hospitals: a qualitative systematic review of associated factors and practical strategies for improvement. *BMC Health Serv Res*. 2015;15:244. https://doi.org/10.1186/s12913-015-0879-z
46. Langabeer JR, DelliFraine JL, Heineke J, Abbass I. Implementation of Lean and Six Sigma quality initiatives in hospitals: a goal theoretic perspective. *Oper Manag Res*. 2009;2:13-27. https://doi.org/10.1007/s12063-009-0021-7
47. Liu HC, Zhang LJ, Ping YJ, Wang L. Failure mode and effects analysis for proactive healthcare risk evaluation: a systematic literature review. *J Eval Clin Pract*. 2020;26(4):1320-1337. https://doi.org/10.1111/jep.13317
48. Vilhelmsson A, Cofina IP, Wolodarski M, Alfvén T. Developing a guide for sustainable healthcare practice: a case study from the Swedish Society of Medicine. *J Clim Chang Health*. 2025:100413. https://doi.org/10.1016/j.joclim.2025.100413
49. Alshehhi A, Nobanee H, Khare N. The impact of sustainability practices on corporate financial performance: literature trends and future research potential. *Sustainability*. 2018;10(2):494. https://doi.org/10.3390/su10020494
50. Eckelman MJ, Sherman J. Environmental impacts of the US healthcare system and effects on public health. *PLoS ONE*. 2016;11(6):e0157014. https://doi.org/10.1371/journal.pone.0157014
51. Gray O, McCance T, Brown D. Exploring how key performance indicators influence nursing and midwifery practice: a mixed-methods study. *J Adv Nurs*. 2021;77(12):4900-4918. https://doi.org/10.1111/jan.15049
52. Fernandes O, Gorman S, Slavik R, et al. Development of clinical pharmacy key performance indicators for hospital pharmacists using a modified Delphi approach. *Ann Pharmacother*. 2015;49(6):656-669. https://doi.org/10.1177/1060028015577445
53. Conroy T, Grimmett J, Boylan S, Feo R. Identifying the contributors to nursing caring success stories. *J Clin Nurs*. 2024;33(9):3659-3668. https://doi.org/10.1111/jocn.17197
54. Gu X, Itoh K. Performance indicators: healthcare professionals' views. *Int J Health Care Qual Assur*. 2016;29(7):801-815. https://doi.org/10.1108/ijhcqa-12-2015-0142
55. Hoyer E, Padula W, Brotman D, et al. Patterns of hospital performance on the hospital-wide 30-day readmission metric: is the playing field level? *J Gen Intern Med*. 2017;33(1):57-64. https://doi.org/10.1007/s11606-017-4193-9
56. Pandey A, Patel K, Li L, et al. Association of hospital performance based on 30-day risk-standardized mortality rate with long-term survival after heart failure hospitalization. *JAMA Cardiol*. 2018;3(6):489. https://doi.org/10.1001/jamacardio.2018.0579
57. Pandey A, Keshvani N, Vaughan-Sarrazin M, et al. Evaluation of risk-adjusted home time after hospitalization for heart failure as a potential hospital performance metric. *JAMA Cardiol*. 2021;6(2):169. https://doi.org/10.1001/jamacardio.2020.4928
58. Mentias A, Desai M, Keshvani N, et al. Ninety-day risk-standardized home time as a performance metric for cardiac surgery hospitals in the United States. *Circulation*. 2022;146(17):1297-1309. https://doi.org/10.1161/circulationaha.122.059496
59. Horstman M, Li Y, Almenoff P, et al. Denominator doesn't matter: standardizing healthcare-associated infection rates by bed days or device days. *Infect Control Hosp Epidemiol*. 2015;36(6):710-716. https://doi.org/10.1017/ice.2015.42
60. Horwitz L, Wang Y, Altaf F, et al. Hospital characteristics associated with postdischarge hospital readmission, observation, and emergency department utilization. *Med Care*. 2018;56(4):281-289. https://doi.org/10.1097/mlr.0000000000000882
61. Datta S, Staicu M, Brundige M, et al. Days of therapy avoided: a novel method for measuring the impact of an antimicrobial stewardship program to stop antibiotics. *J Hosp Med*. 2018;13(5):326-327. https://doi.org/10.12788/jhm.2927
62. Rego I, Coelho S, Semedo P, et al. 360 health analysis (H360)—a comparison of key performance indicators in breast cancer management across health institution settings in Portugal. *Curr Oncol*. 2023;30(7):6041-6065. https://doi.org/10.3390/curroncol30070451

63. Shawahna R. Development of key performance indicators for capturing impact of pharmaceutical care in Palestinian integrative healthcare facilities: a Delphi consensus study. *Evid Based Complement Alternat Med*. 2020;2020:7527543. https://doi.org/10.1155/2020/7527543
64. Lloyd G, Singh S, Barclay P, et al. Hospital pharmacists' perspectives on the role of key performance indicators in Australian pharmacy practice. *J Pharm Pract Res*. 2016;47(2):87-95. https://doi.org/10.1002/jppr.1156
65. Cossart AR, Kennedy E, Yong FR, et al. Consumer perceptions of direct-to-consumer electronic prescription services in Queensland, Australia. *Digit Health*. 2024;10:1-10. https://doi.org/10.1177/20552076241294184
66. Lewis AK, Harding KE, Snowdon DA, Taylor NF. Reducing wait time from referral to first visit for community outpatient services may contribute to better health outcomes: a systematic review. *BMC Health Serv Res*. 2018;18(1):869. https://doi.org/10.1186/s12913-018-3669-6
67. De Jong K, Delgadillo J, Barkham M. *Routine Outcome Monitoring and Feedback in Psychological Therapies*. Maidenhead, United Kingdom: McGraw-Hill Education; 2023.
68. Tisminetzky M, Nepomuceno R, Kung JY, et al. Key performance indicators in extracorporeal membrane oxygenation (ECMO): protocol for a systematic review. *BMJ Open*. 2023;13(12):e076233. https://doi.org/10.1136/bmjopen-2023-076233
69. Bleustein C, Rothschild DB, Valen A, et al. Wait times, patient satisfaction scores, and the perception of care. *Am J Manag Care*. 2014;20(5):393-400. PMID: 25181568
70. Janssen S, Moeller K, Schlaefke M. Using performance measures conceptually in innovation control. *J Manag Control*. 2011;22(1):107-128. https://doi.org/10.1007/s00187-011-0130-y
71. Khare S, Batist G, Bartlett G. Identification of performance indicators across a network of clinical cancer programs. *Curr Oncol*. 2016;23(2):81-90. https://doi.org/10.3747/co.23.2789
72. Healthcare Information Management Systems Society (HIMSS). *What Is Interoperability?* http://nationalcapitalarea.himss.org/resources/interoperability-healthcare. Accessed March 4, 2026.
73. Perugu B, Wadhwa V, Kim J, et al. Pragmatic approaches to interoperability–surmounting barriers to healthcare data and information across organizations and political boundaries. *Telehealth Med Today*. 2023;8(4):1-22. https://doi.org/10.30953/thmt.v8.421
74. Rusanov A, Weiskopf NG, Wang S, Weng C. Hidden in plain sight: bias towards sick patients when sampling patients with sufficient electronic health record data for research. *BMC Med Inform Decis Mak*. 2014;14:51. https://doi.org/10.1186/1472-6947-14-51
75. Bhartiya S, Mehrotra D, Girdhar A. Issues in achieving complete interoperability while sharing electronic health records. *Procedia Comput Sci*. 2016;78:192-198. https://doi.org/10.7759/cureus.47731
76. Torab-Miandoab A, Samad-Soltani T, Jodati A, Rezaei-Hachesu P. Interoperability of heterogeneous health information systems: a systematic literature review. *BMC Med Inform Decis Mak*. 2023;23(1):18. https://doi.org/10.1186/s12911-023-02115-5
77. Cohen DJ, Dorr DA, Knierim K, et al. Primary care practices' abilities and challenges in using electronic health record data for quality improvement. *Health Aff (Millwood)*. 2018;37(4):635-643. https://doi.org/10.1377/hlthaff.2017.1254
78. De Mello BH, Rigo SJ, da Costa CA, et al. Semantic interoperability in health records standards: a systematic literature review. *Health Technol (Berl)*. 2022;12(2):255-272. https://doi.org/10.1007/s12553-022-00639-w
79. Bundi DG, Mutua SM, Karume SM. Mitigating factors affecting secure interoperability of medical systems using DLTs in healthcare. *Int J Comput Appl Technol Res*. 13(1):1-6. https://doi.org/10.7753/IJCATR1301.1001
80. Tariq MU. Revolutionizing health data management with blockchain technology: enhancing security and efficiency in a digital era. In: *Emerging Technologies for Health Literacy and Medical Practice*. Hershey, PA: IGI Global; 2024:153-175. https://doi.org/10.4018/979-8-3693-1214-8.ch008
81. Isgut M, Gloster L, Choi K, et al. Systematic review of advanced AI methods for improving healthcare data quality in post COVID-19 era. *IEEE Rev Biomed Eng*. 2023;16:53-69. https://doi.org/10.1109/RBME.2022.3216531
82. Mehta S, Grant K, Ackery A. Future of blockchain in healthcare: potential to improve the accessibility, security and interoperability of electronic health records. *BMJ Health Care Inform*. 2020;27(3):e100217. https://doi.org/10.1136/bmjhci-2020-100217

83. Reegu FA, Abas H, Gulzar Y, et al. Blockchain-based framework for interoperable electronic health records for an improved healthcare system. *Sustainability*. 2023;15(8):6337. https://doi.org/10.3390/su15086337

84. Nazer LH, Zatarah R, Waldrip S, et al. Bias in artificial intelligence algorithms and recommendations for mitigation. *PLoS Digit Health*. 2023;2(6):e0000278. https://doi.org/10.1371/journal.pdig.0000278

85. Singh K. Artificial intelligence & cloud in healthcare: analyzing challenges and solutions within regulatory boundaries. *Int J Comput Sci Eng*. 2023;10(9):1-9. https://doi.org/10.14445/23488387/IJCSE-V10I9P101

86. Watson SE, Smith P, Snowden J, et al. Facilitators and barriers to pediatric clinical trial recruitment and retention in rural and community settings: a scoping review of the literature. *Clin Transl Sci*. 2022;15(4):838-853. https://doi.org/10.1111/cts.13220

87. Moy AJ, Schwartz JM, Chen R, et al. Measurement of clinical documentation burden among physicians and nurses using electronic health records: a scoping review. *J Am Med Inform Assoc*. 2021;28(5):998-1008. https://doi.org/10.1093/jamia/ocaa325

88. Gelman A, Carlin J. Beyond power calculations: assessing type S (sign) and type M (magnitude) errors. *Perspect Psychol Sci*. 2014;9(6):641-651. https://doi.org/10.1177/1745691614551642

89. Eng J. Sample size estimation: how many individuals should be studied? *Radiology*. 2003;227(2):309-313. https://doi.org/10.1148/radiol.2272012051

90. Hedges LV, Pigott TD. The power of statistical tests in meta-analysis. *Psychol Methods*. 2001;6(3):203-217. PMID: 11570228

91. Topp SM, Schaaf M, Sriram V, et al. Power analysis in health policy and systems research: a guide to research conceptualisation. *BMJ Glob Health*. 2021;6(11):e007268. https://doi.org/10.1136/bmjgh-2021-007268

92. Miles J. A framework for power analysis using a structural equation modelling procedure. *BMC Med Res Methodol*. 2003;3:27. https://doi.org/10.1186/1471-2288-3-27

93. Salas E, Almeida SA, Salisbury M, et al. What are the critical success factors for team training in health care? *Jt Comm J Qual Patient Saf*. 2009;35(8):398-405. https://doi.org/10.1016/s1553-7250(09)35056-4

94. Stange KC, Etz RS, Gullett H, et al. Metrics for assessing improvements in primary health care. *Annu Rev Public Health*. 2014;35:423-442. https://doi.org/10.1146/annurev-publhealth-032013-182438

95. Al Ani M, Garas G, Hollingshead J, et al. Which electronic health record system should we use? A systematic review. *Med Princ Pract*. 2022;31(4):342-351. https://doi.org/10.1159/000525135

96. Gray CP, Yakir M, Hung DY. Physician engagement with metrics in Lean primary care transformation. *Qual Manag Health Care*. 2018;27(3):117-122. https://doi.org/10.1097/QMH.0000000000000182

97. Berenson RA, Pronovost PJ, Krumholz HM. Achieving the potential of health care performance measures. *Timely Anal Immed Health Pol*. 2013; 2:1-31.

98. Chee TT, Ryan AM, Wasfy JH, Borden WB. Current state of value-based purchasing programs. *Circulation*. 2016;133(22):2197-2205. https://doi.org/10.1161/CIRCULATIONAHA.115.010268

99. Kachalia A, Mello MM, Nallamothu BK, Studdert DM. Legal and policy interventions to improve patient safety. *Circulation*. 2016;133(7):661-671. https://doi.org/10.1161/CIRCULATIONAHA.115.015880

100. Menard AR, Hentel K, Raja AS, et al. A way forward for the imaging appropriate use criteria program: aligning quality metrics. *Health Aff Forefront*. August 26, 2021. https://doi.org/10.1377/forefront.20210819.144848

101. Barber CE, Patel JN, Woodhouse LJ, et al. Development of key performance indicators to evaluate centralized intake for patients with osteoarthritis and rheumatoid arthritis. *Arthritis Res Ther*. 2015;17(1):1-12. https://doi.org/10.1186/s13075-015-0843-7

102. Mottes TA, Goldstein SL, Basu RK. Process-based quality improvement using a continuous renal replacement therapy dashboard. *BMC Nephrol*. 2019;20(1):1-7. https://doi.org/10.1186/s12882-018-1195-8

103. del Castillo J, Lopez-Herce J, Cidoncha E, et al. Circuit life span in critically ill children on continuous renal replacement treatment: a prospective observational evaluation study. *Crit Care*. 2008;12(4):R93. https://doi.org/10.1186/cc6965

104. Eiro N, Torres A. Comparative study: total quality (TQ) and Lean production ownership models in health services. *Rev Lat Am Enfermagem*. 2015;23(5):846-854. https://doi.org/10.1590/0104-1169.0151.2605

3 Observational Study Designs

Elinor G. Borgert, PhD, MSc

INTRODUCTION

Case-control, cohort, and randomized controlled trials all focus on comparisons of individuals. Information for these analyses is often gathered through interviews or medical records and is specific for each person included in the sample. These individual-level approaches can be labor-intensive and expensive, but they are routinely conducted because they allow researchers to predict risk or odds. This chapter will describe various study designs employed frequently in clinical and epidemiologic studies, with a primary focus on case-control, cohort, and ecologic study designs. Randomized controlled trials will be covered in more detail in Chapter 5.

CASE REPORT AND CASE SERIES

A clinician who observes and reports a clinical finding regarding a patient has conducted an observational study called a case report. A case series differs from a case report in that it reports the findings regarding several patients. These two study designs describe the finding with respect to person, place, time, and other relevant variables, and their primary value is that they are hypothesis-generating. For example, a clinician may describe a patient whose blood pressure increased subsequent to the use of a particular medication. The clinician presents demographic and clinical information about the patient, as well as the time sequence of events. This provides information about a possible association between the drug and clinical outcome, potentially motivating others to test the proposed relationship with a stronger study design.

CROSS-SECTIONAL STUDIES

Cross-sectional studies provide useful information about the prevalence of a condition or disease at a particular point in time. Data can be collected from a variety of sources, including surveys, chart reviews, and large database analyses. A critical shortcoming of this approach is that it does not establish a temporal sequence between the variables examined. For example, a cross-sectional study can provide valuable information about the prevalence of antidepressant use in a population. Likewise, it can provide prevalence data regarding suicide ideation in a community. However, because temporal sequence cannot be established within the context of a cross-sectional design, the researcher and reader cannot infer that suicide ideation is the result of antidepressant use. Cross-sectional studies cannot answer the question of whether antidepressants precede or follow suicide ideation, because both are assessed simultaneously. But it can provide valuable information in support of further investigation.

CASE-CONTROL STUDIES

Case-control studies and cohort studies include the significant design improvement of a control group. The presence of a control group helps to address threats to validity, such as confounding. No longer can a distant clinical outcome be attributed to the aging of the

DOI: 10.37573/9781585287666.003

study population as a plausible alternative explanation, because such changes would have occurred in the control group as well. Because both groups are affected in a similar fashion, the effect of aging or other potential confounders is essentially negated. The introduction of a control group gives the reader increased confidence in the reported results.

In a case-control study, subjects are selected on the basis of an outcome or disease of interest. Subjects who have the disease are called cases. Subjects who do not have the disease are called controls. Cases can be either incident (newly diagnosed) or prevalent (current but previously diagnosed). Cases and controls are then compared with respect to an exposure of interest. The selection of subjects begins with case or control status (ie, whether the subject has the disease), and then the researcher looks back in time to assess everyone's exposure status. If subjects with the disease have a markedly different level of historic exposure (to a drug, surgical technique, diet, method of counseling, etc.) than those without the disease, it is considered evidence of an association between the exposure and outcome.

Cases are identified based on a clear disease diagnosis. The control group is drawn from subjects who are comparable to the source population for cases and so could have been recruited into the study as cases if they had developed the disease. For example, a case-control study examining the relationship between a new pain medication and the development of ulcers subsequent to surgery may identify cases from the orthopedic service of a hospital. Controls might then be selected from people who had general surgery within the same hospital. The critical aspect of selecting controls is not that the general surgery patients are the same as the orthopedic patients or that they represent all people who have had surgeries. The control group must simply come from the same source population (admitted to the hospital) so that they would have been identified as a case if, in fact, they instead had orthopedic surgery and developed an ulcer.

Researchers have several possible sources to consider in building their control group, including hospital patients, the general population, and friends/relatives of cases. Each source offers particular advantages and disadvantages. Although hospitalized patients can be most easily identified, they are also usually very ill. General population controls can be obtained via random-digit dialing, population registers, or voting lists/poll information, but this approach to obtaining controls can be costly and time-consuming. A more detailed discussion of the advantages and disadvantages of the different sources of control groups can be found in Hennekens and Buring.[1]

The number of subjects in the control group depends on the availability of subjects for inclusion, as well as the time and cost associated with identifying them and collecting information about them. Where cases and controls are plentiful and the cost of obtaining information about cases and controls is similar, a ratio of 1:1 is desirable. However, if the number of cases is small and the time and money cost of obtaining information on additional controls is not excessive, additional subjects in the control group may be desirable. Increasing the number of subjects in the control group will give the study additional power by reducing estimate variability. But beyond a 4:1 control to case ratio, any increased power resulting from expanding the number of subjects in the control group is negligible.[1]

Determining exposure status in cases and controls can involve a variety of sources. Examples include pharmacy records (to determine drug exposure), diet surveys and diaries (to determine nutritional exposure), and school records (to determine whether subjects were immunized). To avoid bias, the method used to obtain exposure information should be similar for all subjects—both cases and controls. It generally works best if a subject's case status is not known by the person collecting or recording information about the subject's exposure.

Measures of association are point estimates of the relationship between an exposure and disease or outcome. In case-control studies, this association is assessed by calculating an odds ratio (OR). The odds of exposure among cases are compared with the odds of exposure among controls. Dividing the respective odds yields an OR. An OR of 1.0 indicates that the odds of exposure among cases are equal to the odds of exposure among controls; this is the null value, indicating that there is no association between the exposure and outcome. A value greater than 1.0 indicates that the odds of exposure among cases are greater than the odds of exposure among controls. A value less than 1.0 indicates that the odds of exposure among cases are less than the odds of exposure among controls.

In their simplest form, case-control studies can be summarized using a 2 × 2 table that categorizes individuals by disease status (yes or no) and exposure status (yes or no). In **Table 3-1**, "a" represents individuals who both had the disease and were exposed, while "c" represents those who had the disease but were not exposed. The odds of exposure among the cases are calculated as the ratio of exposed to unexposed cases, or a/c. Similarly, among the controls (those without the disease), "b" represents the exposed and "d" the unexposed, giving an odds of exposure of b/d.

$$OR = (a/c) / (b/d)$$

which simplifies to

$$OR = ad / bc$$

Case-control designs typically involve investigations into multiple potential exposures suspected of contributing to the disease. These variables may not be the main variable of interest, but they are included because they might influence the association between the exposure variable of interest and the outcome variable. If these variables are related to the outcome and are present to different degrees in the two exposure groups, then the variables may be confounders in that they can distort the observed relationship between the exposure and outcome. Investigators have several strategies to control for confounding, including stratification, restriction, and multivariate analysis. A full description of the other methods is beyond the scope of this chapter on designs, and the reader is referred to Hennekens and Buring,[1] Gordis,[2] or Rothman.[3]

As an example, suppose a pharmaceutical company accumulated evidence from case reports and case series suggesting that its drug for hypertension is protective against developing glaucoma. A case-control study was conducted in which community-based cases of glaucoma were identified. An appropriate control group of subjects without glaucoma was created. The distribution of cases and controls with and without exposure to the hypertension drug is reported in **Table 3-2**.

$$OR = (a/c) / (b/d)$$
$$ad / bc$$
$$(100 \times 1{,}600) / (300 \times 800)$$
$$160{,}000 / 240{,}000$$
$$0.67$$

Glaucoma patients (the cases) were two-thirds as likely to have been exposed to the hypertension drug as people who did not have glaucoma (the controls). This case-control study provides additional evidence to support the hypothesis developed from the case reports and case series, namely, that exposure to the hypertension drug is protective against developing glaucoma.

The confidence placed in the estimate of an OR is determined by the *p*-value and confidence interval (CI), the latter of which establishes low and high bounds within which the true point estimate lies. A large CI indicates a low level of precision of the OR, whereas a small CI indicates a higher precision of the OR. If the 95% CI includes the null value of 1, then the association would not be considered

TABLE 3-1. 2 × 2 Cross-Tabulation of Exposure and Disease in a Case-Control Study

Exposure	Disease	No Disease
Present	a	b
Absent	c	d

TABLE 3-2. Hypothetical Example of Glaucoma Potentially Resulting From Medication for Hypertension

Exposure	Glaucoma	No Glaucoma
Took Medication	100	300
Did NOT Take Medication	800	1,600

TABLE 3-3. Strengths and Limitations of Case-Control and Cohort Study Designs

Case-Control Designs

Strengths

- Quicker and less expensive than cohort or experimental studies
- Well-suited for evaluating diseases with long latency periods
- Optimal for evaluating rare diseases
- Allow for examination of multiple etiologic factors for a single disease

Limitations

- Inefficient for the evaluation of rare exposures
- Prone to bias, especially recall bias and selection bias
- Do not allow for direct calculation of incidence rates
- Temporal sequence of exposure and outcome not always known

Cohort Designs

Strengths

- Appropriate for evaluating rare exposures
- Temporal sequence of exposure and outcome is clear
- Selection and recall bias are minimized
- Allow for direct calculation of incidence rates

Limitations

- Time and cost tend to be greater than case-control studies
- Subjects are lost to follow-up over the course of the study
- Not efficient for evaluating rare diseases

statistically significant and $p > 0.05$. Conversely, if the CI does not cross the null threshold of OR = 1, then the results are statistically significant and the $p < 0.05$. If the 95% CI for the OR calculated above is 0.52 to 0.85, then odds of prior medication use in glaucoma patients are statistically significantly less than the odds of prior medication use in people without glaucoma.

Odds ratios are only an approximation of relative risk (RR), which will be discussed in detail later in the chapter. But the two measures become (nearly) indistinguishable when the disease under consideration is rare. The 2 × 2 tables in Table 3-1 and **Table 3-3** can help to provide a separate mathematical explanation for why this is the case and why case-control studies are ideally suited for rare diseases. If a disease is very rare, then the numbers in cells a and c become very small in value, so that (a + b) approximates b alone and (c + d) approximates d alone. When the values of b and d overwhelmingly dominate the denominator, ORs are essentially equivalent to RR. The formula for RR, which is (a/a + b)/(c/c + d), essentially reduces to the formula for the OR, which is (a/b)/(c/d).

Case-control studies have several important strengths and limitations (Table 3-3). They are relatively quick and inexpensive compared with experimental or cohort studies. They are often the best/only study design suited to the evaluation of very rare diseases or those with especially long latency periods. Both of these strengths are derived from the fact that case-control studies do not require the investigator to follow subjects over time to determine whether the disease or outcome develops. Case-control designs allow the investigator to begin at a point in time when disease status is already known.

However, this also results in limitations. Case-control studies are retrospective, meaning that they look back in time to assess exposure after the outcome or disease has occurred, which can lead to recall bias. Subjects who have a disease may be more motivated to recall exposures in the past than subjects who do not have the disease. If cases remember exposures differently than controls, the misclassification bias or differential accuracy in information between the exposed and unexposed groups could lead to either an underestimation or overestimation of the OR. In contrast, nonrandom or nondifferential misclassification tends to bias the OR towards the null value.

Case-control studies are also inefficient for the study of the relationship between a disease and especially rare exposures. Because the size of the population at risk is never known, researchers are unable to directly calculate incidence rates. The OR serves as only an approximation of the RR, although as noted above, the distinction is moot when case-control studies are used for very rare diseases.

COHORT STUDIES

In contrast to the case-control study design, a cohort study identifies disease-free subjects based on their exposure status and then follows them forward for a specific time frame to assess the occurrence of disease.[4] They can be categorized as prospective or retrospective, depending on the point in the analytical process that the study begins. When the cohort's exposure status is defined at study start, and they are then followed into the future to see if and when a disease develops, the cohort study is referred to as prospective study (**Figure 3-1A**). A drawback of this approach is that it can take a long time for a disease to develop, which can be quite costly and result in subjects lost to follow-up.

When a cohort is identified and assembled in the past based on existing records and then followed to the point when the study is started, the cohort study is referred to as retrospective or historical. In this type of cohort study, both the exposure and outcome/disease occurred at the start of the study (**Figure 3-1C**). Retrospective studies generally require a shorter time commitment and are less expensive than prospective studies. They also tend to be better suited for the assessment of diseases with longer time periods between exposure and disease manifestation. They are especially useful when records can be linked to other registries and public information data sources, such as when occupational/work records can be linked to mortality and cancer registries.[4] Because they are dependent on information collected prior to the planning of the study, the quality of exposure or outcome data is sometimes not the most ideal for addressing the research questions posed.

Designs representing a combination of prospective and retrospective cohorts have also been constructed and utilized (**Figure 3-1B**).[1] The advantage of this type of hybrid cohort study design is its ability to explore both the possible short- and long-term effects of an exposure.

Cohort studies are especially well-suited to assess associations when rare and potentially harmful exposures are of interest, such as can occur with occupational exposures or industrial accidents. Because all participants are clearly

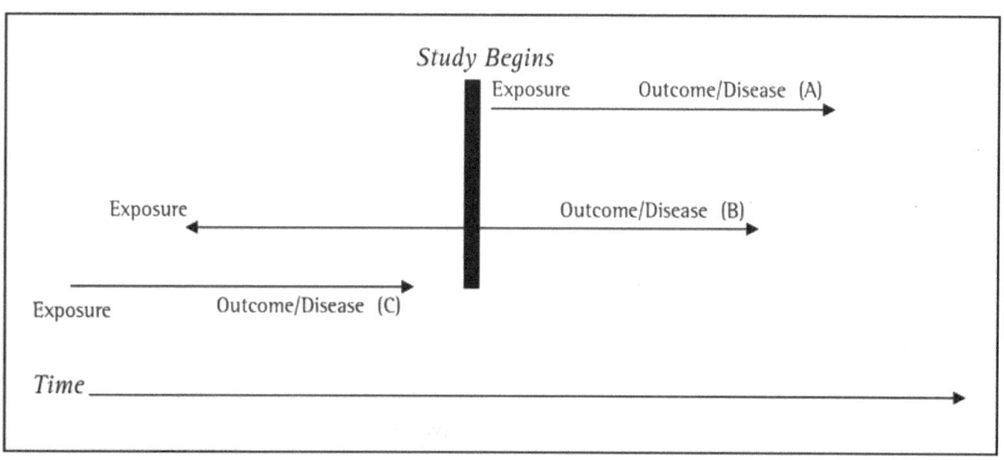

FIGURE 3-1. **Difference in cohort categorization: (A) prospective cohort design, (B) combination of prospective and retrospective design, and (C) retrospective cohort design.**

disease-free when their exposure status is defined, the temporal sequence between exposure and outcome is clear, which minimizes selection bias. Also, because exposure is measured at baseline, misclassification bias from incorrectly assessing an individual's exposure status is also less likely to be a concern.

However, other types of biases remain a concern. Attrition bias is more common in longitudinal studies and occurs when individuals who are lost to follow-up differ from those who remain in ways related to the outcome, or when losses to follow-up are different in the exposed and unexposed groups. Nonresponse bias is a related concern but occurs at the beginning of a study if the individuals who choose not to participate (or drop out early) differ meaningfully from participants, particularly in ways related to both the exposure and the outcome. Cohort studies also tend to be more expensive than case-control studies in terms of both time and money. Table 3-3 summarizes some of the key strengths and limitations of both study designs.

A key assumption in calculating incidence or risk rates in a cohort study is that individuals lost to follow-up are similar to those who remain with regard to characteristics affecting the outcome of interest. To quantify the association between exposure and outcome, the incidence in each group is calculated as the number of people who developed the disease divided by the number of people in the group. When data are tabulated as in **Table 3-4**, the formulas are as follows:

Incidence in the exposed group = a/(a + b)

Incidence in the unexposed group = c/(c + d)

Researchers can then use these estimates of risk to calculate a measure of association as either the absolute difference (attributable risk or attributable risk reduction) or relative difference (RR). Attributable risk (AR) measures the excess risk of disease associated with the exposure of interest. As such, it is simply the difference between the incidence or risk estimates in the two groups, calculated by subtracting the incidence estimate in the unexposed group from the incidence estimate in the exposed group.

AR = Incidence in the exposed group − Incidence in the unexposed group

$$AR = a/(a + b) - c/(c + d)$$

Attributable risk represents the number of cases of disease within the exposed group that is attributed to the exposure. If there is no additional risk, its value is 0. Values greater than 0 indicate that a certain number of cases can be attributed to the exposure. Values less than 0 would indicate that the exposure is in some way protective against developing the disease.

As mentioned previously, the RR of developing the disease is expressed as the ratio of the risk (incidence) in exposed individuals to that in unexposed.

RR = Incidence in the exposed group / Incidence in the unexposed group

$$RR = a/(a + b) \,/\, c/(c + d)$$

If the RR is 1.0, then the incidence in the exposed population is equal to the incidence in the unexposed population, and there is no evidence of an association between exposure and disease. If the RR is greater than 1.0, the incidence in the exposed is greater than the incidence in the unexposed, suggesting a positive relationship between exposure and outcome. This means that the exposed group is at greater risk of developing the disease compared with the unexposed group. Conversely, if the RR is less than 1.0, then the incidence in the exposed group is less than the incidence in the unexposed, a negative relationship, which indicates that the exposure is protective against developing the disease.

In a hypothetical example shown in **Table 3-5**, the exposure of interest is a new drug indicated for the treatment of cardiovascular disease that is suspected of contributing to liver disease.

$$RR = a/(a + b) \,/\, c/(c + d)$$

$$RR = 400/\,20{,}000 \,/\, 100/\,20{,}000$$

$$RR = 4.0$$

TABLE 3-4. 2 × 2 Cross-Tabulation of Exposure and Disease in a Cohort Study

Exposure	Disease	No Disease	Total Number
Present	a	b	a + b
Absent	c	d	c + d

TABLE 3-5. Hypothetical Example of New Cardiovascular Drug with Liver Disease Presenting as an Adverse Effect

Exposure	Liver Disease	No Liver Disease	Total Number
Present	400	19,600	20,000
Absent	100	19,900	20,000

An RR = 4 means that the risk of developing liver disease is four times greater in people who were taking the cardiovascular disease drug than in the unexposed group who were not taking the drug.

As with ORs discussed above, the confidence placed in the estimate of RR is determined by the CI and *p*-value. If the 95% CI includes the null value of 1, then the association would not be considered statistically significant. For example, if the estimate of RR = 4 above has a 95% CI of 0.8 to 7, then the risk of developing the outcome in the exposed group is not statistically significantly greater than the risk of developing the outcome in the nonexposed group. A broad interval also reflects a lack of precision of the point estimate, as the true point estimate of RR may be quite different than the calculated point estimate within the CI.

As simple as the calculations for AR and RR appear, they are often either confused or selectively deployed to confuse others.[10] Researchers or advertisers wanting to imply the maximum impact for otherwise modest findings might be tempted to focus attention on the RR rather than AR. If a really expensive new drug reduces the risk of death from 0.2% to 0.1%, they could rightly trumpet an impressive-sounding RR reduction of 50%. Because the difference or the AR reduction was just 0.1%, this means that a patient's chance of surviving would increase from 99.98% to 99.99%. This reflects only a very small improvement for which few would be willing to pay a great deal.

Fortunately, there is an alternative but related statistic that is intuitively understandable by patients and policy makers alike. The number needed to treat (NNT) is the number of patients who would need to be treated to prevent one additional bad outcome, such as death or stroke. It is calculated as the inverse of the AR, rounded up to the nearest whole number.

$$\text{NNT} = 1/\text{AR}$$

For example, if a new drug reduces the risk of a stroke from 40% to 20%, then:

$$\text{AR} = \text{Incidence in the exposed group} - \text{Incidence in the unexposed group} = 0.4 - 0.2 = 0.2$$

$$\text{NNT} = 1/\text{AR} = 1/0.2 = 5$$

Therefore, five patients would need to be treated with the new drug to prevent one stroke.

In disclosing information about the risks and benefits of therapeutic alternatives, NNT is often the easiest to understand/share and can be used to generate patient-specific estimates of the outcome event.

ECOLOGIC STUDIES

Case-control, cohort, and randomized controlled trials (see Chapter 5) all focus on comparisons of individuals. Information for these analyses is specific for each person included in the sample, often gathered through individual interviews or medical records. These individual-level approaches are relatively labor-intensive and expensive, but they are routinely conducted because they allow researchers to predict individual risk or odds.

In contrast, ecologic studies focus on comparisons of groups. Typically, the groups are derived from geographically defined areas, such as nations, states, or counties, and the analyses combine existing datasets on large populations. Ecologic analyses look at aggregated data, such as percentages, rates, and means. These data may be classified into three main types:[5]

1. Aggregate measures or summaries of observations derived from individuals in a group (eg, national literacy rates, state cancer rates, county employment rates, or class average SAT scores)

2. Environmental measures or characteristics of the place in which the individuals in the group live or work (eg, average environmental toxin levels or mean hours of sunlight)
3. Global measures (eg, the existence of a specific law, the type of healthcare system, and population density)

Ecologic analyses use these data to predict group rates of outcomes, such as disease. The most common method of analysis for ecologic data is linear regression.[5] The dependent variable (Y) is the group-specific disease rate or prevalence, and the independent variables (Xs) are group-specific exposure prevalences.

For example, an analysis by Gross and colleagues examined the relationship between the increased consumption of refined carbohydrates and the prevalence of type 2 diabetes in the United States between 1933 and 1997.[4-6] Their linear regression model found a strong and statistically significant association between an increasing trend in the prevalence of type 2 diabetes and both an increased consumption of refined carbohydrates in the form of corn syrup ($\beta = 0.013$, $p = 0.038$) and a decreased consumption of dietary fiber ($\beta = -13.86$, $p < 0.01$) (**Table 3-6; Figure 3-2**). For further information on interpreting the results of linear regression analyses, refer to Chapter 9.

Ecologic analyses have several practical advantages that make them especially appealing for certain types of research and have led to their widespread use in epidemiology:

1. *They are quick, convenient, and inexpensive*. Because they are often based on existing (ie, secondary) data that are publicly available, such as the two datasets employed by Gross and colleagues,[5] ecologic analyses are generally less expensive and take less time than individual-level analyses.
2. *They are ideally suited to generate hypotheses*. Because they are so quick and inexpensive, they are often used to explore potential relationships between diseases and exposures and provide theoretical support for individual-level studies of the same issue.
3. *They avoid some of the measurement limitations of individual-level studies*. There are many variables that are difficult to accurately measure at an individual level and are far easier to get on an aggregated level. For example, obtaining accurate annual carbohydrate consumption figures for individuals in a study population would be an extraordinarily complex, expensive, and time-consuming undertaking. By contrast, Gross and colleagues used a readily available estimate of per capita carbohydrate consumption based on national food disappearance data.[5] In fact, many individual level studies are now routinely incorporating some ecologic or

TABLE 3-6. Linear Regression Model Examining the Associations Between Trends in Nutrients and the Prevalence of Type 2 Diabetes in the United States Between 1933 and 1997

Nutrient Contribution	β Coefficient	*P*
Dietary fiber (% of energy)	−13.86	0.0083
Corn syrup (% of energy)	0.0132	0.038
Protein (% of energy)	−3.58	0.084
Fat (% of energy)	0.00196	0.79
Total energy (kcal)	0.00011	0.28

A positive β coefficient indicates an increased risk of type 2 diabetes, whereas a negative coefficient indicates a decreased risk of type 2 diabetes.

Source: Reproduced with permission by the American Journal of Clinical Nutrition. *Am J Clin Nutr.* © American Society for Clinical Nutrition.

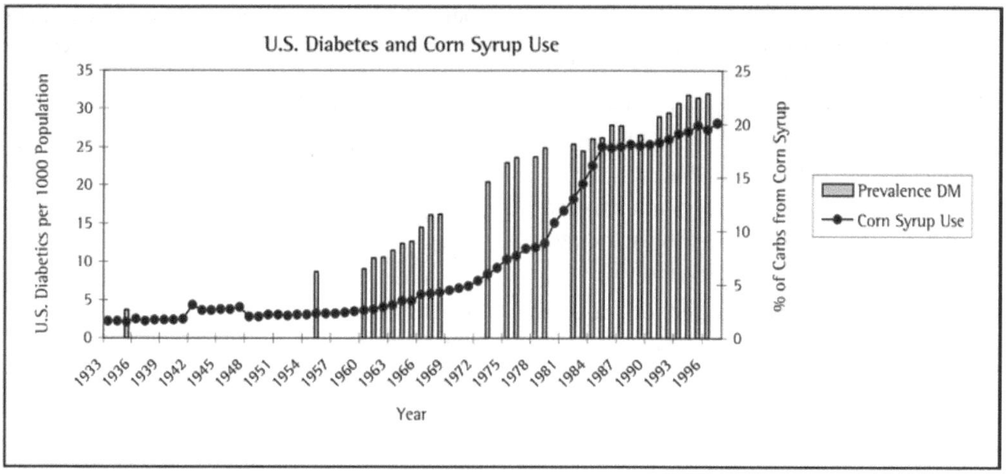

FIGURE 3-2. **Increasing prevalence of type 2 diabetes (vertical bars) in the United States between 1933 and 1997 with increasing per capita percentage of carbohydrate intake from corn syrup.**

Source: Reproduced with permission by the American Journal of Clinical Nutrition. *Am J Clin Nutr.* © American Society for Clinical Nutrition.

group-level measurements in their analyses.[6] This is especially true in environmental epidemiology, where researchers are unable to accurately measure relevant exposures or doses at the individual level for large numbers of subjects—at least not with available time and resources. Thus, an ecologic measurement may be the only practical way to approximate a measure of the exposure of interest.[5,7]

4. *They are ideally suited to evaluate the population effect of public policies, programs, and legislation*. Ecologic analyses are especially well-suited for evaluating issues from a public health perspective, such as policy analyses evaluating the effectiveness of a community intervention. Because legislation is applied to an entire population, it is actually more informative to analyze the effect on the group. For example, researchers could use an ecologic analysis to assess the effect of gun safety laws on state murder rates or the effect of flu vaccine clinics on employee workdays missed.

Still, it is especially important to keep in mind the limitations of an ecologic analysis.

1. *The ecologic fallacy is the mistaken conclusion that because an association exists between exposure and disease at the group level, it also exists at the individual level.* It is the failure of ecologic effect estimates to reflect biologic effects at the individual level. Because the data in ecologic studies are measurements aggregated over individuals, the associations between exposure and disease at the group level do not necessarily reflect individual-level associations. The basic problem is heterogeneity within groups. Suppose a researcher finds that national breast cancer mortality rates tend to be higher in countries with high-fat diets using ecologic data. If, based on this analysis alone, he or she were then to infer that individuals with high-fat diets are more likely to have breast cancer, he or she would be committing an ecologic fallacy. Because only group-level variables were used in the analysis, the researcher would have no way of knowing whether the breast cancer observed occurring in nations with high fat consumption was actually occurring among women who are consuming a lot of fat.
2. *They are restricted to available data.* Another chief limitation of ecologic analyses is that they are restricted to available data. For example, the analysis of type 2 diabetes by Gross and colleagues used

data from the National Nutrition Databank.[5] These nutrient data are based on annual food disappearance in the United States over the past century and are the foundation of essentially all public and private work in the field of human nutrition.[2] However, food disappearance data at the population level is only an indirect measure of individual consumption.

As in the previous section, suppose that a researcher finds that national breast cancer mortality rates tend to be higher in countries with high-fat diets using ecologic data. It would be important to note that the researcher used readily available mortality data, instead of the preferred incidence data. Because treatment and access can vary dramatically across countries, it is possible that disease rates were actually the same between the countries but that different levels of healthcare led to higher detection or death rates in some countries.

3. *Overall correlations can mask important differences in subgroups*. As in the previous sections, suppose that the same researcher noted a number of important outliers in the analysis of national breast cancer mortality rates and dietary fat. In particular, perhaps the Mediterranean countries tended toward a relatively high per capita fat consumption; yet their breast cancer mortality rates were much lower than would be expected based on the cross-national data. The fact that olive oil is the predominant source of fat in these countries has helped to fuel the notion that the type as well as the amount of dietary fat typical of a nation's diet may be an important determinant of future public health.

Wary of the ecologic fallacy, early epidemiologists and public health researchers at first tended to shy away from ecologic analyses and data altogether. Later, they used ecologic analyses to generate hypotheses and tended to trust the results only when they were supported by individual-level analyses, such as a case-control study.

Today, there is a growing appreciation for the merits of ecologic analyses, especially given the increased awareness in the research community that not all disease determinants can be conceptualized as individual-level attributes.[8] Ecologic or group-level variables may be used as proxies for unavailable individual-level data.

Increasingly, they are also being used because of the potential health effects of group-level constructs, such as income inequality, neighborhood characteristics, environmental factors, and the presence of certain public health policies.[8] Many individual-level analyses now routinely incorporate some ecologic measurements. These multilevel analyses extend beyond the study of individual epidemiologic factors by simultaneously incorporating different levels of variables (ie, individual, workplace, neighborhood, community, or region) that might influence an individual's state of health.[9] They can then assess whether individual health is shaped by group-level variables, such as household income, or population characteristics, such as the proportion of people living in poverty.[9]

CONCLUSION

The study designs most frequently employed in clinical and epidemiologic research—case-control, cohort, and ecologic studies—each offer unique strengths and limitations that must be considered when designing or interpreting a study.

Case-control studies are particularly efficient for studying rare diseases or outcomes with long latency periods. Because they begin with known disease status, they are less time- and resource-intensive than cohort or experimental studies. A key measure of association in case-control studies is the OR, which compares the odds of exposure among cases to the odds among controls. While ORs do not directly estimate risk, they approximate RR when the disease is rare, making them especially useful in such contexts.

In contrast, cohort studies are ideal for evaluating the effects of rare or potentially harmful exposures, such as occur with industrial accidents. Because exposure status is defined before the outcome occurs, they are able to establish a clear temporal relationship and allow for the direct calculation of RR, showing how much more (or less) likely the outcome is in the exposed group.

Ecologic studies offer a cost-effective and efficient way to explore hypotheses at the population level, especially when individual-level data are unavailable or unreliable. While they are limited by the potential for ecologic fallacy, they remain valuable tools for public health research, particularly in evaluating the impact of policies or environmental exposures.

Together, these observational study designs provide a comprehensive toolkit for investigating associations between exposures and outcomes. Understanding how to interpret and apply measures, such as OR, RR, and NNT, enhances the ability to draw meaningful conclusions from research and to translate findings into actionable health interventions.

REFERENCES

1. Hennekens MD, Buring JE. *Epidemiology in Medicine*. Boston: Little, Brown and Company.
2. Gordis L. *Epidemiology*. 2nd ed. Philadelphia: W.B. Saunders Company; 2000.
3. Rothman KJ. *Epidemiology: An Introduction*. New York: Oxford University Press; 2002.
4. Morgenstern H. Ecologic studies. In: Rothman KJ, Greenland S, eds. *Modern Epidemiology*. 2nd ed. Philadelphia: Lippincott; 1998:459-480.
5. Gross LS, Li L, Ford ES, et al. Increased consumption of refined carbohydrates and the epidemic of type 2 diabetes in the United States: an ecologic assessment. *Am J Clin Nutr*. 2004;79(5):774-779. https://doi.org/10.1093/ajcn/79.5.774
6. Centers for Disease Control and Prevention, National Center for Health Statistics, Division of Health Interview Statistics. Census of the population and population estimates. Hyattsville, MD: Centers for Disease Control and Prevention; 1997.
7. Roux AVD. The study of group-level factors in epidemiology: rethinking variables, study designs, and analytical approaches. *Epidemiol Rev*. 2004;26:104-111. https://doi.org/10.1093/epirev/mxh006
8. Morgenstern H. Uses of ecological analysis in epidemiologic research. *Am J Public Health*. 1982;72(12):1336-1344. https://doi.org/10.2105/ajph.72.12.1336
9. Krieger N. A glossary for social epidemiology. *J Epidemiol Community Health*. 2001;55(10):693-700. https://doi.org/10.1136/jech.55.10.693
10. Saver JL, Lewis RJ. Number needed to treat: conveying the likelihood of a therapeutic effect. *JAMA*. 2019;321(8):822-823. https://doi.org/10.1001/jama.2018.21971

Quasi-Experimental Study Designs

4

Annie N. Simpson, PhD, and Kit N. Simpson, DrPH, MPH

Quasi-experimental designs (QEDs) represent a set of study of designs that attempts to minimize the effects of selection bias common to observational data, which can affect the internal validity of the study results.[1] The use of these types of designs is becoming quite common. They are our main resource when it is not possible to use randomization to minimize the effects of selection bias on study outcomes. The word *quasi-* means seemingly; apparently but not experimental. Quasi-experimental designs are not new, but recent research has increased our understanding of how best to use them in real-world evidence studies. There are many great resources that explain QEDs. In this chapter, we will describe the six main types of QEDs and provide references to papers that provide in-depth theoretical and practical points related to using and interpreting a specific design. It is important to remember the classical epidemiologic rules for inferring causation. In epidemiology, we check the causal logic to differentiate between causation and association by asking, (1) Does the cause precede the effect; (2) Is the effect plausible; (3) How strong is the association; and (4) Is there a dose effect? These questions should be kept in mind as we consider the outcomes of QEDs. In this chapter, we will examine the following methods: (1) interrupted time series, (2) difference-in-differences, (3) regression discontinuity, (4) propensity score stratification or matching, (5) inverse-probability weighting, and (6) designs using instrumental variables. We will discuss each design and its potential future role in generating causal inferences from observational data.

INTERRUPTED TIME SERIES

The interrupted time series (ITS) design examines outcomes in a population before and after an intervention, with the interruption being the time period when the intervention occurs. This minimizes selection bias that would be present if outcomes were compared with a control group. The design may be most powerful when it is used to examine natural experiments, such as the implementation of a new policy or program. However, it is still subject to confounding owing to other time-dependent changes in the environment of the population. To examine the presence of such contemporaneous factors, Lopez Bernal and colleagues[2] discuss adding a control time series that might be expected to show the impact of external factors affecting outcomes around the time of the interruption. Barwise and colleagues[3] use an ITS to examine the difference in the effect of COVID-19 vaccine on hospital admissions and mortality for 5,837 non-Hispanic and 605 Hispanic patients in Mayo Clinic hospitals in Minnesota, Florida, Arizona, and Wisconsin. The authors took advantage of the effect of rolling out the COVID-19 vaccine to compare monthly rates of hospital admissions, intensive care unit admissions, and deaths in the prevaccine rollout time (April 2020 through December 2020) compared with the postvaccine rollout time (January 2021 through December 2021). The authors examined disparities by ethnicity by analyzing the difference in the mortality using an interaction term for Hispanic patient rates in the time-series model. The monthly

DOI: 10.37573/9781585287666.004

mortality rate was fourfold greater (8.3%) for Hispanic patients versus (2.2%) non-Hispanic patients, but this difference was not related to vaccine rollout but to differential risk factors in the populations. The vaccine rollout reduced monthly admissions similarly for both ethnic groups, but the Hispanic group had a higher adverse event rate both before and after the vaccinations started. This study shows how implementation of a new intervention can be used as a natural experiment to examine differences in outcomes by using an ITS design.

DIFFERENCE-IN-DIFFERENCES DESIGN

This design can be considered a variation of the ITS design that compares time-related treatments for the group of interest compared with trends observed for a "treatment as usual" group. It subtracts an observed trajectory of the "usual" group from the trajectory of the "intervention" group. This subtraction essentially isolates the effect of the intervention on the health outcomes of interest. Both the ITS and difference-in-differences (DiD) designs generate summary data of sample populations over weeks, months, or years as the unit of measurement. A good example of this design was published by Bian and colleagues.[4] They examined the effect of school telehealth on emergency department (ED) use in South Carolina. They used a DiD with multivariable modeling to compare ED visit rates in Williamsburg County, which had school telehealth, with the rates in four neighboring counties without the telehealth program. The Medicaid data from 2012 to 2014 was designated as the preintervention period and data from 2015 to 2017 as the postintervention period. For children with asthma, they found a 21% relative decrease in ED visits compared with the control counties that saw an increase over the postintervention period, becoming strongest during the third year of the program. The program did not show a significant reduction in ED visits during the first 2 years postintervention, but a statistically significant reduction of 1.1 ED visits per 100 children per month (a 35% relative decrease) during year 3. This study is a good example of the potential power of a DiD design to detect differences even in small samples and particularly when the impact of an intervention may be gradual.

REGRESSION DISCONTINUITY DESIGN

The regression discontinuity design requires time series data similarly to the first two designs. In this design, a trend over time is examined that looks for an interruption or jump in the estimated outcome. This is quite similar to the two designs described previously, but it can be applied to slightly different types of data. One simple example was published by Mims and colleagues who examined the "July effect" by using the Healthcare Cost and Utilization Project National Inpatient Sample (HCUP NIS) data for 2011.[5] To minimize effects of case mix heterogeneity, they selected admission for acute myocardial infarction (AMI), heart failure (HF), or pneumonia (PNA) and compared outcomes for the first academic quarter with the other three quarters in teaching versus nonteaching hospitals, controlling for comorbidity burden. The "July effect" is associated with the first quarter (ie, July, August, and September) in academic medicine when new trainees enter clinical training. The authors hypothesized that two process measures (length of stay and total cost) and one outcome measure (mortality) would be worse in patients during the July quarter compared with the other quarters in the year. They tested a regression discontinuity in process and outcome measures for the July quarter by using an interaction term. Models were adjusted for sex, age, race, admission type (AMI, HF, or PNA), Charlson comorbidity score, hospital location (rural vs. urban), and patients' insurance status, as well as correlation within each hospital. They found that 544,617 patients with a primary diagnosis code of AMI who were admitted to academic medical centers had a higher risk-adjusted mortality (1.22), patients with HF had $584 higher mean cost per admission, and longer length of stay compared with similar patients admitted to a nonacademic medical center. However, these effects were not observed for patients with a primary diagnosis of PNA. They concluded that PNA admissions may not be sensitive to the July effect and that it is possible that a PNA effect is obscured by seasonal variation in PNA cases. This small study provides a nice example of how the regression discontinuity design can be used to untangle complex variations in care processes.

PROPENSITY SCORE DESIGNS

The designs described to this point have all required longitudinal data. The propensity score design is often used with cross-sectional data. This design, of all the QEDs discussed up to this point, is the one closest to a randomized clinical trial. It replaces the randomization with a detailed matching scheme that uses all non-outcome measures in the dataset to predict being in the treatment group. There are three different design subtypes: (1) propensity score stratification, (2) propensity score matching, and (3) inverse probability weighting. The first step in each of these designs is to estimate the likelihood of being in the treatment group for both the treated and control (or practice as usual) patients by using a logistic regression approach. This is a study design step where a new variable, "the probability of being treated," is added to each observation in the study dataset by using logistic regression to estimate the probablity of being treated given a set of baseline characteristics (as a set of independent variables in the regression model). This variable captures the likelihood of being in the treatment group, for *both* the treated and control patients. Once that is accomplished, this score is either divided into categories or strata (propensity score stratification) from lowest chance to highest probability of being treated, used for matching treated and control patients with similar scores (propensity score matching), or used as an inverse probability weight in a regression model to weigh observations' contributions to outcomes so that the probability of being treated is equal between the treated and control groups. This stratification, matching, or weighting methodology may be considered a "pseudo-randomization" that helps control for bias associated with baseline differences between those who were treated and controls, similarly to the goal of randomizing individuals at baseline in randomized controlled trials (RCTs).

The evolution of study designs that use a pseudo-randomization approach to observational studies goes back nearly 30 years to early work by Rubin[6] who made the use of propensity score stratification easily understandable to clinical audiences. Over the three decades since this important work, a number of researchers have added to our understanding and approach to this type of QED. In 2005, Professor Thomas Love presented a workshop at the 6th International Conference for Health Policy Research in October 2005, presenting numerous papers showing applications of the design, both for studies where an effect is found and for one where an effect could not be identified, despite a strong propensity score model.[7-9] The slides from this workshop may represent the most parsimonious, understandable, and comprehensive early training of propensity score design (see reference 9 for link to slide set). Two other authors contributed enormously to the diffusion of the QED into healthcare research. In 2010, Elizabeth Stuart published a statistical review paper of the approach,[10] and in 2011 Peter Austin published an extensive introductory paper aimed at behavioral scientists.[11] These three contributions made the design accessible to many health services researchers, and the use of the propensity score as a QED for observational studies accelerated greatly. The key points accentuated by Rubin, Love, Stuart, and Austin for these designs are (1) the balance of the baseline covariates between the groups is paramount for maximum bias control; (2) the treatment prediction model should include all available independent variables as measured before the time of intervention (not a parsimonious model); (3) overlapping propensity scores are needed for treatment and control populations to have valid results; (4) covariate balance should be measured before and after application of propensity scores calculating standardized differences in means or proportions of each covariate included in the propensity model; (5) residual confounding should be corrected using double-robust multivariable modeling by including those covariates in multivariable regression models on the outcomes; and (6) sensitivity analysis can be used to quantify the potential impact that unmeasured confounders may play on the results. There are key points to remember when reading a report of an observational study that uses any type of propensity design. The most important thing is that all observational studies are potentially affected by hidden bias owing to unmeasured confounders. The authors must use sensitivity analysis in any such study. Furthermore, the omitted variable is most likely to affect conclusions about the treatment effect if it is (1) closely related to the outcome(s), (2) imbalanced for the treatment and control group, and (3) not correlated with any of the variables included in the propensity score model.

Propensity score stratification is usually performed by the propensity scores five strata. The effect is then estimated for each stratum. This is helpful for identifying heterogeneity in effect across the population, because the effect of the intervention may be strongest in the groups that are most or least likely to receive the treatment and, thus, unevenly across the population. However, it has the disadvantage that it produces five effect size results, which can be confusing; it requires the researcher to calculate the weighted mean effect across the strata to get a population effect measure. Using more than five strata increases the granularity of the results but may make the reporting even more complicated. An early example of the use of propensity score stratification that was responsible for rapid uptake of this approach for healthcare studies examined effects of lipid-lowering medication on early mortality after acute coronary syndromes. The study by Aronow and colleagues[12] found that 180-day survival after myocardial infarction for patients on lipid-lowering drugs at discharge was associated with a 33% lower risk of death at 6 months after accounting for differences between groups using propensity scores.

An example of propensity score matching is the study on measurement of the impact of frailty on cost of care for Medicare beneficiaries, which is also used in Chapter 11, showing that cost of care for Medicare patients with frailty is much higher than the cost for nonfrail patients, even after controlling for a large number of covariates.[13] Indeed, this study provides a good example of how one can "enrich" a dataset with constructed measures to enhance the propensity scoring model. We show the many composite variables that can be constructed from billing data to bolster the propensity score model to decrease the likelihood of omitted-variable bias. In this study, we included age, race, sex, polypharmacy, use of prescription drugs listed on Beer's Criteria, Charlson score, Elixhauser score, and rural or urban residence. These were all used to predict being in the "treatment" (frailty) group compared with the controls (not frail). This type of variable enrichment approach is a desirable feature of any design that uses propensity scoring in billing data.

Inverse probability weighting, also known as inverse probability of treatment weighting, or propensity score weighting, is the third way to use propensity scoring as a study design approach. This design is usually used when observational data are sparse or when all patients may be likely to receive the treatment. It is ideal to use for quality improvement or for pilot studies for planning randomized clinical trials by using electronic health record (EHR) or registry data from settings where patients are treated differently as a natural practice variation. We use this approach to examine the effect of managing systolic blood pressure (SBP) control in patients with acute ischemic stroke admitted to stroke units for endovascular therapy (EVT).[14] One perennial problem with this type of data is that of missing data, where certain key variables are missing in a significant proportion of the sample. This makes it difficult to capture all patients of interest in the propensity score model. Thus, we combined the inverse probability weighting design with multiple imputation approach in our study. We found that SBP goals of between 140 and 160 mmHg following EVT treatment appear to be associated with better clinical outcomes for patients post-EVT than SBP of higher than 180 mmHg. Inverse probability weighting is an ideal approach to these kinds of clinical studies that have small patient numbers and require many clinical measures to be included in the modeling.

INSTRUMENTAL VARIABLE DESIGN

The instrumental variable design (IVD) is powerful in its ability to prevent bias in observational studies particularly because it can control for bias associated with both measured and unmeasured confounders, but it is often difficult to operationalize in a healthcare setting. It is not that the design will not work well, but that it may be quite difficult to find a good instrumental variable (IV) measure that fits the population, the setting, and the data available. Love briefly discusses the IVD in his slide presentation pointing out two situations when IVD may have an advantage over a propensity score method. Instrumental variable designs are especially useful to consider when (1) treatment is not the most important issue, but adherence to the treatment varies greatly and is the most important effect on the outcome; or (2) the observational dataset does not contain a substantial collection of variables that are useful for predicting the treatment. In the first example, to examine the effect of a chronic drug regimen, such as antiretrovirals in human immunodeficiency virus, it is the adherence to the drug regimen that is associated with improved health outcomes, not so much the prescription of the specific drug combination that prevents acquired immunodeficiency syndrome events. In the second case, if there is a meager choice of variables in a dataset that minimally predict treatment assignment often identified with a limited range of propensity scores, then your propensity score model may provide little insight into the population differences and thus may be unable to control for the confounding effects of differences between groups. When either of these two conditions hold, then an IV, such as a variable denoting distance from patients' home to the medical center, may be a better choice than a propensity scoring method for controlling for the effects of selection bias on health outcomes.

Garabedian and colleagues provide a great overview of the issues related to the use of IVD in their paper discussing studies that use IV to manage bias.[15] They list the most common IVs by category as (1) distance to facility from patient's residence, (2) regional variation in the use of the treatment, (3) facility variation in practice, and (4) physician variation in treatment use. It is important to know that IVD relies on several study and data assumptions, some of which may be difficult to meet or to verify in the data. The most serious bias in the results may stem from a confounder that is associated with the IV and directly affect the outcome but is not known to the researcher, also called an "instrument–outcome confounder." In a later publication, Garabedian[16] provides a great example of an IVD that compares effectiveness of bariatric surgery to other weight-loss methods. Thus, IVD is a valuable QED, but the difficulty in its use is related to meeting the assumptions required for application of a good IV.

SUMMARY OF QEDs

Quasi-experimental designs are essential for using the large volumes of observational data generated by EHR systems, patient registries, and billing processes to examine potential causal effects, particularly in comparing treatment choices that already exist in regular healthcare practice or where randomization is infeasible. These data constitute a "gold mine" for comparative effectiveness studies aimed at discovery of what works best in current practice, for whom it works best, and where care gaps or population disparities in access, use, and outcomes exist. The QEDs differ, and choice of approach should be assessed, considering the sample size, type of data available, richness of variables present, intervention type, and time horizon of the study. **Table 4-1** summarizes some of the important characteristics of the QEDs discussed in this chapter.

Quasi-experimental designs provide the designs that we need to guard against bias in observational studies comparing treatments that have not or cannot be randomized; however, they usually require complex statistical approaches, such as multivariable regression models, to work as intended. It is important for the reader to recognize that QEDs are considered designs, not statistical approaches, even if they use statistical methods, such as regression, in their application. It is also important to stress that, particularly in propensity methods, the rules for fitting a good propensity score model are vastly different from the rules for analyzing differences in outcomes using regression models as is discussed in the statistical analysis chapter. Quasi-experimental designs are valuable designs that are especially useful for examining differences in effectiveness of how we treat patients under real practice conditions. However, they do not replace RCTs, which are needed to show efficacy. However, they are less expensive to undertake than large clinical trials and may produce evidence more rapidly. Just like any type of healthcare research design, they are subject to limitations

TABLE 4-1. Characteristics to Consider in Choosing a QED

Design Type	Sample Size Required	Time Span Needed	Timing of Treatment Applied	Unique Timing	Number of Covariates	Other Issues
Interrupted time series	Large	Long	Clear time demarcation before and after	Natural experiment	Not important	Subject to bias from time-varying policy changes
Difference-in-differences	Large	Long	Clear time demarcation before and after	Intervention and control populations	Not important	Subject to bias from subtle geographic policy variation
Regression discontinuity	Large	Long	Clear time demarcation before and after	Intervention and control populations	Not important	The underlying relationships must be measured using continuous variables
Propensity score stratification	Medium to large	Any length	Baseline and intervention demarcation	Intervention and control populations	Rich variable mix needed	Easy method; results are presented as effect by strata
Propensity score matching	Medium to large	Any length	Baseline and intervention demarcation	Intervention and control populations	Rich variable mix needed	Results may be impacted by unmeasured confounders
Inverse probability weighting	Any size	Any length	Baseline and intervention demarcation	Intervention and control populations	Rich variable mix needed	Difficult to understand compared to matching
Instrumental variable	Any size	Any length	Baseline and intervention demarcation	Intervention and control populations	Low variable need	Difficult to find a good instrument

QED = quasi-experimental design.

and can be done well or poorly. However, this is the case with all research studies; even RCTs have issues that affect internal and external validity of results (poor randomization, cross-over cases, dropouts). As explained so eloquently by Dr. Thomas Love, the only perfect study design is to (1) take a population and treat them and wait X years for results to mature, (2) then turn time back to the start, (3) then do NOT treat those same individuals and then wait the same X years, and (4) then measure the difference in outcomes between the patients when they were treated and when they were not treated. Because this scenario is not possible, we need to use good substitutes: RCTs to measure efficacy, and QEDs to measure effectiveness. Neither design is perfect, so we need to examine every study result for internal and external validity and identify any biasing factors.

REFERENCES

1. Capili B, Anastasi JK. An introduction to types of quasi-experimental designs. *Am J Nurs*. 2024;124(11):50-52. https://doi.org/10.1097/01.NAJ.0001081740.74815.20
2. Lopez Bernal J, Cummins S, Gasparrini A. The use of controls in interrupted time series studies of public health interventions. *Int J Epidemiol*. 2018;47(6):2082-2093. https://doi.org/10.1093/ije/dyy135
3. Barwise A, Tekin A, Domecq Garces JP, et al. Impact of SARS-CoV-2 vaccine rollout on Hispanic and non-Hispanic admission and mortality trends: an interrupted time series analysis. *Chest*. 2024;165(6):1341-1351. https://doi.org/10.1016/j.chest.2023.12.025
4. Bian J, Cristaldi KK, Summer AP, et al. Association of a school-based, asthma-focused telehealth program with emergency department visits among children

enrolled in South Carolina Medicaid. *JAMA Pediatr.* 2019;173(11):1041-1048. https://doi.org/10.1001/jamapediatrics.2019.3073

5. Mims LD, Porter M, Simpson KN, Carek PJ. The "July effect": a look at July medical admissions in teaching hospitals. *J Am Board Family Med.* 2017;30(2):189-195. https://doi.org/10.3122/jabfm.2017.02.160214
6. Rubin DB. Estimating causal effects from large data sets using propensity scores. *Ann Intern Med.* 1997;127(Part 2):757-763. https://doi.org/10.7326/0003-4819-127-8_part_2-199710151-00064
7. Strategies for Using Propensity Scores Well—A Workshop given by Thomas E. Love, Ph.D. Center for Health Care Research and Policy Case Western Reserve University. 6th International Conference for Health Policy Research Friday, October 28, 2005, Boston Park Plaza Hotel and Towers. https://chrp.org/propensity/ICHPR/ICHPR_final.pdf. Accessed February 9, 2026.
8. Moore HJ, Wu WC, Heidenreich PA, et al. Higher risk of kidney failure associated with angiotensin receptor blockers vs ACE inhibitors in patients with heart failure. *Am J Med.* 2025:S0002-9343(25)00314-6. https://doi.org/10.1016/j.amjmed.2025.05.024
9. Sheriff HM, Thogaripally MR, Panjrath G, et al. Digoxin and 30-day all-cause readmission in long-term care residents hospitalized for heart failure. *J Am Med Dir Assoc.* 2017;18(9):761-765. https://doi.org/10.1016/j.jamda.2017.03.016
10. Stuart EA. Matching methods for causal inference: a review and look forward. *Stat Sci.* 2010;25(1):1-21. https://doi.org/10.1214/09-STS313
11. Austin PC. An introduction to propensity score methods for reducing the effects of confounding in observational studies. *Multivariate Behavior Res.* 2011;46:399-424. https://doi.org/10.1080/00273171.2011.568786
12. Aronow HD, Topol EJ, Roe MT, et al. Effect of lipid-lowering therapy on early mortality after acute coronary syndromes: an observational study. *Lancet.* 2001;357(9262):1063-1068. https://doi.org/10.1016/S0140-6736(00)04257-4
13. Simpson KN, Seamon BA, Hand BN, et al. Effect of frailty on resource use and cost for Medicare patients. *J Comp Eff Res.* 2018. https://doi.org/10.2217/cer-2018-0029
14. Anadani M, Arthur AS, Tsivgoulis G, et al. Blood pressure goals and clinical outcomes after successful endovascular therapy: a multicenter study. *Ann Neurol.* 2020;87(6):830-839. https://doi.org/10.1002/ana.25716
15. Garabedian LF, Chu P, Toh S, et al. Potential bias of instrumental variable analyses for observational comparative effectiveness research. *Ann Intern Med.* 2014;161(2):131-138. https://doi.org/10.7326/M13-1887
16. Garabedian LF. Potential bias of instrumental variable analysis in comparative effectiveness research for bariatric surgery. *JAMA Netw Open.* 2022;5(8):e2225970. https://doi.org/10.1001/jamanetworkopen.2022.25970

Randomized Controlled Trials

5

Sherry Livingston, PhD, and Patrick Mauldin, PhD

Randomized controlled trials (RCTs) are considered the "gold standard" in clinical research for establishing cause and effect. Participants in an RCT are randomly assigned to one of two or more treatment groups. Typically, one group serves as the control, which is compared with one or more clinical interventions. The control group typically receives either a placebo or (more often now) the current standard of care to ensure that differences between the groups are truly the result of the intervention. If possible, blinding is used to limit the biases of the investigators and expectations of the participants. The goal of randomization is to ensure that baseline characteristics between the groups are similar, allowing for better isolation of the treatment effect, with minimal influence from other factors that also could affect the study outcome. Participants are followed for a prespecified amount of time to capture the treatment effect or outcome. Depending on the treatment, these outcomes can be measured immediately after administration or over months/years. A clear definition of endpoints and the methods for gathering and measuring such data must be detailed in the RCT protocol before the trial begins. This protocol is a document that serves as a guideline for the conduct of the trial, describing in a clear and detailed manner the endpoints, objectives, methodology, and analytical methods of the study, and serving as a historical document of the trial. Components of a standard protocol are listed in **Table 5-1**, with more description provided in this chapter.

PHASES OF CLINICAL TRIALS

Clinical trial designs are based on the specific research question of interest. There are four phases of clinical trials (**Figure 5-1**).[1] Phase I studies are designed to assess the metabolism, absorption, toxicity, and pharmacologic effects of a new drug in human studies. Participants of Phase I studies typically include healthy volunteers, and side effects are monitored to see whether they are related to increasing dosage. Phase II studies are designed to test safety and efficacy in a larger population of patients who have the disease that the drug was designed to treat. After evaluating pharmacologic activity from Phase I results and observing safety and efficacy in Phase II, Phase III studies are conducted on larger populations of sick patients, typically comparing the effectiveness of a new treatment to the standard therapy currently used for the disease in question. Information from Phase III trials provides a basis for Food and Drug Administration (FDA) approval. Phase IV studies are conducted following FDA approval of the drug or device and are considered postmarketing studies. These studies aim to gain further information on the treatment's effect within various populations and to assess side effects, benefits, and optimal administration associated with long-term use. Phase III trials are usually randomized; on occasion, Phase II trials may also be randomized when a control group is needed, particularly for critical

DOI: 10.37573/9781585287666.005

TABLE 5-1. Protocol Components

- Primary and secondary objectives
- Background of disease and drug/device
- Rationale of study
- Study design, population, sites, and duration
- Inclusion/exclusion criteria
- Prohibited therapy during study
- Participant recruitment methods and screening logs
- Eligibility assessment; presentation of informed consent; randomization or registration; registration log procedure, central registration procedure, or central randomization procedure
- Baseline assessments and treatment procedures
- Drug dosage, administration, and adjustments
- Concomitant or ancillary therapy
- Clinical guidelines
- Follow-up procedures
- Notification of death
- Procedure for unblinding
- Data collection schedule/schema
- Participant withdrawal
- Primary and secondary outcomes definitions
- Site monitoring
- Data processing, security, and confidentiality
- Data quality assurance
- Statistical considerations, sample size and power estimation, stratification, covariates, randomization, safety outcomes, missing data, interim analysis, final analysis
- Definitions of adverse events
- Regulatory and ethical obligations, informed consent, institutional review board (IRB)
- Study termination, study documentation and storage, publication policy; steering committee, executive committee, and data safety and monitoring committee
- References
- Master informed consent

diseases, such as acquired immunodeficiency syndrome (AIDS) or cancer.[2,3]

Clinical trials might also be categorized as explanatory or pragmatic. Explanatory trials confirm whether an intervention works in a carefully controlled setting, and they are often Phase II and III trials. Pragmatic trials, conversely, aim to show effectiveness in broad patient populations and in real-world practice settings, and they might be Phase III or IV.[4,5]

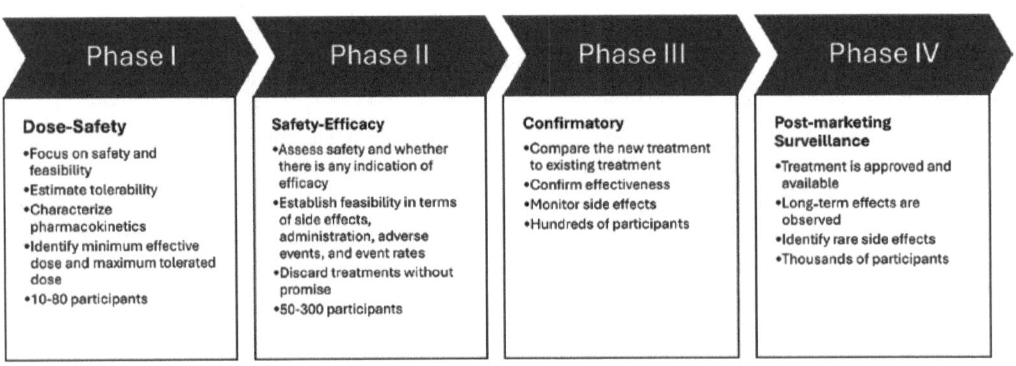

FIGURE 5-1. **Phases of clinical trials.**

Most trial designs lie on a spectrum between explanatory and pragmatic, with increasing emphasis on the importance of including pragmatic elements in trials. These elements include broad eligibility requirements, application in a usual care setting, flexibility in delivery and adherence of the treatment, and routine follow-up, ideally through healthcare databases.[6] Pragmatic trials are best for comparing existing treatment alternatives or evaluating a new approach for delivery of an existing treatment, but they are not a good fit for evaluating new drugs or devices.

TRIAL DESIGNS

Most RCTs use a standard parallel design, where treatment and control groups are followed simultaneously from randomization.[7-9] For example, if a participant is randomized to treatment X, then it will be the only treatment this participant receives during the course of the trial. A similar group would receive a different therapy or placebo, with the outcomes of the two groups analyzed for comparison. Parallel designs are highly versatile, and the analysis and interpretation of results is generally straightforward.

A crossover design lets each participant receive both available treatments at different time periods, separated by a washout period between the treatments.[1,10] Statistically, this design allows for the estimation of the within-patient treatment difference. The main advantages of crossover designs are that they (1) will not hinder recruitment, as all participants will receive each study treatment, and (2) can increase accuracy as each participant serves as his or her own control. However, care should be taken with the design and interpretation of a crossover trial.[10,11] There may be a "carryover effect" of the first treatment that could influence the second treatment. For example, if the first treatment significantly alters the state of (or even cures) the disease in the participant before the second treatment is administered, then the treatment effect will be skewed. As a result, crossover designs are more appropriate for chronic rather than acute conditions.

The stepped-wedge design is a type of crossover design where a treatment is rolled out at staggered time points to clusters of participants (**Figure 5-2a**).[12] A cluster might be a site, community, or region. This approach offers the advantage that all participants will

a. Stepped-wedge design

Cluster 1	Control	Treatment	Treatment	Treatment	Treatment
Cluster 2	Control	Control	Treatment	Treatment	Treatment
Cluster 3	Control	Control	Control	Treatment	Treatment
Cluster 4	Control	Control	Control	Control	Treatment

time →

b. 2 x 2 Factorial design

	Treatment A	**Placebo for A**
Treatment B	Group 1: Both A and B	Group 2: B only (placebo for A)
Placebo for B	Group 3: A only (placebo for B)	Group 4: placebo / placebo

FIGURE 5-2. **(a) Example of a stepped-wedge design with 4 clusters and 5 time periods. (b) Example of a 2 × 2 factorial design with treatments A and B.**

receive the treatment before the end of the trial, and it is particularly useful in cases where it is impractical to deliver the treatment simultaneously to all of the clusters.[13] For example, when distributing a limited resource, such as a newly developed vaccine, a stepped-wedge design might be the most feasible approach.

Factorial designs test two or more treatments (or factors) and their interactions simultaneously, where participants are randomized to receive different combinations of the available treatments.[14] The most common is a 2 × 2 factorial design, with two treatments and their corresponding placebos, where participants are randomized to one of four groups: A only; B only; A and B; or placebos only (**Figure 5-2b**). This design can be very efficient for testing multiple treatments and their interactions. However, it may become impractical when there are numerous factors or levels, or when interactions are weak or not of primary interest.

Proper planning and statistical design should ensure a true assessment of the treatment effect from each alternative therapy. The choice of design is based on the question being asked, so it is crucially important that the objectives are clearly defined ahead of time.

RANDOMIZATION

Randomization reduces the chance for selection bias, which can cause the experimental group to differ from the control group based on certain characteristics.[1,7,15] In nonrandomized studies, selection bias might occur if investigators choose the intervention for each participant, because they could potentially be influenced by any number of factors, including the patient's prognosis. Another example of selection bias might result from studying the effects of a new treatment in an adult patient population and assuming the effect is the same for pediatric patients. Selection bias may cause difficulty in the interpretation of results, as the sample participants may not be representative or able to be generalized for the intended patient population.[9,16]

When participants are randomly allocated to treatment groups in an RCT, it means that they have a specified chance of being assigned to each treatment choice in the trial. The most basic design has two groups with an equal chance of being randomized into each group, or an allocation ratio of 1:1. Sometimes this chance is 2:1 or some other unequal ratio, and there may also be more than two groups. Response-adaptive designs are becoming increasingly common, where the allocation ratio might be adjusted during the trial based on outcomes at predetermined points. For example, the allocation might be increased for a treatment that shows better results at an interim analysis, or treatments with poor outcomes might be dropped from the trial.[17]

Various methods allow for the proper randomization of participants.[7,9,17-23] A simple randomization design might use a random number generator to assign each participant a random number between 0 and 1, where treatment A is assigned if the number is less than 0.5 and treatment B is assigned if the number is greater than 0.5.

Another common randomization scheme is the permuted block design. This method generates an allocation sequence of assignments based on "blocks" of a prespecified size.[21] For example, if the block size is 6 and the allocation ratio is 2:1, then each block would consist of a random arrangement of four A and two B participants, such as AABABA or BAAABA. At the end of each block, the groups will always be balanced with the desired allocation ratio, and then a new block (with another random arrangement) will be started. The full sequence of random assignments may be pregenerated at the beginning of the trial when using this design.

A simple random design can lead to imbalanced groups at the end of a trial, reducing the power of the analysis. The permuted block design prevents such imbalance but could lead to selection bias, because an investigator might be able to predict assignments, particularly at the end of each block. Other randomization designs have been proposed to attempt to maintain good balance while limiting predictability of assignments. Many of these designs base each assignment on the current imbalance at that point in the trial and define a maximum tolerated imbalance (MTI).[23] The Big Stick design is completely random until the MTI is reached, at which point the next assignment is forced to the smaller arm. Urn models and biased coin designs increase the allocation probability for the smaller arm when there is an imbalance.

If a particular characteristic or prognostic factor is important to the analysis, it may also be important to maintain a balance between groups for that variable. Covariate balancing methods, including stratification, aim to balance these factors between the treatment arms of RCTs. For example, if gender is a potentially important prognostic factor, then the treatment allocation should ensure that the proportion of men and women is comparable between treatment groups.

BLINDING

If either the participant or clinician is aware of the treatment assigned to the participant, bias could result if actions taken by either party, even unknowingly, influence the true treatment effect. For example, if the participant knows that he or she has been randomized to active medical therapy for blood pressure management rather than placebo, the participant may not adhere to the scheduled exercise and diet recommendations as closely as they would if assigned to the placebo arm of the trial. Similarly, a clinician who knows that a participant is receiving the treatment may choose not to emphasize exercise and diet factors as heavily. The converse of both of these scenarios may also be true. Blinding is particularly important for "soft" outcomes, such as those that are self-reported by the participant or based on a subjective scale by an investigator.

Double blinding keeps the treatment assignment unknown to all parties of the RCT. If only the participants are kept unaware of the treatment assignment, this is referred to as single blind. Partial blinding allows for the identification of study participants by their treatment group without revealing the treatment by name. For example, participants will be listed as being in Group A or B, but whether A (or B) is the experimental treatment or control is unknown. This format is commonly used for data reports to the Data Safety and Monitoring Committee (explained below).

Individuals whose conduct could affect the results of the interpretation of the results should be blinded as necessary.[24] Many factors could lead to the accidental unblinding of a study participant. These include pill appearance, packaging, treatment side effects, and patient appearance (eg, surgical scars). Careful attention should be given to the planning of the RCT to avoid these disclosures. In addition, circumstances and methods for planned or emergent unblinding should be clearly described in the study protocol.

ENDPOINTS

Clinical trial endpoints are the measurements that allow study hypotheses to be tested, and they can be either quantitative or qualitative in nature. Depending on the underlying clinical issue, examples of clinical endpoints include the improvement in symptoms, presence or absence of disease, changes in quality of life or resource utilization/costs, and time-to-event endpoints, such as tumor progression, repeat hospitalizations, or death. Ideal endpoints should be clinically relevant and clearly reflect the study objectives.[25] In addition, endpoints should be both valid and reliable. Validity assures that the endpoint being measured truly reflects the relevant treatment effect. Reliability addresses the extent to which the measurement obtained is reproducible; it is a measure of the randomness of the measurement process itself. Endpoints should be capable of being accurately measured regardless of the treatment assignment, and they should be void of bias.

Endpoints can be quantified as continuous, categorical, or time-to-event. Continuous outcomes include variables that are measured on a continuous scale, such as blood pressure, number of colon polyps, weight, or lipid levels. For example, to assess the efficacy of a daily treatment of drug X on multiple sclerosis, an appropriate endpoint would be the change in the mean number of lesions seen on pretreatment and posttreatment magnetic resonance imaging (MRI). Categorical endpoints are typically measured as success/failure or the qualitative grouping of endpoints, such as scale scores. These scores are often ordinal endpoints; examples include angina class (rated from I to IV, reflecting the degree of chest pain), cancer stage (rated from I to IV reflecting the progression of cancer), and number of vision lines lost (for macular degeneration). Unfortunately, the changes from one category to another are often not necessarily scaled equally; ie, a change from category I to II may not equal the change from categories II to III. Finally, time-to-event endpoints are appropriate when analyzing overall survival, tumor progression, or time to relapse. For example, if the protocol assesses the efficacy of a particular treatment on participants with advanced esophageal cancer, an appropriate endpoint would be time to dysphagia relapse.

When a defined endpoint cannot be measured (for clinical or possibly financial reasons), a surrogate endpoint can be substituted.[26] A surrogate endpoint is used as a proxy for the "true" or final biological or clinical outcome. Examples include the number of MRI lesions for progression of multiple sclerosis or prostate-specific antigen for prostate cancer. The benefits of surrogate endpoints include earlier measurement and increased frequency of observations as well as an independence from potential covariates likely to affect the true endpoint.[27] The surrogate must yield a predictive ability for the clinical outcome in question and be responsive to the treatment alternatives in the RCT,[28] but they must be used with care.[29] Each surrogate endpoint requires validation to ensure appropriate measurement. As quoted in Senn, "the difference between a surrogate endpoint and a true endpoint is like the difference between a check and cash. You may get a check earlier, but it may bounce."[26]

Measurement of a surrogate endpoint may be clinically misleading. For example, prior to 1989, the efficacy of antiarrhythmic agents was usually determined by the drug's ability to suppress premature ventricular complexes (PVCs). The Cardiac Arrhythmia Suppression Trial (CAST) included a placebo arm and used mortality as an endpoint.[30] In CAST, participants who received drugs that were known to decrease PVCs had a higher mortality rate than those participants given a placebo. Although the drugs decreased the number of PVCs, they did not improve patient outcomes. Until then, it had been widely assumed that suppressing PVCs would lead to better cardiac outcomes, but CAST disproved this hypothesis. This scenario demonstrated that an improvement in a surrogate endpoint (the number of PVCs) was not a reliable measure for long-term survival, underscoring the need for RCTs to explore even widely accepted medical theories.

CLINICAL TRIAL HYPOTHESES

Most clinical trials aim to show that a new treatment results in better outcomes for patients than the current standard of care, and these hypotheses reflect a superiority trial.[9] For example, if the outcome is recurrent stroke, the null hypothesis (H_0) might be: There is no difference in the rates of recurrent stroke between the treatment group and the control group; the alternative hypothesis (H_1) might be: The treatment group has a lower rate of recurrent stroke than the control group. To be conservative, the alternative hypothesis is usually two-tailed, so the trial is also testing whether the control group is better than the treatment group, even though this is not expected to be the case.

Noninferiority trial designs have recently become quite common in RCTs, and they aim to show that a novel treatment A is not worse than preexisting treatment B.[9,31,32] This might be the case if treatment A does not offer better efficacy than treatment B but is preferable in some other way, such as lower cost, less intensive treatment, more convenient dosing, or fewer side effects. The noninferiority margin is the predefined value that establishes the threshold for the novel treatment to be considered noninferior. In other words, it specifies the degree to which the new treatment can be deemed "acceptably worse" than the standard treatment. For example, noninferiority hypotheses might be as follows: H_0: Physical therapy conducted via teleconference results in worse outcomes than physical therapy conducted in person by more than the noninferiority margin; H_1: Physical therapy conducted via teleconference is not worse than physical therapy conducted in person by more than the noninferiority margin. With continuous improvements in health technologies, standard care, and clinical outcomes, the incremental benefits of newly developed treatments over existing treatments may be only marginal at best, so this really comes down to the concept of a good substitute: Noninferiority trials compare a novel treatment to an active treatment with a view of demonstrating that it is not clinically worse with regards to a specified endpoint.

Futility designs are sometimes employed in Phase II trials to discard treatments that do not show sufficient promise for further study in a larger Phase III study.[33] The futility threshold is the minimum clinically relevant improvement in outcome. An example of hypotheses for a futility trial might be the following: H_0: The difference in the proportion of good outcomes between the treatment group and control group is greater than or equal to the futility threshold; H_1: The difference in the proportion of good outcomes between the treatment group and control group is less than the futility threshold. Here, H_1 demonstrates futility, and H_0 assumes the treatment is not futile.

SAMPLE SIZE AND POWER

Sample size calculations vary depending on trial factors, such as study design, patient population, and type of endpoint. As discussed further in Chapter 8, there are generally four components to a sample size calculation: (1) Type II error (false-negative rate), which occurs when one fails to reject H_0 when H_1 is true (for determination of power); (2) Type I error (false-positive rate), which occurs when one falsely rejects H_0 when it is true; (3) the clinically relevant difference; and (4) the variance within each group.[34] With these four components prespecified, a standard sample size calculation can be made to estimate how many participants should be enrolled into each arm of the trial to ensure a specific significance level at a specific level of power.

As mentioned earlier, clinical trial endpoints are the quantitative or qualitative measurements that correspond to the study objectives. The basic goal of any RCT protocol is to make sure there is sufficient statistical power so that a proper interpretation of the endpoints can occur. Power is the probability of detecting a treatment effect if indeed there is one. Under traditional superiority testing, H_0 assumes there is no difference between groups. If H_0 is rejected based on a certain significance level (often 0.05), then there is sufficient evidence in favor of H_1 that there is a difference between the groups. Type II error (false-negative rate) is defined as (1 – power). Thus, the smaller the false-negative rate, the higher the power of the study. Although there are no rigid guidelines, most RCTs seek to achieve a power of at least 80% (ie, a 20% chance of failing to reject H_0 when H_1 is true).

A larger sample size always enhances the power of a study, increasing the probability of detecting a difference if one exists. However, financial or practical constraints often limit the feasible sample size.

Sample size calculations should be inflated to account for unforeseen circumstances. Depending on the illness, treatment, or follow-up period, participants can be lost to follow-up or may voluntarily withdraw from the study. Participants in the treatment group may not adhere to the treatment protocol due to side effects, or participants in the control group might find a way to "cross over" and receive a conventionally available treatment, resulting in a dilution of the treatment effect. Should either of these circumstances occur, an adequate sample of participants might not be available at the end of the study to achieve the expected power. Thus, depending on the type of illness, study design, or the experience of the investigator or clinical center with these types of clinical trials, an appropriate inflation factor should be considered for the final estimation of sample size.

INTERIM ANALYSES

Randomized controlled trial designs often include one or more interim analyses, where the accumulated data from the ongoing trial is evaluated. These analyses guide decisions on trial modifications, such as stopping early or adjusting the sample size.[35] While a trial might be stopped at any point if there are safety concerns, the statistical analysis plan can also define boundaries for stopping the trial early owing to evidence of overwhelming efficacy or futility at an interim analysis. If an interim analysis finds that the treatment effect is substantially larger than expected, the trial may be stopped early so that all patients have the opportunity to access a promising treatment. Conversely, if interim findings show that a significant result at the end of the study is highly unlikely, the trial may be stopped early to reduce both costs and patient burden for a trial with a low chance of success. These stopping boundaries should be carefully defined before the trial begins (and the sample size is appropriately inflated) using group sequential methods to ensure that multiple analyses of the data do not result in inflated Type I error rates or loss of power.

PARTICIPANT RECRUITMENT

Recruitment strategies to enroll patients into RCTs should be free from any actions that may be interpreted as intimidation or persuasion.[36] Unless justified in the protocol, recruitment should be open to all patients without regard to age, gender, or ethnic characteristics. It should be noted that specific considerations are required to evaluate certain populations, such as pregnant women, human fetuses and neonates (45 CFR 46 Subpart B), prisoners (45 CFR 46 Subpart C), and children (45 CFR 46 Subpart D).[37] The objective in RCTs is to recruit participants who will adhere to the protocol requirements.[38] During the assessment of potential participants, the study investigator must provide a detailed and understandable presentation of the protocol so that a fully informed decision can be made by the potential participant to agree to the protocol requirements. Patients with a high probability of noncompliance (for reasons such as difficulties returning to the clinical center owing to large geographic distances, development of a new clinical condition, or an inability to read and/or complete the self-administered forms) should not be entered into the RCT. The clinical investigator must thoroughly assess patients' understanding of the protocol and provide an atmosphere that encourages ongoing compliance.[39]

If, for any reason, a participant chooses to voluntarily withdraw from the RCT, they have the right to do so without influencing their future medical care. For those who withdraw consent (explained below), documentation should include the date and reason for consent withdrawal, and their data should be included in the analysis up to that point in time. For participants who do not withdraw consent yet miss some clinic visits or fail to complete forms, documentation should be made for the missing data, and the participants should continue to be followed according to protocol requirements. All follow-up data for these participants should be included in the analysis.

ELIGIBILITY CRITERIA

The RCT protocol specifies eligibility criteria that determine who can participate in the trial, defining the patient population of interest. Limiting the population allows trial investigators to capture patients who have greater potential to benefit and exclude patients who may be harmed or are unlikely to benefit or for whom it is not likely that the outcome variable can be easily assessed. While strict eligibility criteria might reduce heterogeneity and increase the probability of finding a treatment effect, they are at odds with the goal of obtaining results that are generalizable to the broad patient population who will ultimately be treated.[40]

In order to improve representation, the National Institutes of Health (NIH) Revitalization Act of 1993 mandated that all NIH-funded clinical research must include women and members of minority groups as subjects.[41] However, older patients and patients with other chronic conditions often remain excluded owing to concerns about negative impacts from comorbidities. Children, adolescents, and pregnant women may be excluded owing to ethical concerns. However, these exclusions result in no information about potential benefits or risks for these patients, even though they might be treated with the trial drug if it is approved.

It is often the case that early-phase (I and II) trials aim to show internal validity in an explicitly defined homogeneous population, whereas late-phase (III and IV) and pragmatic trials enroll a broader and more diverse patient population who more closely resembles clinical practice. This remains an active topic of discussion and consideration for clinical trial researchers.

INFORMED CONSENT

Informed consent is a process of communication between the clinical investigator and patient that ensures the complete understanding of the RCT (including risks, costs, and other treatment options), allowing the potential participant to make an informed decision about whether or not they wish to participate. Patients must be considered competent to understand and process the information so that they can make an appropriate decision, and the consent must be voluntary and in accordance with US FDA regulations (21 CFR 50) and guidelines.[36] The investigator must obtain consent from the participant or the participant's legally authorized representative following a thorough explanation of the purpose, potential benefits, risks, and responsibilities of the study. No RCT screening procedures should be performed for the purpose of research until consent has been obtained. All questions regarding therapy and the protocol should be answered and clearly understood prior to signing the consent, and an observer should witness the informed consent process.

STATISTICAL ANALYSIS POPULATIONS

In order to minimize bias in the analysis of data, a statistical plan should be devised prior to looking at the data.[42] The plan should include the rules to decide which data will be excluded from the planned statistical analysis, including ways of dealing with missing outcome and covariate data. The primary components in the statistical analysis plan are listed in **Table 5-2**.

Typically, RCTs are designed utilizing the intention-to-treat (ITT) principle.[43,44] This means that following randomization to a specific treatment group, each participant's data should be included in the primary analysis regardless of compliance with the protocol-specified intervention or follow-up requirements. In addition to ITT, investigators may want to assess the treatment effect when participants are compliant with protocol procedures. For example, an investigator may be interested in evaluating the treatment effect for participants who took the intervention as assigned. This type of analysis is referred to as "per protocol." Per protocol analyses should be conducted secondary to ITT analyses for RCTs. If conclusions are the same for both analyses, then the interpretation of study results is strengthened. If there is a discrepancy, reasons for the difference can be explored. However, it is the ITT analyses that support the primary hypothesis. Intention to treat reduces or avoids biases (such as selection bias) that may result from excluding randomized participants who are not compliant with the protocol.

MULTICENTER TRIALS

A high priority of all RCTs is the rapid and appropriate recruitment of participants into the clinical trial. If meeting the recruitment target is improbable by screening patients from only one clinical center, then more sites may be necessary. The necessity of multiple sites may be attributed to the fact that the clinical condition under investigation is relatively rare, and one site cannot screen enough patients to achieve the targeted enrollment.[45] Similarly, if the investigator or sponsor desires a very rapid recruitment of participants into the trial for FDA approval of their drug or device, or if the trial is a large screening study that requires a great number of participants to test the hypothesis, an RCT involving several centers may be desired. Whatever the reason, opening

TABLE 5-2. Components of a Statistical Analysis Plan

- Definition of target population and study samples (target population, intent-to-treat sample, per protocol sample)
- General statistical considerations (participant accountability, randomization and blinding, missing data, treatment group(s), comparability at baseline and study conclusion, preliminary analysis, site effects, participant compliance)
- Efficacy analyses
- *Primary outcome:* parameter description, handling of missing outcome and covariate data, statistical hypotheses, interim analysis method, final analysis method, additional analyses
- *Secondary outcome(s):* description of analysis methods for secondary outcome variable(s)
- Safety analyses (overview, definition and categorization of adverse events, descriptive statistics of adverse events, inferential statistics of adverse events, description of laboratory measures, descriptive statistics of laboratory measures, inferential statistics of adverse events, and other safety variables)
- Data to be excluded from analysis

the trial to more than one center may increase the speed of recruitment and generalizability of the results, at a potential cost of added complexity.[26] Ensuring adherence to the protocol from geographically dispersed locations, different hospital types (public or private), or even different countries and cultures requires very careful management and oversight of the study. A strong organizational infrastructure must be in place so that appropriate protocol, ethical, financial, and data management issues can be addressed with expedience.

In RCTs, particularly multicenter RCTs, the coordinating center (CC) has responsibility for all aspects of the day-to-day conduct of the clinical trial.[46] From the preparation of the operations manual and data collection instruments to the collection of data and final statistical analysis, the CC assumes the primary role in assisting the clinical centers with the appropriate implementation and conduct of the RCT. For multicenter RCTs, central randomization is usually performed at the CC, ensuring better control of the randomization process by providing a central location to which all screening and randomization data is sent. Centralized data management at the CC provides consistent data queries and clarifications as well as proper storage and management of all case data collection instruments. The CC has the responsibility of coordinating the central medical review and overseeing quality assurance, including regular site visits to clinical centers. Finally, given the centralized data management and project coordination, it is most efficient for the statistical responsibilities to reside with the CC. Having biostatisticians involved with each aspect of the RCT, from the protocol and forms design to the final analysis and report generation, saves time and resources and ensures that all clinical and scientific questions are answered with appropriate statistical methods.

INSTITUTIONAL REVIEW BOARD

In accordance with US FDA regulations (21 CFR 56) and guidelines, all research involving human subjects and changes to the research plan must be reviewed and approved by an institutional review board (IRB).[36] A copy of the protocol, proposed informed consent form, other written participant information, and any proposed advertising material must be submitted to the clinical center's IRB for written approval. Before recruitment of participants, the investigator must receive a copy of the IRB approval of the protocol and informed consent form. If amendments to the protocol are ever made following the initiation of the study, the investigator must submit all protocol amendments and revisions to the informed consent document to the IRB for approval. The IRB approval must be received before the amendment can be implemented. Furthermore, IRB protocol renewals must be received annually.

ADVERSE EVENTS AND SAFETY MONITORING

Because the safety of participants during an RCT is of primary importance, detailed monitoring of adverse events is required.[36] An adverse event is a serious or more prevalent event occurring during a research study that may or may not be related to trial participation. Adverse events may involve drugs, biologics, devices, loss of confidentiality, privacy issues, or harm to others. "An adverse event can therefore be any unfavorable and unintended sign (including an abnormal laboratory finding), symptom, or disease temporally associated with the use of a medicinal (investigational) product, whether or not related to the medicinal (investigational) product."[36]

Serious adverse events include "any adverse therapeutic experience occurring at any dose (of a drug) that results in any of the following outcomes: death, a life-threatening adverse drug experience, inpatient hospitalization or prolongation of existing hospitalization, a persistent or significant disability/incapacity, or a congenital anomaly/birth defect."[36] Other important medical events may be considered serious adverse drug experiences if they jeopardize the participant and require medical or surgical intervention to prevent death or hospitalization.

The data safety monitoring committee (DSMC, or data safety monitoring board [DSMB]) meets on a periodic basis to review all interim data relating to the RCT.[42] The DSMC typically consists of at least three members external to the conduct of the study with expertise in RCT methodology, epidemiology, ethics, quality-of-life evaluation for clinical trials of this nature, and clinical treatments for the types of patients under investigation. The study biostatistician can participate in the DSMC meetings as a nonvoting member. The DSMC responsibilities include the following: (1) review all adverse effects or complications related to the trial interventions, (2) review interim data on the primary and secondary outcomes according to prespecified guidelines, (3) monitor participant enrollment, (4) review the compliance of clinical centers, and (5) recommend to the investigators and/or sponsor whether the RCT should continue as usual, be modified, or stopped. In general, clinical investigators are not present at the "closed sessions" of the DSMC but may on occasion be requested to present or provide information to assist the DSMC in performing its functions appropriately.

REPORTING RESULTS OF CLINICAL TRIALS

The International Council for Harmonisation's Guideline for Good Clinical Practice (ICH GCP) sets an international standard for the design, conduct, recording, and reporting of clinical trials involving human participants. It details the responsibilities of those conducting the trial in order to safeguard the rights, safety, and well-being of trial participants, while ensuring the integrity of trial data.[36]

The Consolidated Standards of Reporting Trials (CONSORT) Group was established in 1996 in an effort to standardize reporting of clinical trials worldwide. The group introduced the CONSORT statement (https://www.consort-spirit.org/), revised in 2001, 2010, and 2025, which includes a 30-item checklist and flow diagram to provide guidance for reporting RCTs.[47]

CONCLUSION

If designed and implemented appropriately, RCTs provide the strongest type of data from which clinical practice guidelines derive their recommendations. Efforts must be made to avoid bias in all steps of the process, including recruitment, randomization, treatment, and analysis. Trial design and mathematical requirements for needed statistical analysis determine the number of participants needed for the study. Once the appropriate study design has been determined, the investigator must abide by the regulations designed to protect the human subjects who will participate. Successful research requires careful consideration of study design before embarking on the endeavor.

REFERENCES

1. Piantadosi S. *Clinical Trials: A Methodologic Perspective*. 4th ed. New York: Wiley; 2024.
2. Katz DG, Dutcher GA, Toigo TA, et al. The AIDS Clinical Trials Information Service (ACTIS): a decade of providing clinical trials information. *Public Health Reports*. 2002;117(2):123-130. https://doi.org/10.1093/phr/117.2.123
3. National Institutes of Health (NIH). *Cancer Clinical Trial Information for Patients and Caregivers*. Rockville, MD: National Cancer Institute; 2005. https://www.cancer.gov/research/participate/clinical-trials. Accessed February 11, 2026.
4. Patsopoulos NA. A pragmatic view on pragmatic trials. *Dialogues Clin Neurosci*. 2011;13(2):217-224. https://doi.org/10.31887/DCNS.2011.13.2/npatsopoulos
5. Schwartz D, Lellouch J. Explanatory and pragmatic attitudes in therapeutical trials. *J Chronic Dis*. 1967;20(8):637-648. https://doi.org/10.1016/0021-9681(67)90041-0
6. Ford I, Norrie J. Pragmatic trials. *N Engl J Med*. 2016;375(5):454-463. https://doi.org/10.1056/NEJMra1510059
7. Rosenberger WF, Lachin JM. *Randomization in Clinical Trials: Theory and Practice*. 2nd ed. New York: Wiley; 2016.
8. Lachin JM, Matts JP, Wei LJ. Randomization in clinical trials: conclusions and recommendations. *Controlled Clin Trials*.1988;9:365-374. https://doi.org/10.1016/0197-2456(88)90049-9
9. Friedman LM, Furberg CD, DeMets DL, et al. *Fundamentals of Clinical Trials*. 5th ed. Berlin: Springer Nature; 2015.
10. Cleophas TJM, Tavenir P. Clinical trials in chronic diseases. *J Clin Pharm*. 1995;35:594-598. https://doi.org/10.1002/j.1552-4604.1995.tb05016.x
11. Jones B, Donev AN. Modelling and design of cross-over trials. *Stat Med*. 1996;15:1435-1446.

https://doi.org/10.1002/(SICI)1097-0258(19960715)15:13%3C1435::AID-SIM278%3E3.0.CO;2-Y

12. Hussey MA, Hughes JP. Design and analysis of stepped wedge cluster randomized trials. *Contemporary Clin Trials*. 2007;28(2):182-191. https://doi.org/10.1016/j.cct.2006.05.007
13. Brown CA, Lilford RJ. The stepped wedge trial design: a systematic review. *BMC Med Res Methodol.* 2006;6:1-9. https://doi.org/10.1186/1471-2288-6-54
14. Smalheiser N. *Data Literacy: How to Make Your Experiments Robust and Reproducible*. Cambridge, MA: Academic Press; 2017.
15. Schechtman KB. Clinical trials. In: Chung-Chow S, ed. *Encyclopedia of Biopharmaceutical Statistics*. New York: Marcel Dekker; 2000.
16. Berthet V. The impact of cognitive biases on professionals' decision-making: a review of four occupational areas. *Front Psychol*. 2022;12:802439. https://doi.org/10.3389/fpsyg.2021.802439
17. Rosenberger, WF, Sverdlov O, Hu F. Adaptive randomization for clinical trials. *J Biopharm Stat*. 2012;22(4):719-736. https://doi.org/10.1080/10543406.2012.676535
18. Jadad AR, Enkin MW. *Randomized Controlled Trials: Questions, Answers and Musings*. 2nd ed. London: BMJ Publishing Group; 2007.
19. Lachin JM. Properties of simple randomization in clinical trials. *Control Clin Trials.* 1988;9:312-326. https://doi.org/10.1016/0197-2456(88)90046-3
20. Lachin JM. Statistical properties of randomization in clinical trials. *Control Clin Trials.* 1988;9:289-311. https://doi.org/10.1016/0197-2456(88)90045-1
21. Matts JP, Lachin JM. Properties of permuted-block randomization in clinical trials. *Control Clin Trials*. 1988;9:327-344. https://doi.org/10.1016/0197-2456(88)90047-5
22. Zelen M. The randomization and stratification of patients to clinical trials. *J Chron Dis.* 1974;27:365-375. https://doi.org/10.1016/0021-9681(74)90015-0
23. Berger VW, Bour LJ, Carter K, et al. A roadmap to using randomization in clinical trials. *BMC Med Res Methodol.* 2021;21:1-24. https://doi.org/10.1186/s12874-021-01303-z
24. Day SJ, Altman DG. Statistics notes: blinding in clinical trials and other studies. *Br Med J*. 2000;321(7259):504. https://doi.org/10.1136/bmj.321.7259.504
25. Terrin ML. Efficient use of endpoints in clinical trials: a clinical perspective. *Stat Med*. 1990;9:155-160. https://doi.org/10.1002/sim.4780090122
26. Senn S. *Statistical Issues in Drug Development*. New York: Wiley; 1997.
27. Herson J. The use of surrogate endpoints in clinical trials (an introduction to a series of four papers). *Stat Med*.1989;8:403-404. https://doi.org/10.1002/sim.4780080403
28. Prentice RL. Surrogate endpoints in clinical trials: definition and operational criteria. *Stat Med*. 1989;8:431-440. https://doi.org/10.1002/sim.4780080407
29. Fleming TR, Demets DL. Surrogate end points in clinical trials: are we being misled? *Ann Intern Med*. 1996;125:605-613. https://doi.org/10.7326/0003-4819-125-7-199610010-00011
30. Cardiac Arrhythmia Suppression Trial (CAST) Investigators. Preliminary report: effect of encainide and flecainide on mortality in a randomized trial of arrhythmia suppression after myocardial infarction. *N Engl J Med*. 1989;321:406-412. https://doi.org/10.1056/NEJM198908103210629
31. Lesaffre E. Superiority, equivalence, and non-inferiority trials. *Bull NYU Hosp Jt Dis*. 2008;66(2):150-154. PMID: 18537788
32. Leung JT, Barnes SL, Lo ST, Leung DY. Non-inferiority trials in cardiology: what clinicians need to know. *Heart.* 2020;106(2):99-104. https://doi.org/10.1136/heartjnl-2019-315772
33. Yeatts SD, Palesch YY, Coffey CS, et al. Futility designs. In: *Principles and Practice of Clinical Trials.* New York: Springer; 2022:1067-1082.
34. Lachin JM. Introduction to sample size determination and power analysis for clinical trials. *Control Clin Trials*. 1981;2:93-113. https://doi.org/10.1016/0197-2456(81)90001-5
35. Jennison C, Turnbull BW. Group sequential methods with applications to clinical trials. New York: CRC Press; 1999.
36. Department of Health and Human Services, Food and Drug Administration. International Council for Harmonisation's Guideline for Good Clinical Practice (ICH GCP) 2018. https://www.fda.gov/media/93884/download. Accessed February 11, 2026.
37. Department of Health and Human Services, Office for Human Research Protections, Title 45 of the Code of Federal Regulations, Part 46, Protection of Human Subjects, 2018. https://www.hhs.gov/ohrp/

regulations-and-policy/regulations/45-cfr-46/index.html. Accessed February 11, 2026.

38. Spilker B, Cramer JA, eds. *Patient Recruitment in Clinical Trials*. New York: Raven Press; 1992.
39. Cramer JA, Spilker B, eds. *Patient Compliance in Medical Practice and Clinical Trials*. New York: Raven Press; 1991.
40. Food and Drug Administration. Evaluating inclusion and exclusion criteria in clinical trials. *Workshop Report*. Washington DC: The National Press Club; 2018.
41. NIH Revitalization Act, Subtitle B, Part 1, Sec. 131-133, June 10, 1993.
42. Department of Health and Human Services. *Statistical Principles for Clinical Trials* (E9). Rockville, MD: Food and Drug Administration; 1998. https://www.fda.gov/media/71336/download. Accessed February 11, 2026.
43. Fischer LD, Dixon DO, Herson J, et al. Intention-to-treat in clinical trials. In: Pearce KE, ed. *Statistical Issues in Drug Research and Development*. New York: Marcel Dekker; 1990.
44. Lee YJ, Ellenberg JH, Hirtz DG, Nelson KB. Analysis of clinical trials by treatment actually received: is it really an option? *Stat Med*. 1991;10:1595-1605. https://doi.org/10.1002/sim.4780101011
45. Huster WJ. Multicenter trials. In: Chung-Chow S, ed. *Encyclopedia of Biopharmaceutical Statistics*. New York: Marcel Dekker; 2000.
46. Meinert CL. *Clinical Trials: Design, Conduct, and Analysis*. Oxford: Oxford University Press; 1986.
47. Hopewell S, Chan AW, Collins GS, et al. CONSORT 2025 statement: updated guideline for reporting randomised trials. *Lancet*. 2025;405:1633-1640. https://doi.org/10.1016/S0140-6736(25)00672-5

Systematic Literature Reviews and Meta-Analyses

6

Heather Shaw Bonilha, PhD, CCC-SLP

THE IMPORTANCE OF SYSTEMATIC LITERATURE REVIEWS

Systematic literature reviews play a crucial role in research, and, when done well, are widely considered to provide the highest level of scientific evidence. By synthesizing multiple studies, they identify common findings, highlight differences, and often explain the reasons behind discrepancies. A well-conducted systematic review offers a comprehensive summary of the state of the science on a given topic. This chapter aims to help readers evaluate the quality of systematic reviews while also serving as a guide for those interested in conducting their own reviews.

Systematic reviews are valuable in any field, as they consolidate existing knowledge and pinpoint gaps in research. They are particularly beneficial for newcomers, such as students or researchers exploring a novel area, as well as for professionals who require an overview of the current state of science for decision-making purposes. A well-crafted review allows readers to quickly grasp key concepts, historical context, limitations, and potential applications of research. Additionally, systematic reviews often serve as the foundation for clinical practice guidelines and policy statements, making them an essential resource for busy clinicians and policymakers seeking reliable evidence to inform their decisions.

For authors, conducting a systematic literature review provides an opportunity to thoroughly engage with the existing body of research. Review guidelines ensure that key studies are included, research rigor is assessed, and conclusions are drawn from well-supported findings. A systematic review is often a researcher's first publication on a topic, helping to establish their presence in the field and build a publication record. Moreover, these reviews frequently serve as a precursor to research grant submissions, offering a solid foundation for decisions regarding study design, inclusion/exclusion criteria, treatment approaches, and outcome measures. A published review can also demonstrate collaboration among co-investigators, strengthening a grant proposal.

In healthcare, systematic literature reviews can be particularly impactful in advocating for practice or policy changes. If a professional identifies concerns regarding a specific practice, they can consult an existing systematic review to provide a robust, evidence-based argument for change. If no existing systematic reviews exist, they may embark on a line of scientific inquiry to collaborate on a review. By presenting high-quality scientific evidence, systematic literature reviews can be instrumental in influencing decision-making and contribute to the advancement of their field.

TYPES OF SYSTEMATIC LITERATURE REVIEWS

Systematic literature reviews are a specific type of review conducted with methodological rigor, adhering to established guidelines for both execution and reporting. The most widely recognized guideline is the Preferred Reporting Items for Systematic Reviews and Meta-Analyses (PRISMA).[1] Unlike general reviews,

DOI: 10.37573/9781585287666.006

which may lack methodological structure and fail to include all relevant publications, systematic literature reviews are designed to minimize bias, particularly in article selection, by following strict inclusion criteria.

Scoping reviews are often conducted as a preliminary step before a systematic literature review. Their purpose is to assess the breadth of available literature on a given topic and provide a broad overview of existing research.[2] The key distinction between scoping reviews and systematic literature reviews lies in their objectives. When the goal is to inform practice or policy implementation, a full systematic review, complete with a critical appraisal of the methodological rigor of included studies, is necessary. Conversely, the goal of the scoping review is to achieve an overview of a specific topic to summarize the extent and nature of the publications available on the topic. Scoping reviews do not typically include critical appraisals of the included articles.

A Cochrane review is a specialized form of systematic literature review conducted under the Cochrane Collaboration and published in the Cochrane Database of Systematic Reviews.[3] These reviews focus on healthcare and health policy research and follow strict methodological standards outlined in Cochrane handbooks. They differ from general systematic reviews that adhere to PRISMA guidelines in four key ways[1]: (1) authors must submit a proposal to the Cochrane Collaboration; (2) there is a strong emphasis on randomized controlled trials (RCTs); (3) the review must include all available data, including from unpublished material; and (4) the review process is subject to rigorous oversight by the Cochrane Collaboration. This chapter focuses on non-Cochrane systematic literature reviews, which follow PRISMA guidelines.[1]

PREREQUISITE SKILLS, PREPARATION, AND COLLABORATIVE TEAM

Systematic literature reviews are an excellent way to gain in-depth knowledge of a field, but they require specific skills, preparation, and a team with diverse expertise to be conducted effectively. Essential skills include a strong understanding of the field to formulate a relevant research question, proficiency in using article databases, such as PubMed, and familiarity with reference management systems. Additionally, organizational skills, collaboration, critical thinking, and the ability to interpret findings meaningfully are crucial for a successful review.

The preparation process for a systematic literature review mirrors that of any research project. Collaborators must define the review's focus and objectives, establish a timeline, and determine each member's contributions, including authorship roles and order for the planned publication. Authorship follows standard research publication guidelines, such as those outlined by the International Committee of Medical Journal Editors (ICMJE).[4] It is also important to identify potential journals for submission, keeping in mind that not all journals accept systematic literature reviews, and some only publish solicited submissions.

A minimum team for a systematic literature review should include a subject matter expert and a reference librarian. Additional collaborators may be necessary to distribute the workload and demonstrate validity of the review via interrater reliability. The subject matter expert is vital throughout the process, particularly in refining the research topic, selecting relevant search terms and databases, and interpreting results. The reference librarian plays a crucial role in developing a robust search strategy, ensuring that all relevant studies are included, and ultimately strengthening the validity of the review's conclusions.

STEP 1: BRAINSTORM TOPICS

Selecting a Topic

Selecting a topic for a systematic literature review can be either one of the easiest or most challenging steps in the process. If the review is intended to synthesize evidence for clinical practice or policy decisions, the need is clear, making topic selection relatively straightforward. However, for early-career researchers using a review to identify potential research directions, this step can be more difficult but highly valuable. In this case, working closely with a mentor to define the research question(s) is essential.

An ideal topic should align with both personal research goals and the needs of the broader field, ensuring that it is relevant and publishable. Because systematic literature reviews serve a wide audience, their ability to be published and disseminated is crucial. During topic brainstorming, it is important to continuously assess both the team's objectives and the topic's relevance. To determine whether a review on the topic is publishable, conduct an early literature search to check for recent systematic reviews on the subject. As a general guideline, systematic reviews on the same topic should be published roughly every 10 years or sooner if a significant number of new studies have emerged. Given the lengthy process of conducting and publishing a review, the feasibility of a new review should be based on the date of the literature search, not the publication dates of existing reviews (as these may be years apart). Additionally, searching systematic review registries, such as PROSPERO, can help to identify ongoing reviews by other research teams.

Assessing a topic's feasibility is an iterative process. A viable systematic review topic should have enough published studies to justify synthesis but not so many that the review becomes unmanageable. Generally, topics with at least 10 relevant studies warrant a review, whereas those with more than 100 may be too broad and labor-intensive. Besides the number of studies to be included, researchers should consider the total number of search results, because all articles will need to be screened at least at the title and abstract level. As a result, topic selection may evolve as more information is gathered about existing reviews, available search terms, and the volume of relevant publications.

STEP 2: SEARCHING, REFINING THE TOPIC, AND DRAFTING THE INTRODUCTION

As with other types of research, pilot studies are essential for refining the design of a systematic literature review. This involves selecting appropriate databases, identifying search terms, and applying filters to optimize the search. Conducting this preliminary step ensures the review is both relevant and feasible before finalizing the methodology.

An initial task involves identifying relevant databases. In health-related research, commonly used databases include PubMed/MEDLINE, Embase, and Scopus, with additional options, such as PsycINFO and CINAHL, depending on the topic. A reference librarian is invaluable in selecting the most appropriate databases. The number of databases chosen affects the workload, because including nonessential databases may yield only a small number of additional relevant articles while significantly increasing the screening burden. Often, these extra articles can be identified through citation tracking rather than expanding the search to less relevant databases.

Once databases are selected, the next step is developing a search strategy. The validity of the review depends on identifying all relevant studies; otherwise, conclusions drawn from an incomplete dataset will be flawed. Thus, a valid search strategy requires that all important concepts be included in the search incorporated with the matching search terms relevant to the field. This is another step of the process where it is necessary to have one or more experts in the field participate in brainstorming concepts and search terms. One method to identify the main concepts is forming a PICO question.[5] PICO questions help to ensure inclusion of some of the key concepts related to participant/patient description, intervention, control group, and outcome measure(s) of interest.

Each database has a unique indexing system, requiring tailored search terms while maintaining consistent core concepts. For example, PubMed/MEDLINE uses Medical Subject Headings (MeSH), meaning that search terms in this database may differ from those in others with different organizational structures. Additionally, search terms need to be combined into search strings with the appropriate Boolean operators. Given this complexity, involving a research librarian is strongly recommended to ensure a comprehensive and accurate search. A useful way to validate a search strategy is by cross-checking it against a list of key articles already known in the field to ensure that they appear in the results.

Often, an initial search yields too many results to manage. When this happens, database filters can help narrow the scope. One common approach is restricting the publication date range, which is useful updating a previous review or when older studies are less relevant because of advancements in technology or practice. Another common filter limits results to specific study designs, such as controlled clinical trials, excluding lower levels of evidence, such as observational studies. However, when filters alone are insufficient to refine the scope, adjusting the topic and search terms may be necessary.

STEP 3: FIRST DRAFT OF THE INTRODUCTION

Once the pilot and feasibility testing are complete, the topic of the systematic literature review will be clearly defined. At this stage, drafting a brief introduction is useful to ensure that the design decisions made in the methods section align with the review's purpose. This initial draft should prioritize content over writing style, as it will be revised extensively after the review is completed to reflect the final findings.

A three-paragraph structure is sufficient for this draft. The first paragraph should highlight the broader significance of the topic within the field. The second paragraph should provide more specific details, including the justification for conducting a systematic review. The third paragraph should clearly state the research question and hypothesis, along with the anticipated impact of the review, such as informing clinical practice, influencing policy, or identifying research gaps. As with other scientific writing, starting with an outline can help structure this section effectively, ensuring that each paragraph includes focused and relevant information.

STEP 4: WRITING THE METHODS SECTION

The methods section of a systematic literature review, like that of other research articles, outlines how the study will be conducted. Unlike the introduction, this section must be finalized with minimal revisions before proceeding with the full literature search, article screening, methodological evaluation, and conclusion formation. Establishing methods *a priori* is crucial to maintaining the validity of the review.

Systematic literature review methods follow the PRISMA guidelines and checklist.[1] Once the methods are finalized, the authors should register the review with a registry, such as PROSPERO.[6] Registration enhances the review's rigor by making the *a priori* methods publicly available and helps prevent duplication of efforts in the field.

Search Procedures

The search procedures, including the search date, databases searched, and inclusion/exclusion criteria, must be clearly specified to ensure replicability. The search date is essential for reproducibility, and all information sources used to identify articles must be listed. These sources typically include article databases, such as PubMed/MEDLINE, although some systematic reviews also incorporate grey literature, such as conference abstracts. In addition to searching major databases, researchers often screen the reference lists of included articles and identify studies that have cited them.

Both the general search concepts and the specific search strategies (ie, search strings) for each database should be detailed. These search strings are typically presented in a table within the main text or as an appendix or supplement. It is also helpful to describe how search terms and strings were validated, including the set of articles used for verification.

Another critical component of the search process is defining the eligibility criteria (ie, inclusion and exclusion criteria). These criteria guide researchers in determining whether an article should be included in the review. Common inclusion/exclusion factors include publication date, language, study design (eg, level of evidence), and topic-specific elements, such as patient/population/problem, intervention, comparison, or outcome measures. Additionally, it is important to note whether exclusion criteria were applied through database filters (eg, limiting results by language, publication date, or study type).

Selection Process

This section of the methods should detail the article selection process, which typically follows a three-step approach: (1) an initial title and abstract screening, (2) a full-text review, and (3) a citation search to identify additional relevant studies. In addition to outlining these steps, this section should describe how articles will be organized, deduplicated, and processed before screening. Information about the software used, whether a basic spreadsheet (eg, Excel) or specialized systematic review software (eg, Covidence systematic review software, Veritas Health Innovation, Melbourne, Australia. https://www.covidence.org/), should be provided, along with details on whether deduplication is performed manually or automatically.

Each step of the screening process must be described in detail. The title and abstract screening involve reviewing all identified articles to classify them as: (1) clearly irrelevant, (2) clearly relevant, or (3) uncertain due to insufficient information. Articles in the latter two categories proceed to full-text review. The full-text review process should be explicitly detailed, including how inaccessible articles will be handled, such as attempts to contact authors and criteria for deciding when to exclude an article due to unavailability. Once eligible articles are identified, the citation search is conducted by screening both the reference lists and studies that have cited the included articles, with details of this process also documented.

To ensure rigor, at least two independent screeners must be involved in both title/abstract and full-text reviews. The methods should specify how discrepancies between screeners will be managed. At minimum, intrarater reliability should be assessed by having the primary screener reevaluate approximately 10% to 20% of articles, whereas interrater reliability should be assessed by a second screener. The number of articles assessed should be sufficient to establish confidence in screening reliability. If agreement is below 90%, the screening process may need refinement, and this section should specify how modifications will be handled.

For discrepancies, a discussion among screeners and collaborators should be conducted to resolve differences. During title and abstract screening, any unresolved doubts should default toward inclusion in the full-text review. For full-text screening, if consensus cannot be reached, the methods should define how final decisions will be made regarding article inclusion.

Data Collection Process

The data collection process begins once all articles for the systematic literature review have been identified. This section should list the data elements to be extracted and provide definitions, if necessary. These elements should include both study-specific factors relevant to the research question and general study descriptors, such as participant characteristics and study design details. When planning data extraction, it is helpful to consider the tables that will be included in the manuscript and the key information needed for the results and discussion sections. A trial extraction on a subset of studies identified during the pilot search can help refine the data elements.

Some studies may lack certain data elements, or there may be concerns about participant duplication across publications from the same research group. The methods section should specify how these situations will be addressed, for example, whether authors will be contacted or how overlapping cohorts will be handled (eg, selecting the most comprehensive or recent study). This strategy is similar to how missing data are accounted for in intervention studies and should be explicitly stated in the methodology.

Article Critique Procedures

The article critique process in a systematic literature review typically involves evaluating the level of evidence, assessing methodological rigor, and conducting a bias assessment. These steps are essential to understanding the study's value and determining the weight its findings should carry in the discussion and conclusion sections. At a minimum, one reviewer evaluates each article for these factors, with an additional reviewer assessing a subset of studies (typically 10% to 20%) to establish and report reliability.

If the review includes studies with varying designs, the first step is to classify each study's level of evidence. This is based on study design (eg, RCTs, cohort studies) and is commonly assessed by using the Oxford Centre for Evidence-Based Medicine (OCEBM) classification system.[7] If only RCTs are eligible for inclusion, this step is unnecessary.

Methodological rigor is evaluated using published, validated tools or checklists. For systematic literature reviews that focus on RCTs, these include assessments of randomization, blinding, reporting of dropouts, as well as other aspects of research rigor. Several options exist for RCTs, including the Jadad Scale, Van Tulder Scale, and Physiotherapy Evidence Database (PEDro) Scale.[8-10] The Consolidated Standards of Reporting Trials (CONSORT) checklist also can be used but does not produce a quantitative score.[11] For non-RCTs, fewer validated tools are available, but the Critical Appraisal Skills Programme (CASP) and Strengthening the Reporting of Observational Studies in Epidemiology (STROBE) checklists are commonly used.[12,13] These tools address aspects of research rigor related to nonrandomized trials, such as inclusion criteria, sample size calculation, statistical analyses, etc.

Bias assessment is crucial for determining a study's internal validity and the reliability of its findings. Articles should be evaluated for selection, performance, detection, attrition, and reporting bias. Tools, such as the Downs and Black Checklist and the Cochrane Collaboration Risk of Bias Tool, can aid in this assessment.[14,15] Critical appraisal, including analysis of methodological rigor and bias assessment, is necessary per PRISMA guidelines.[1] Authors and readers of systematic literature reviews should carefully attend to the quality of the included articles and give more weight to results of high-quality studies.

STEP 5: COMPLETING THE LITERATURE REVIEW AND WRITING THE RESULTS SECTION

Organizing Search Results

Once the methods are finalized, the next step is to run the search. The search results must be organized into a unified database to facilitate deduplication, because duplicates are common across the databases used. This can be done using Excel, a reference manager, or software designed specifically for systematic literature reviews. An important aspect of this step is to track the number of articles from each database that are included in the first-level screening (title/abstract). This information is essential for creating the PRISMA flowchart, which will be included as a figure in your manuscript.[1]

Screening Search Results

Screening articles occurs in two stages: the initial title and abstract screening, followed by the more in-depth full-text screening. Both stages require at least two individuals to ensure reliability in the inclusion/exclusion judgments. Reporting reliability is a key feature of systematic literature reviews, adding to their methodological rigor and ensuring the validity of the conclusions drawn. Before starting the screening process, all collaborators should review the eligibility criteria and their definitions. It is often necessary to revisit this topic during the process to clarify any unanticipated scenarios.

During the initial title and abstract screening, screeners make two key decisions: whether to pass an article to full-text review or exclude it. Articles passed to full-text review may either clearly meet the inclusion criteria based on the title and abstract or provide insufficient information to make a determination. To facilitate this, it can be useful to have a third category: (1) meets criteria, (2) unclear, and (3) does not meet criteria. Articles in categories 1 or 2 proceed to full-text review. This level of detail aids in resolving discrepancies during screenings and does not add significant time to the process. Articles that do not meet criteria should have the exclusion reason recorded, because this information will be included in the PRISMA flowchart (**Figure 6-1**).[1] The workload at this stage depends on how specific the search terms are. Broad search terms may result in many articles to screen, although many will clearly be irrelevant, making the screening process faster for each individual article. However, the challenge is managing a large volume of articles. Additionally, articles may need to be passed to full-text screening when titles and abstracts are insufficient or when the focus of the review is different from the article's scope, such as in a review of a specific patient population or methodology.

Full-text screening involves obtaining the full text of articles and evaluating them against the inclusion/exclusion criteria. This stage also

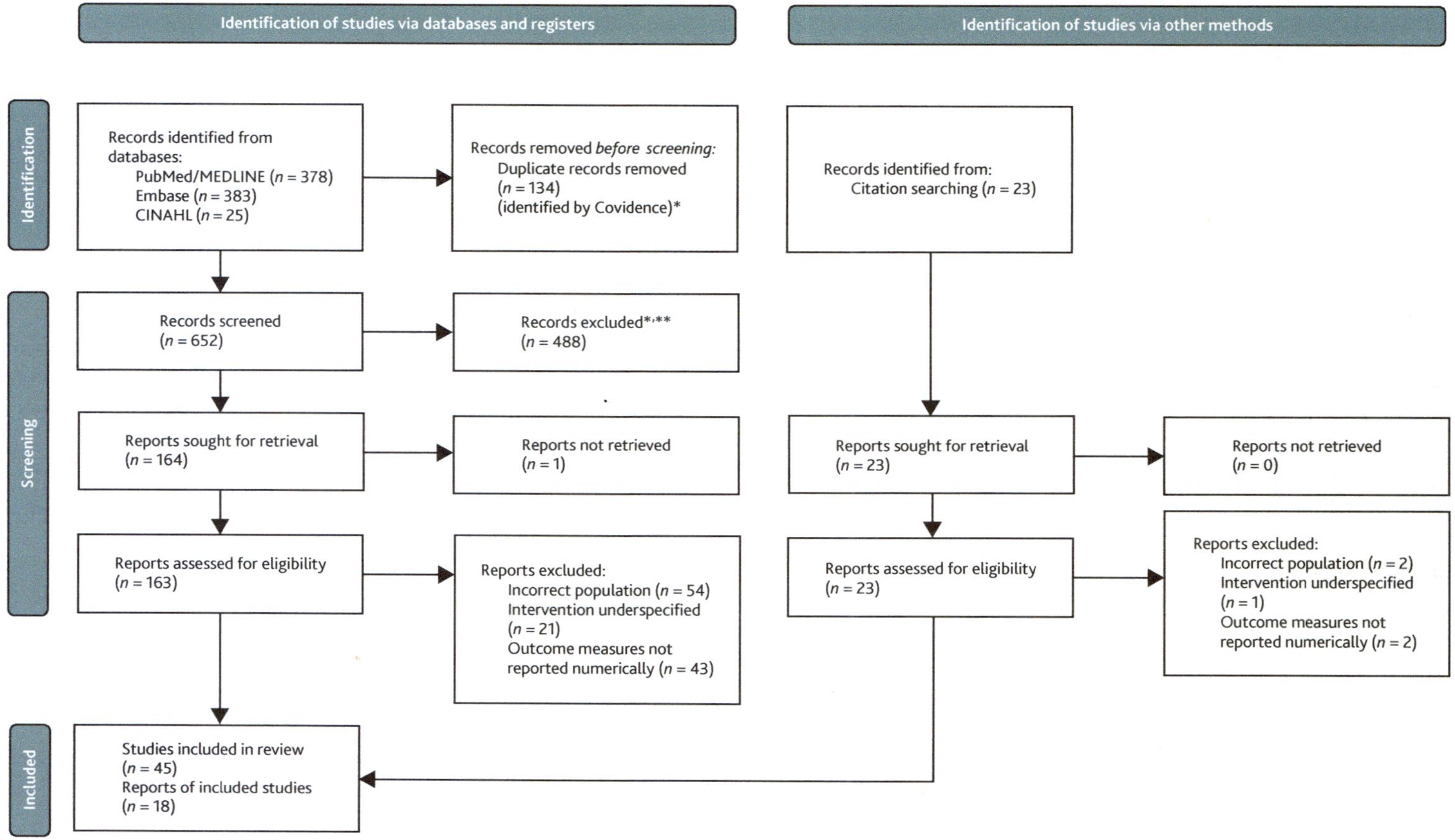

FIGURE 6-1. **PRISMA 2020 flow diagram for new systematic reviews, which included searches of databases, registers, and other sources.**
*Keep a record of reasons even though they do not need to be included in the flowchart.

**If automation tools were used, indicate how many records were excluded by a human and how many were excluded by automation tools.

Source: Page MJ, McKenzie JE, Bossuyt PM, et al. The PRISMA 2020 statement: an updated guideline for reporting systematic reviews. *BMJ.* 2021;372:n71. doi: 10.1136/bmj.n71.

requires a second reviewer, calculation of reliability, and discussions to resolve any discrepancies. Before full-text screening, it is essential to gather all relevant full-text articles. If articles are inaccessible, they should be excluded, and the reason for exclusion should be noted in the PRISMA flowchart.[1] Before beginning full-text screening, the eligibility criteria should be re-reviewed. Screeners should focus on the specific information relevant to the eligibility criteria without assessing the article's methodological rigor at this stage. If articles are excluded but may be useful in the introduction or discussion sections, it is helpful to mark them for later reference. The rationale for excluding any article during full-text screening also should be recorded for inclusion in the PRISMA flowchart.

Articles identified through reference and citation searches should be tracked in the PRISMA flowchart, initially placed in a unique section indicating their source, and then incorporated into the main flow. It is important to track how many articles were screened (title/abstract and full text) through these processes.

In this section of the results, intrarater and interrater reliability should be reported, typically as percent agreement. Additionally, any changes made to the screening process to improve reliability, as well as how discrepancies were managed, should be detailed here.

Extracting Data

Once the articles to be included in the review have been selected, the next step is to extract data from these articles, as outlined in the Methods section. At a minimum, data extraction should be completed by one person, with another person performing accuracy spot checks. It is common for the process to be refined after extracting data from the first five to 10 articles to ensure consistency and accuracy across the full set of articles.

Summarizing Data

Once data have been extracted and organized, typically into a large spreadsheet, the next task is to consider how to structure the results section. This section will usually include a narrative synthesis, tables, and the PRISMA flowchart at a minimum. Given that systematic literature reviews often cover multiple subtopics, it is helpful to use subheadings in both the results and discussion sections to improve clarity and organization for both the writer and the reader.

The narrative portion of the results should summarize key findings relevant to the research question and any other notable findings that will be discussed later. This part of the results is useful for providing a broad summary of the outcomes (eg, "75% [15/20] of the articles reviewed revealed that . . ."). It should also highlight outlier results that might not fit within the general trends. However, it is crucial not to duplicate the information already presented in the tables in the narrative portion of the results.

In terms of tables, there are typically at least three in a systematic literature review:

- Table 1 often provides an overview of the articles included in the review, including key details, such as participant characteristics, intervention details, outcome measures, and study designs.
- Table 2 usually summarizes the information from the article critique procedures (detailed above in Step 4), such as methodological rigor of the studies, including the level of evidence and the results of any bias critiques.
- Table 3 and beyond typically present the results relevant to the research question, summarizing the findings of each study included in the review.

Having these organized tables ensures clarity and allows readers to quickly grasp the key details of the included studies without having to sift through dense narrative descriptions.

STEP 6: WRITING THE DISCUSSION SECTION

The discussion section of a systematic literature review is essential for interpreting the key findings in relation to the research question and hypotheses while contextualizing them within existing literature. It is here that authors provide actionable insights for research, practice, and policy. The section begins by reviewing the results, comparing them with previous studies, identifying trends, and addressing discrepancies or outliers. It then highlights research gaps, offering future directions for studies, and discusses how the findings can influence practice, such as clinical or educational applications, as well as potential policy changes. Authors must also address the limitations found in the studies reviewed, such as methodological flaws, biases, or inconsistencies, and consider how these affect the validity of the findings. Additionally, the review process itself has limitations, such as exclusion of certain databases or sources, or potential biases in selection and data extraction. The section concludes with a summary of the main findings and their broader implications, stressing areas for further investigation and adjustments to research, practice, or policy.

Highlighting and Interpreting Key Results

The discussion section primarily focuses on highlighting the key results of the systematic literature review and addressing how these findings align with the research question and the initial hypotheses. This includes restating the main results and examining whether the hypothesis was supported by the evidence gathered. Additionally, the discussion should incorporate any surprising or unexpected insights that emerged during the review process, which may not have been anticipated at the outset. The authors' expertise is essential for interpreting these results, providing a deeper understanding of their relevance, and contextualizing them within the broader field of study. Furthermore, the results should be compared with existing literature to highlight similarities, discrepancies, or new perspectives that the review has uncovered.

Highlighting Actionable Insights and Implications

From the discussion of the results, the authors must determine whether there is enough evidence to offer actionable insights or to guide practice or policy changes or if more research is necessary before implementation can occur. This decision is crucial. It is often valuable for the authors to consult with trusted experts in the field to ensure a well-rounded perspective on the findings and their readiness for implementation. Factors, such as the amount and quality of the available research, the consistency of the results, and the potential risks and benefits of premature implementation, should all be carefully considered. If the literature is deemed insufficient to support immediate implementation, the focus of the actionable insights can shift to identifying areas where further research is needed before implementation can be confidently pursued.

Acknowledging Limitations

In all systematic literature reviews, there are limitations related to both the articles available in the field and the review process itself. Limitations of the articles in the field may arise from factors, such as the inclusion/exclusion criteria, measurement issues, variability in study design, inconsistent terminology, or differences in how outcomes are reported. These factors can limit the ability to draw broad conclusions. Additionally, systematic literature reviews themselves often face limitations, including the exclusion of articles written in different languages, the possibility that the search strategy did not capture all relevant articles, or that the included studies had too much variability in methods and measurements, preventing the use of meta-analysis. These limitations should be clearly acknowledged, because they can affect the validity and generalizability of the review's conclusions.

STEP 7: WRITING THE CONCLUSION, REFINING THE INTRODUCTION, AND REVIEWING THE MANUSCRIPT

Conclusion

The conclusion of a systematic literature review provides a concise summary of the key findings related to the research question, emphasizing the value of the review in advancing knowledge in the field. It highlights the main results and their implications, while ensuring that these conclusions are directly supported by the evidence presented in the review. The conclusion also suggests future directions, whether it be recommendations for implementation, identification of gaps that warrant further research, or both. It is crucial that no new information is introduced in the conclusion and that the conclusions drawn are rooted in the findings of the review, rather than personal opinions of the authors.

Reviewing and Revising the Entire Manuscript for Accuracy and Clarity

Once the conclusion is finalized, the authors proceed to write the abstract, summarizing the key elements of the systematic review in a concise manner. Following this, the manuscript is carefully reviewed and revised for coherence, accuracy, and clarity. The introduction is revisited and expanded upon, as it has served its initial purpose of guiding the authors. Now, it is developed to introduce the systematic review to the reader, justifying its relevance, and setting expectations for the content of the article. The rest of the manuscript is also thoroughly reviewed and refined to ensure that it accurately reflects the methods used, maintains clarity, and adheres to a consistent and clear writing style.

Adding a Meta-Analysis

When the studies included in a systematic review are confirmed to be of high quality, with similar designs and outcome measures, further analysis may be possible. A meta-analysis is a quantitative method that applies statistical techniques to combine (or "pool") the results of multiple studies included in a systematic review. By mathematically merging data from multiple studies, the overall sample size increases, leading to more precise estimates of the effect being studied. Meta-analyses are most commonly used in systematic reviews on interventions, aiming to determine whether definitive evidence supports a particular treatment approach.

Meta-analyses are particularly valuable in fields where large clinical trials are uncommon. When individual studies have small sample sizes, pooling multiple trial results can help to identify a treatment effect that might not have been statistically significant in each separate study. Conversely, meta-analysis may reveal that no true treatment effect exists—indicating that the lack of statistical significance in individual studies was not simply due to small sample sizes.

Because meta-analyses rely on statistical tests, they help to minimize bias in conducting and reporting results. However, they are still subject to biases present in the original studies or the systematic review used to select them. Not all studies from a systematic review may be of sufficient quality or appropriate design to be included in a meta-analysis. Additionally, meta-analyses require consistency across studies in terms of patient population, study design, intervention(s), and outcome measures. For outcome measures, studies must not only use the same measurement tool but also report results in a way that allows meaningful combination. For instance, if one study reports only an average without a standard deviation and another reports only a total score without subscale breakdowns, their data may not be compatible for pooling.

The first step in conducting a meta-analysis, as an extension of a systematic literature review, is defining the outcome of interest. Next, relevant studies from the systematic review that meet the inclusion criteria are identified. Before pooling results, it is crucial to assess heterogeneity, or variation, among study results. This can be done by using statistical tests, such as the chi-square test, and visually through forest plots. If the results show homogeneity, meaning the variation is likely due to random error, a fixed-effects model can be used. However, if heterogeneity is high, a random-effects model is needed to account for differences between studies. It is important to understand the limitations related to both fixed-effects and random-effects models.[16] Fixed-effects models assume that all studies are similar, which is often an oversimplification. In contrast, random-effects models account for variability across studies but do not explain why variability exists. Furthermore, random-effects models are less likely to produce statistically significant results compared with fixed-effects models. To quantify heterogeneity, researchers often use the I^2 statistic, which helps determine how much variability among studies may influence the meta-analysis results. Additional analyses, such as subgroup analyses and regression analyses, may be performed to explore factors that influence the results or identify potential moderators affecting the treatment effect.[16] Meta-analyses can be conducted by using major statistical software packages, as well as specialized tools designed for this purpose, such as Cochrane's RevMan or Comprehensive Meta-Analysis (CMA) https://www.meta-analysis.com/.

CONCLUSION

Systematic literature reviews and meta-analyses are essential tools for synthesizing research evidence, identifying trends, and informing decisions in practice, policy, and future research. They require careful planning, methodological rigor, and collaboration among experts to ensure validity and reliability. From topic selection and search strategy development to data extraction and critical appraisal, each step contributes to producing a comprehensive and trustworthy synthesis of existing knowledge.

These reviews not only consolidate findings across studies but also highlight gaps in the literature, offering direction for future investigations. When appropriate, meta-analyses enhance the precision of conclusions by statistically combining results from multiple studies. Ultimately, systematic reviews and meta-analyses provide a foundation for evidence-based decision-making and contribute meaningfully to the advancement of knowledge across disciplines.

REFERENCES

1. Page MJ, McKenzie JE, Bossuyt PM, et al. The PRISMA 2020 statement: an updated guideline for reporting systematic reviews. *BMJ*. 2021;372:n71. https://doi.org/10.1136/bmj.n71
2. Munn Z, Peters MDJ, Stern C, et al. Systematic review or scoping review? Guidance for authors when choosing between a systematic or scoping review approach. *BMC Med Res Methodol*. 2018;18:143. https://doi.org/10.1186/s12874-018-0611-x
3. Higgins JPT, Thomas J, Chandler J, et al., eds. *Cochrane Handbook for Systematic Reviews of Interventions*, version 6.5. Updated August 2024. Cochrane; 2024.
4. International Committee of Medical Journal Editors (ICMJE). Recommendations for the conduct, reporting, editing, and publication of scholarly work in medical journals. Updated January 2025. *ICMJE*; 2025.
5. Richardson WS, Wilson MC, Nishikawa J, Hayward RS. The well-built clinical question: a key to evidence-based decisions. *ACP J Club*. 1995;123(3):A12-3. PMID: 7582737
6. International Prospective Register of Systematic Reviews (PROSPERO). https://www.crd.york.ac.uk/PROSPERO/home. Accessed March 26, 2026.
7. OCEBM Levels of Evidence Working Group. The Oxford 2011 Levels of Evidence. Oxford Centre for Evidence-Based Medicine. https://www.cebm.net/. Accessed March 26, 2026.
8. Jadad AR, Moore RA, Carroll D, et al. Assessing the quality of reports of randomized clinical trials: is blinding necessary? *Control Clin Trials*. 1996;17(1):1-12. https://doi.org/10.1016/0197-2456(95)00134-4
9. van Tulder M, Furlan A, Bombardier C, Bouter L; Editorial Board of the Cochrane Collaboration Back Review Group. Updated method guidelines for systematic reviews in the Cochrane collaboration back review group. *Spine*. 2003;28(12):1290-1299. https://doi.org/10.1097/01.BRS.0000065484.95996.AF
10. Physiotherapy Evidence Database (PEDro). Centre for Evidence-Based Physiotherapy, School of Physiotherapy, The University of Sydney. https://pedro.org.au/. Accessed March 26, 2026.
11. Schulz KF, Altman DG, Moher D; CONSORT Group. CONSORT 2010 Statement: updated guidelines for reporting parallel group randomised trials. *BMC Med*. 2010;24:8-18.
12. Critical Appraisal Skills Programme UK. CASP qualitative studies checklist. Published 2024. https://casp-uk.net/casp-tools-checklists/qualitative-studies-checklist/. Accessed March 26, 2026.
13. von Elm E, Altman DG, Egger M, et tal; STROBE Initiative. Strengthening the reporting of observational studies in epidemiology (STROBE) statement: guidelines for reporting observational studies. *BMJ*. 2007;335(7624):806-808.
14. Downs SH, Black N. The feasibility of creating a checklist for the assessment of the methodological quality both of randomised and non-randomised studies of health care interventions. *J Epidemiol Community Health*. 1998;52(6):377-384. https://doi.org/10.1136/jech.52.6.377
15. Sterne JAC, Savovic J, Page MJ, et al. RoB 2: a revised tool for assessing risk of bias in randomised trials. *BMJ*. 2019;366:l4898. https://doi.org/10.1136/bmj.l4898
16. Hansen C, Steinmetz H, Block J. How to conduct a meta-analysis in eight steps: a practical guide. *Manag Rev Q*. 2022;72:1-19. https://doi.org/10.1007/s11301-021-00247-4

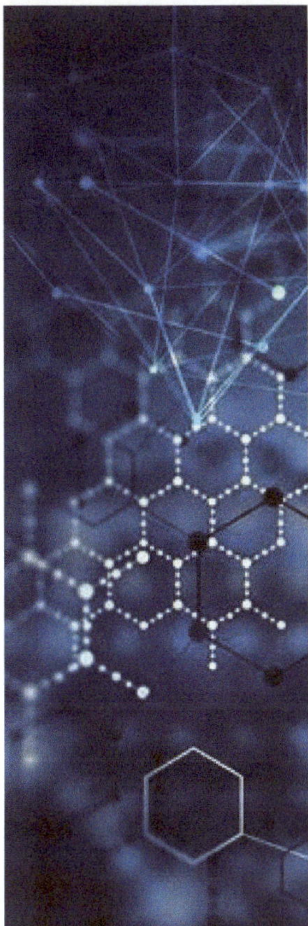

SECTION TWO

Statistical Analyses

DOI: 10.37573/9781585287666.TITLE

7

Introduction to Statistical Analysis

Elinor G. Borgert, PhD, MSc

In the pursuit of evidence-based healthcare, the ability to understand and apply statistical methods is as essential as the clinical knowledge that guides patient care. Just as study design provides the blueprint for rigorous research, statistical analysis provides the tools to interpret data, test hypotheses, and draw meaningful conclusions. This section introduces the foundational concepts of statistical analysis, beginning with univariate methods and progressing to multivariable modeling. Together, these chapters will equip readers with the skills to critically evaluate published research and conduct their own analyses with confidence and clarity.

Drs. Caitlin Koob and Jada M. Johnson begin with a discussion of data types, measurement scales, and distributions, because these determine exactly which types of statistics and statistical tests can be appropriately employed. Descriptive statistics, measures of both central tendency and variability, are used to summarize the data. Hypothesis testing takes things a step further; here, understanding null/alternative hypotheses, *p*-values, power, and Type I and Type II errors are key. Finally, the chapter describes some of the most common statistical tests, both parametric and nonparametric, and concludes with a discussion of correlation, confidence intervals, and the distinction between statistical and clinical significance.

Building on this foundation, Drs. Ralph Ward and Annie N. Simpson guide readers through the more complex terrain of multivariable analysis in Chapter 9. While univariate methods examine the relationship between a single independent variable and an outcome, multivariable models allow researchers to estimate the simultaneous effects of multiple explanatory variables. This is particularly important in healthcare research, where outcomes are rarely influenced by a single factor.

Readers are guided through the data preparation process, including defining variables, handling missing data, and structuring datasets for analysis. Throughout, the authors emphasize the importance of aligning statistical methods with research questions and study design.

Ordinary least squares (OLS) regression is explained in detail as a foundational method for modeling continuous outcomes, followed by logistic regression for binary outcomes. Advanced topics provide a roadmap for readers interested in exploring more sophisticated techniques and highlight the growing role of data science in healthcare research.

Taken together, these chapters provide a comprehensive introduction to statistical analysis in health services research. From basic descriptive statistics to advanced multivariable modeling, they offer readers the tools to interpret data, evaluate evidence, and contribute to the growing body of knowledge that informs healthcare practice and policy. Whether reviewing a published study or designing a new investigation, a solid understanding of statistical methods is essential for making informed, data-driven decisions.

DOI: 10.37573/9781585287666.007

Univariate Analysis

8

Caitlin Koob, PhD, MS, OTR/L, and Jada M. Johnson, MS

AN INTRODUCTION TO STATISTICAL TESTS

A basic understanding of statistics is essential to evaluating peer-reviewed literature relevant to healthcare administration, including healthcare systems research, program evaluation, implementation science, and applications to public health. Practitioners frequently rely on what is published in the literature—or what is "evidence-based"—to guide them in developing the best way to address patient needs, workforce issues, and a myriad of other topics. Those who are involved in designing and conducting research also rely on what has been published previously to provide foundational evidence and direct them in designing investigations that result in new knowledge. To understand how to appropriately digest and apply the results of previous studies, a reader must be able to assess the validity of those investigations, including the statistics that were used. Clear data presentation, rigorous statistical procedures and analyses, and methodological transparency are key factors that affect validity and overall impact of the investigation.

The objective of this chapter is to introduce basic statistical terminology, concepts, and tests commonly used for presenting, analyzing, and interpreting research. It is designed for the reader with a limited knowledge or recollection of statistics, intended to promote an understanding of basic statistical concepts. Rather than perform the work of a statistician, the goal is for readers to be able to (1) determine whether the statistical methods used in the research reports they encounter appear to be appropriate and (2) understand how to interpret them in real-world settings, including healthcare systems and public health organizations.

BUILDING BLOCKS

Statistical methods enable practitioners, researchers, and administrators to use observations made on a subset of a population to better understand the whole. This process is referred to as estimation. In statistics, the term population refers to the whole (ie, the collection of all possible measurements that could be used to answer a study question). The term sample refers to a subgroup of members drawn from a defined population involved in the study. Samples should accurately represent the larger population of interest with comparable proportions of key characteristics, such as age, gender, and race/ethnicity. With a representative sample, study findings are more likely to be both generalizable and replicable.

The measurements that describe a population are called parameters, and those that are computed from a sample are referred to as statistics. Sample statistics are used to predict/estimate the corresponding population parameters. The descriptive statistics and statistical tests that should be used are determined by the types of data under consideration.

TYPES OF DATA

There are two main types of quantitative (or numerically represented) variables: continuous and discrete. Continuous variables are numerical values that can assume any value in a

DOI: 10.37573/9781585287666.008

specified range. These variables can assume an indefinite number of values between two endpoints, including fractions or decimal points. For instance, a person's weight and height can both be measured to a decimal point and are a continuous variable. In contrast, discrete variables can be counted in whole units. Examples might include the number of physicians who work in a clinic or the number of children living in a household.

Variables that are represented by categories are known as categorical variables. Nominal categorical variables have at least two categories without any intrinsic ordering. Eye color (blue, green, brown) is a good example as there is no implied order. If instead the categories of the variable have a natural order, such as small, medium, or large, they are considered ordinal variables.

Health services research often examines associations between specific health exposures; long-term health outcomes; social factors, such as household income; and patient demographics, including age, gender, and race/ethnicity. Researchers can use validated surveys or electronic health records (EHRs) to measure whether individuals are experiencing a specific health exposure or risk factor. Categorical variables with only two response options (yes/no) are called binary variables. Researchers studying the effect of smoking may be interested in how many years a patient has actively smoked (a continuous variable), their weight in pounds (a continuous variable), and whether they have been diagnosed with lung disease (a yes/no, binary variable) or cardiovascular disease (also a yes/no, binary variable). They may also want to explore or control for household income as that may have an effect on a patient's ability to access necessary healthcare services.[1] Household income can be categorized in various ways. It could be measured to a specific dollar amount, such as an annual income of $50,500 per year, or categorized into ranges as an ordinal variable, such as less than $40,000; $40,000 to $80,000; and more than $80,000 per year.

DESCRIPTIVE STATISTICS

Descriptive statistics can help to provide an unbiased, complete, and summarized view of the data obtained. Measures of central tendency include the mean, median, and mode, and measures of variability include the standard deviation, standard error of the mean, and range.

Measures of Central Tendency

The mean is the arithmetic average of individual data points, the sum of all data points divided by the number of data points. It is used to describe continuous data; calculating a mean for ordinal data would be misleading and invalid, because the distance between numeric units is either unequal or unquantifiable. Even when used appropriately with continuous data, the mean can be extremely sensitive to outliers. To illustrate this point, consider the information in **Table 8-1.** Notice that each dataset is comprised of five data points. Changing just one data point in dataset B compared with dataset A resulted in a greater than 7-fold increase in the mean.

To consider a practical application, a healthcare administrator may need to consider the mean length of stay (LOS) for patients in an inpatient rehabilitation facility for a variety of reasons, including insurance coverage and staffing needs. Suppose that seven of the 10 patients stayed for 5 days, two patients stayed for 4 days, and one patient with particularly complex needs stayed for 21 days. In this case, the mean LOS for all patients would be 6.4 days (5 + 5 + 5 + 5 + 5 + 5 + 5 + 4 + 4 + 21 = 64 days

TABLE 8-1. Datasets A, B, and C

Dataset	Data Points	Sum of Data Points	Computation of Mean	Mean (X)	Median	Mode
A	1, 2, 3, 4, 5	15	15/5	3	3	—
B	1, 2, 3, 4, 100	110	110/5	22	3	—
C	1, 2, 2, 2, 3	10	10/5	2	2	2

divided by 10 patients = 6.4 days/patient). If the outlier (21 days) is removed from the dataset, the mean LOS drops to just 4.8 days (43 days/9 patients = 4.8 days per patient), which is more representative of the patients' general experience.

The median is another measure of central tendency that represents the midpoint, the value above (or below) in which half of the data points fall. It can be used to describe both continuous and ordinal data. In the LOS example above, the median is 5 days. It is the 50th percentile value of a distribution and therefore not sensitive to outliers. To further illustrate this point, look again at Table 8-1 and notice that in both datasets the median value is 3. The median in the second dataset was unaffected by the value of the outlier (ie, data point that equaled 100). As illustrated by these examples, the median is more useful than the mean when outliers are present or when continuous data are not normally distributed.

The mode is the most commonly observed value in the distribution. The mode can be used to describe nominal, ordinal, and continuous data. In the LOS example above, the mode is 5 days, because that was the experience of the majority of patients. Referring again to Table 8-1, the mode for dataset C is 2.

Measures of Variability

Measures of variability allow the investigator or reader to assess the variability or spread of the data. Measures of variability include the range, interquartile range, standard deviation, and standard error of the mean (SEM). The range is simply the difference between the largest and the smallest values in the distribution. Because the range is computed based on the lowest and highest values in a distribution, the presence of one outlier can have a tremendous impact.

The interquartile range is a measure of variability directly related to the median. Interquartile range is described by the interval between the 25th and 75th percentile values. It should be used to describe the variability for continuous data that may include outlier values. The interquartile range clearly defines where the middle 50% of measures occur and indicates the spread of the data.

In contrast, variance is a measure that describes how spread or scattered all of the data points are from the mean. It is calculated by taking the difference between each value in and the mean, squaring the differences and dividing it by the number of values within the dataset. The larger the variance, the more spread out the data points are from the mean. Smaller variances indicate that values are more tightly clustered around the mean, indicating more consistency.

The standard deviation (SD) is the most commonly used estimate of variability. It measures the spread of individual measurements about the sample mean. It is important to note that the SD is meaningful only when it is calculated for normally or near-normally distributed continuous data. It is appropriate for describing the subject-to-subject variation within a dataset. The SD is computed by taking the square root of the variance. In a normal distribution, 68% of the data points fall within ± 1 SD of the mean, 95% of the data points fall within ± 2 SD of the mean, and 99.7% of the data points fall within ± 3 SD of the mean. For example, investigators measured systolic blood pressure (SBP) on 100 first-year pharmacy students who were randomly selected. The mean SBP was computed to be 110 mmHg, and the SD was computed to be 10 mmHg. From this information, it is correct to assume that 95 of the first-year pharmacy students included in the sample had SBPs between 90 mmHg and 130 mmHg, whereas five had SBPs that were either less than 90 mmHg or greater than 130 mmHg.

Many decisions in healthcare administration are made based on data—whether determining staffing levels, revising organizational policies, or managing an annual budget. The SEM, or the "margin of uncertainty" from the sample's true mean, indicates the extent of the variability in the data and how reliable it is to make data-driven decisions. The SEM is a statistic computed from the SD, and mathematically, it is equal to the SD divided by the square root of n; where n is the number of subjects in the sample (SEM = SD / n). By looking at the equation for SEM, *it is apparent that SEM is always smaller than the SD, except for the case when n = 1.*

The SEM decreases as the sample size increases, and it increases as the SD increases.

The SEM is a measure of the precision with which a single sample mean estimates the true, but unmeasured, mean in the larger population of interest. The smaller the value of the SEM, the more confident the investigator or reader is about making inferences about what the true, but unmeasured, mean value would be in the larger population of interest. *SEM quantifies the uncertainty in the estimate of the mean obtained.* In our SBP example, the SEM for this sample is equal to the SD (10 mmHg) divided by 100 students. The SEM = 0.1 mmHg, which indicates a high degree of precision.

The concepts of SD and SEM are often confused; however, there is an important distinction between them. Whereas SD is used to describe the subject-to-subject variability within a dataset, SEM is used to describe the sample-to-sample variation among all possible values of the sample mean.

Furthermore, it is not uncommon for investigators to report their findings as a point estimate ± SEM rather than as ± SD. This is often done to make the data appear to have less variation. If readers fail to recognize this important difference, they may be misled. For example, reporting hospital length of stay (LOS) as mean ± SEM (eg, 5 days ± 0.2) can make the data appear more precise than mean ± SD (eg, 5 days ± 2) for the same dataset. The SEM measures the precision of the mean, while SD measures variability between patients. This distinction is crucial to avoid misleading interpretations.

Presentation of Data

A frequency distribution is a graph that demonstrates the number of times a particular measurement was obtained within the sample being studied. As such, frequency distributions vary in shape and size depending on what was measured. A normal, or Gaussian, distribution is shown in **Figure 8-1**.

Notice that the normal distribution is symmetric and bell-shaped about the mean (X), which in this case is also equal to the median and mode. As mentioned, in a normal distribution, 68% of the data points fall within ± 1 SD of the mean, 95% of the data points fall within ± 2 SD of the mean, and 99.7% of the data points fall within ± 3 SD of the mean.

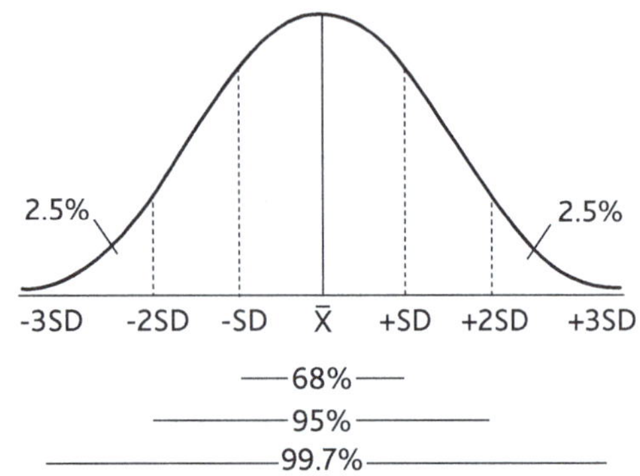

FIGURE 8-1. **Normal distribution.**

To illustrate, a healthcare administrator may be interested in wait times experienced by patients visiting a specific primary care clinic. If the mean wait time is 30 minutes and normally distributed, most patients experience wait times around the mean with fewer patients having very short or very long wait times. If the SD of wait times is 5 minutes, then a majority of patients (68%) can expect to wait 25 to 35 minutes (± 1 SD). A full 95% of patients will wait between 20 to 40 minutes (± 2 SD), and in extreme cases, those few patients may wait as little as 15 minutes or up to 45 minutes (± 3 SD). A healthcare administrator could use this information to improve patient satisfaction, identify inefficiencies in the check-in process, or allocate staff and other resources more effectively.

A bimodal distribution has two peaks that represent areas of data clustering. In a bimodal distribution, neither the mean nor the median provides an adequate representation of the data. For example, imagine if 100 patients in the above-mentioned primary care clinic were weighed at check-in: 50 females and 50 males. The mean and median could both equal 75 kg, but closer evaluation reveals a first peak representing the female body weights and a second peak representing the generally heavier male body weights, as illustrated in **Figure 8-2**. An understanding of data distributions is critical to the next steps of statistical analysis.

HYPOTHESIS TESTING

A well-planned investigation begins with a carefully constructed research question. Experienced researchers routinely involve a statistician throughout the study design process to

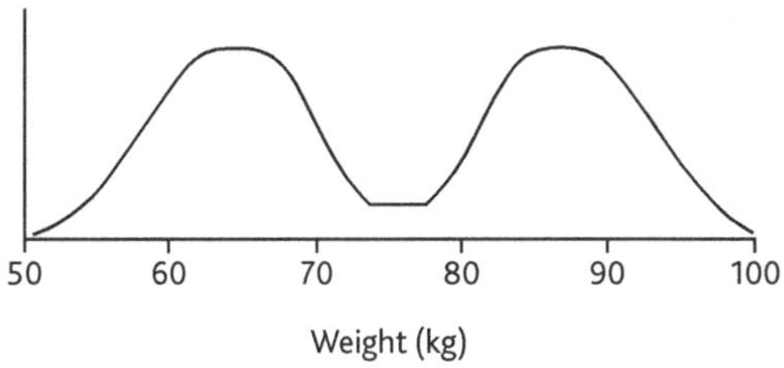

FIGURE 8-2. **Example of a bimodal distribution.**

ensure that after the data have been collected, the question is one that can be answered in a valid and meaningful way. Statistical inference involves hypothesis testing. Statistically, it is the null hypothesis (H_0) that is tested. The H_0 states that there is no difference between treatments with respect to the outcome of interest. The research or alternative hypothesis (H_1) states that there is a difference between treatments with respect to the outcome of interest. The ability to "reject" or "fail to reject" H_0 is dependent upon the statistical analysis of the differences observed between the groups. Hypothesis testing is often approached in a stepwise manner as described in the following steps:

1. Carefully define the research question and restate it in terms of the H_0 and H_1
2. Collect data on the sample subjects
3. Calculate the test statistic, dependent on the type of data collected
4. Evaluate the evidence against H_0
5. State the conclusion—reject H_0 or fail to reject H_0

Following these steps, relative to Figure 8-2, researchers may be interested in the following research question: Is there a statistically significant difference in weight (measured in kg) among male and female patients who receive care at this clinic? To answer the research question, the following hypotheses can be tested:

- H_0: There is no difference in weight between male and female patients.
- H_1: There is a statistically significant difference in weight between male and female patients.

There are two types of errors that may occur with hypothesis testing. A Type I error occurs when researchers falsely conclude that a significant difference exists between the experimental and control groups. It results when the null hypothesis is rejected when, in fact, there is no difference between the two groups. A Type II error occurs when researchers falsely conclude that there is no difference between the two groups when, in fact, there is. Two additional terms are important to this discussion. Alpha (α) is defined as the probability of making a Type I error, whereas beta (β) is defined as the probability of making a Type II error. Alpha is set before data are collected, usually at 0.05. It is the false-positive rate the investigators are willing to tolerate. In contrast, β is the false-negative rate the investigators are willing to tolerate. These concepts will be discussed in more depth in Chapter 9.

P-VALUES

A *p*-value is the probability of obtaining the observed difference between treatments in a study if the H_0 is true and there is no "real" difference between treatments in the larger population of interest. It is the probability of being wrong in asserting that a true difference exists. A *p*-value is calculated after data have been collected, and it is compared to the α level that was previously set to determine whether the findings are statistically significant.

A *p*-value less than or equal to α means that the observed treatment difference is statistically different from 0. If α is set at 0.05, then a *p*-value less than or equal to 0.05 is considered statistically significant, with the understanding that 5 in 100, or 1 in 20, assertions will be wrong. Comparing the *p*-value to the preset α level determines whether the results are deemed statistically significant or not, but the size of the *p*-value also matters. If α is set at 0.05 and the *p*-value is 0.04, then the results are statistically significant, and the probability of observing a difference between treatment groups when there is not one is 1 in 25. If the *p*-value is instead 0.0001, the results are also statistically significant, but now the probability of observing a difference between treatment groups when there is not one is 1 in 10,000. Therefore, the smaller the *p*-value, the more certain one can be that the observed difference in the study is not merely due to chance.

A small *p*-value means that there is strong evidence that some difference between treatments exists—not necessarily that a large difference exists. A small *p*-value means that the observed differences are unlikely to be mistakes in inference due to sampling. The smaller the *p*-value is, the stronger the evidence against H_0.

A *p*-value greater than 0.05 means that there is insufficient evidence to reject H_0 at the 5% level of significance. Although there is insufficient evidence to demonstrate that two treatments are different, that does not mean that the two treatments are the same. This is a key concept. It is also true that results may be statistically significant but not clinically important.

STATISTICAL POWER

Statistical power is the ability of a test statistic to detect a difference of a specified magnitude, if indeed a difference exists in the groups being compared. Power is the probability that a statistical test will reach a correct conclusion (ie, declare that H_1 is true, when it really is true). When designing a study, investigators need to know how many subjects will need to complete the study for it to be adequately powered. They first decide what false-negative rate they are willing to tolerate to determine the necessary sample size. Mathematically, power is equal to $1 - \beta$. Power is expressed as a percentage from 0 to 100, and most studies are powered at the 80% level with $\beta = 0.2$. Given that α is usually set at 0.05 and β is usually set at 0.2, it is apparent that Type II errors (falsely concluding that there is no difference between experimental and control groups) are going to be much more likely in the published literature than type I errors (falsely concluding that there is a difference between groups). One of the first steps a critical reader should take when reviewing a trial that did not achieve statistical significance (ie, a "negative trial") is to evaluate whether the study had sufficient statistical power.

To determine the number of subjects needed to achieve a desired power, investigators must specify the following: α, β, effect size, and the variability of the outcome of interest in the groups studied. Effect size is the difference that would be considered clinically important by practitioners. As the sample size increases, power increases and β decreases. β also decreases as the variability in the outcome of interest in the subjects' studied decreases. As β decreases, α increases. If there is a big difference between the groups being compared, power increases and β decreases, because it is much easier to detect big differences than small differences. While it is generally true that the greater the power of a study the better, it is also important to realize that given a large enough sample size, anything can be statistically significant. Furthermore, simply because the results of an investigation are deemed statistically significant does not mean that they are clinically important. Conversely, just because statistical significance was not detected in an investigation does not mean that the results are not clinically important.

There are several factors that can explain why a statistical test fails to detect a significant difference of a specified effect size between groups studied. These include low power of the statistical test, small sample size, high false-negative rate for the statistical test, and, of course, the possibility that such a difference does not exist.

Sample size determination also depends on whether the test is going to be one-sided or two-sided. A one-sided test assumes that a difference occurs in only one direction; a two-sided test looks for a difference in both the positive and negative directions. A one-sided test is more powerful than a two-sided test, because regardless of the α chosen, a statistical test result need not vary as much from the mean value to achieve significance. For example, if α is set at 0.05 and the test is one-sided, the result must fall in either the top or bottom 5% of the distribution to be declared statistically significant. In contrast, if α is set at 0.05 and the test is two-sided, the result must fall in either the top or bottom 2.5% to be declared statistically significant.

VARIABLES AND MEASUREMENT SCALES

When examining relationships between variables, the dependent variable measures the main outcome of interest and independent variables define the conditions under which the dependent variable is examined. Independent variables are the ones controlled or adjusted for. There may be several independent variables or none, depending on the study design. For example, suppose a study was planned to determine the effect of telehealth (compared with in-person visits) on patient satisfaction among those living in rural communities. In this case, telehealth is the independent variable and patient satisfaction is the dependent variable. Researchers may also want to consider additional independent variables, such as provider type, patient characteristics (age, race/ethnicity, gender), and diagnoses.[2,3] Dependent and independent variables will be discussed at greater length in Chapter 9.

DIFFERENTIATING UNIVARIATE, BIVARIATE, AND MULTIVARIABLE ANALYSES

Depending on the number of variables being examined, researchers may conduct univariate, bivariate, or multivariable analyses. **Univariate analysis** focuses on a single variable and is typically used to describe its distribution, such as the mean number of medication errors in a surgical unit or the proportion of patients experiencing an adverse event.

Bivariate analysis examines the relationship between two variables, which typically involves one independent (predictor) variable and one dependent (outcome) variable. For example, leaders and administrators within a health system may be interested in estimating the association between implementation of a new nursing process and the number of medication errors in a surgical unit. In this case, the nursing process is the independent variable and medication errors are the dependent variable.

When researchers wish to account for additional factors that may influence an outcome, they may use **multivariable analysis**, which includes multiple independent (predictor) variables and a single dependent (outcome) variable. Building on the previous example, researchers may estimate medication errors in the surgical unit while accounting for the new nursing process as well as nurses' years of experience, unit staffing levels, severity of patients' surgeries, and the number of medications administered per patient. Multivariable analyses are commonly used to adjust for potential confounding variables. It is important not to confuse **multivariable** analysis with **multivariate** analysis. Multivariate analysis refers to statistical models that include multiple dependent variables simultaneously, which is beyond the scope of this chapter. See Chapter 9 for more details.

CORRELATION

Correlation measures the strength and direction of the relationship between two variables. Neither variable can be considered the dependent variable in the sense that neither can be considered to cause the other. The correlation coefficient (*r*) defines both the strength and the direction of the linear relationship between two variables and varies from –1 to +1. The sign of *r* indicates the direction of the relationship. A positive sign indicates that as one variable increases, the other variable also increases, and a negative sign indicates that as one variable increases, the other variable decreases. When *r* equals –1, the two variables have a perfectly negative linear relationship (**Figure 8-3**). In this case, all points on a

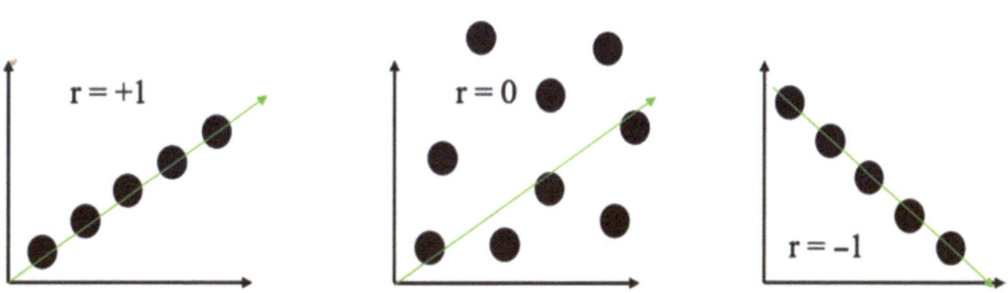

FIGURE 8-3. **Correlation analysis.**

scatter plot would fall exactly on a straight line that slopes downward from left to right. When *r* equals +1, the two study variables have a perfectly positive linear relationship, and all points would fall on a straight line that slopes upward from left to right. When *r* equals 0, there is no linear relationship between study variables. This may mean that the relationship is either nonlinear, or it may be that the two study variables are not related.

Correlation analysis is used in situations where the two variables being measured change together, but neither variable can be the dependent variable. The correlation coefficient is a dimensionless value, because the units in the numerator and denominator cancel. Remember that correlation does not imply causality. The existence of a statistically significant correlation between study variables does not prove that a cause-and-effect relationship exists between variables. Conversely, a statistically significant correlation between two variables does not imply that the association is clinically important.

COMMON TEST STATISTICS

The type of statistical analysis and specific test statistic used depends on several factors, including the type of data collected, the distribution of the data, investigator or statistician preference, the number of groups being compared, and the study design. The type of statistical analysis used varies by the number of groups or samples involved; therefore, **Figures 8-4** and **8-5** are designed to be helpful tools when determining the appropriate statistical test. Refer to Additional Readings for resources on less common test statistics.

Statistical tests are commonly grouped into two broad categories: parametric and nonparametric. Parametric tests are generally more powerful than nonparametric tests, but they require several conditions to be met. The data must approximately follow a normal distribution, and the variability of the data must be approximately equal between groups. The measures of patient response must be independent and unrelated, and the data must be continuous. On the other hand, nonparametric tests can be used for ordinal and nominal data, as well as continuous data if they do not meet the criteria for using a parametric test.

It is important to note that study samples may be either independent or paired. Independent study samples are not related in that the choice of subjects for one sample does not depend on which subjects are in the other sample.

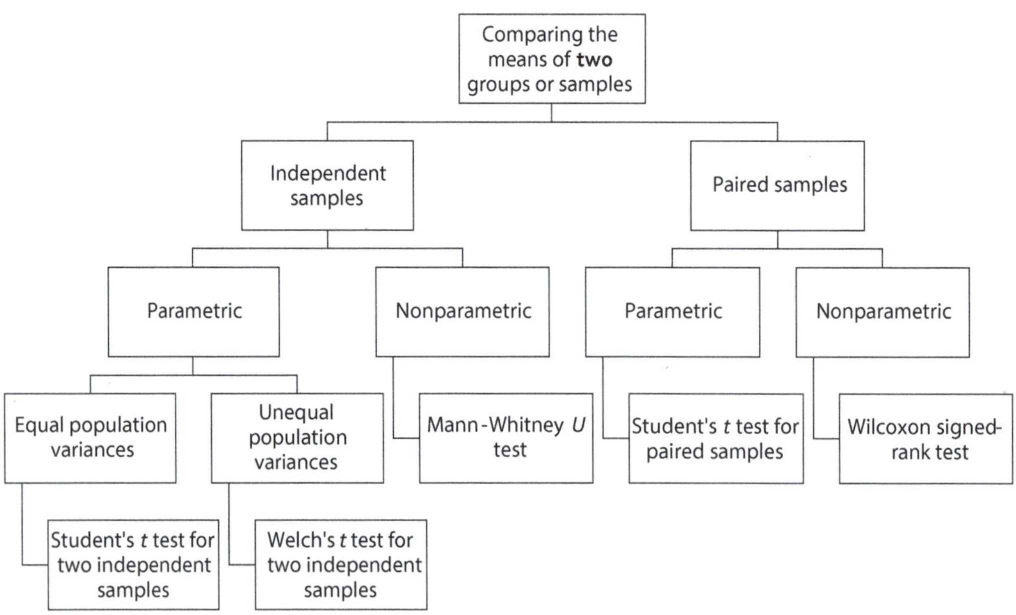

FIGURE 8-4. **Choosing a statistical test to compare the means of two groups.**[4-6]

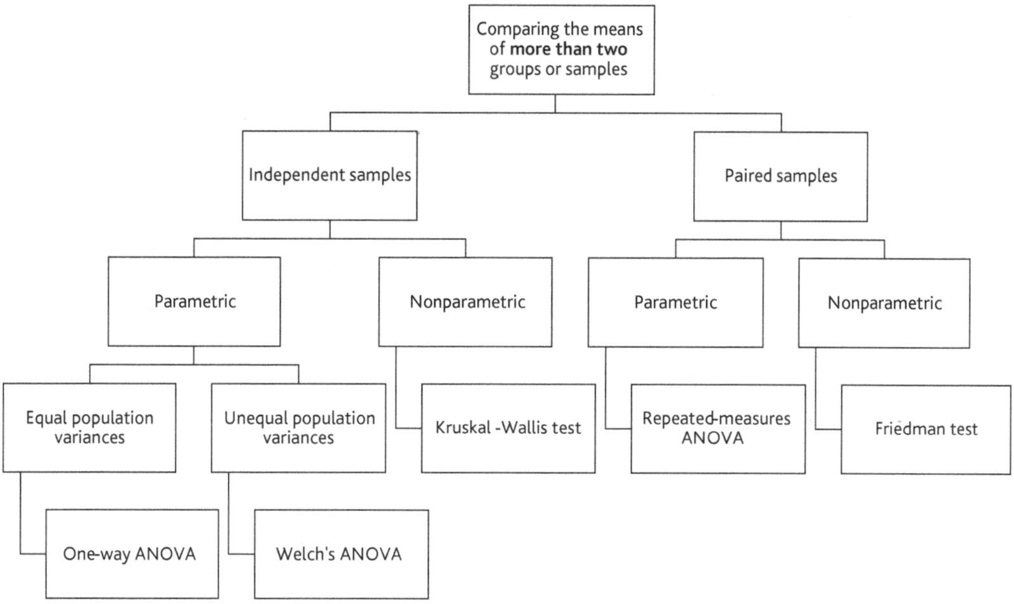

FIGURE 8-5. **Choosing a statistical test to compare the means of more than two groups.**[4-6]

In contrast, paired or matched samples are related. There are a couple different ways in which study subjects can be matched: subjects may serve as their own control, such as in a cross-over trial, or subjects may be matched or paired based on specific factors that may affect the outcome of interest (ie, age, sex, disease severity). In the latter case, one member of the matched pair is assigned to one treatment group, and the other member of the matched pair is assigned to the other treatment group. The distinction between independent and matched or paired samples determines which test statistic is used.

The most commonly used parametric test is the *t* test. The *t* test is used to compare the means from two independent samples (ie, two groups that have different people in each) to determine whether H_0 will be accepted or rejected. When using a *t* test, the H_0 states that the means of the two populations are equal. The paired *t* test is used when comparing the means from a matched or paired sample (eg, cross-over design).

If comparisons need to be made between three or more groups and the conditions for using a parametric test are met, then an analysis of variance (ANOVA) is the preferred test. If the threshold for significant differences between the groups is demonstrated with ANOVA (using an *F* test), the next step is to discern which of the groups are statistically different from each other. Post hoc tests—also known as multiple comparison procedures—are used to compare the means of the groups two at a time to detect where the difference lies. A post hoc test has less error associated with it than performing separate *t* tests. Examples of post hoc tests include Bonferroni, Tukey, and Newman-Keuls.

A chi-square test is a nonparametric test suited for nominal data as it is able to check for a statistically significant association between two variables when the data are in the form of counts. This test can answer research questions about rates, proportions, or frequencies on independent samples. It may also be used to answer questions about differences between proportions. Chi-square should only be used if the sample size is greater than 40. If the sample size is between 20 and 40, the expected frequency for each cell in the matrix must be greater than 5. If either of these conditions fails to hold, the Fisher exact test should be used instead of a chi-square.

McNemar's test is a variant of the chi-square test used when samples are paired. The Mantel-Haenszel chi-square test is another variant of the chi-square test suited for multivariate analysis; it is used to compare nominal data from independent samples while controlling for the effect of a confounder.

The nonparametric equivalents to the *t* test for comparing two groups with independent samples when the data are ordinal include the Mann-Whitney *U* test, also known as the Wilcoxon rank-sum test. These tests are also appropriate when the data are continuous but not normally distributed. It is not appropriate to use the Mann-Whitney *U* test (or Wilcoxon rank-sum test) if the samples are paired or matched. Instead, if the samples are paired, the Wilcoxon signed-rank test is the most appropriate. Similar to the previous tests, the Wilcoxon signed-rank test compares two paired means (such as pre/post measurements on the same individual) and assumes the outcome is ordinal or continuous, but not normally distributed. Lastly, under the same assumptions related to the outcome data as previous tests, the Kruskal-Wallis test is used when comparing three or more treatment groups with independent samples. The Kruskal-Wallis test may be considered a nonparametric alternative to a one-way ANOVA. These tests are used less frequently than some of the previously discussed tests; however, **Figure 8-4** provides support for deciding which test is most appropriate for the available data.

Survival analysis is used when investigators are interested in evaluating the time-to-event of interest for study subjects. This statistical procedure adjusts for the fact that subjects may be followed for different lengths of time. For example, in a clinical trial studying the effect of simvastatin on mortality post myocardial infarction (MI), investigators may follow each patient to one of three endpoints: either the patient suffers another MI (event of interest), is lost to follow-up, or is alive at the conclusion of the study. Censored data refer to those who were either lost to follow-up and those who are alive at the conclusion of the study. For each patient, the time between when they enrolled in the study and when they experience the endpoint is referred to as the patient's survival time. The survival function, when evaluated at time (t) gives the probability that the patient will survive until at least (t) and is depicted using a survival curve, as shown for cancer survival in the paper by Hazra and Gogtay.[7] However, survival analysis often used to evaluate other time-to-event analyses. In **Figure 8-6**, we show how this type of analysis can be used to graphically show time to a 10% weight loss for a cohort of patients who are taking weight-loss medication compared with patients on a prescribed diet for 12 months. In this case, the "good" outcome is the treatment group that decreases most rapidly and has the least censoring owing to dropouts. In both cases of survival and in time-to-event studies, the statistical difference between the curves is tested by using the log-rank test.

CONFIDENCE INTERVALS

Confidence intervals (CIs) provide an objective way to specify how precise a sample estimate is, accounting for both sample size and variability. Because the value of any computed sample statistic varies from sample to sample, there is uncertainty in the estimation process. A CI defines boundaries within which the true population parameter is likely to fall. The most used is the 95% CI, computed as 95% CI = X ± 1.96 (SEM).

Because all the possible values of the sample mean tend to follow a normal distribution (as illustrated in Table 8-1), the true, but unmeasured, mean in the larger population of interest will lie within two SDs about 95% of the time. This means that if someone repeated an experiment 100 times and generated a CI for each time, then 95 of the CIs will contain the true, but unmeasured, mean in the larger population of interest and five of the CIs will not. Confidence intervals are the range of possible values for the true treatment difference that are statistically likely, given the results of a specific trial. Confidence intervals are most commonly used for continuous data that are normally distributed, but they may also be calculated for medians, regression slopes, relative risks, and hazard ratios. These are elaborated on in the Additional Readings at the end of this chapter.

Referring to the example of measuring SBPs in 100 first-year pharmacy students, the calculated SEM equals 0.1 mmHg. It would be correct to state that the researchers may be 95% confident that the true, but unmeasured, mean SBP in all first-year pharmacy students will be contained in the range of 108 mmHg to 112 mmHg. It would be incorrect to state that 95 of the 100 first-year pharmacy students in the sample had SBPs in the range of

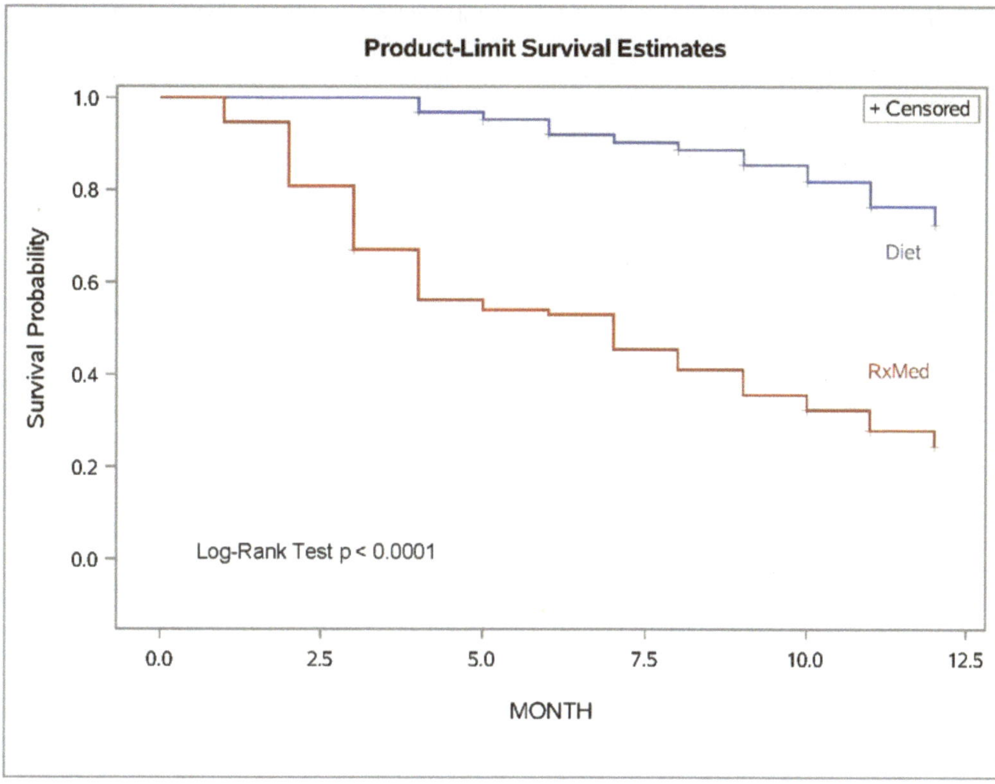

FIGURE 8-6. **Kaplan-Meier survival plots compared by the log-rank test: example of time to 10% loss of body weight on weight-loss medication compared with diet over a 12-month period.**

108 mmHg to 112 mmHg. As mentioned previously, SD is used to describe the subject-to-subject variability with a dataset, and SEM is used to describe the sample-to-sample variation among all possible values of the sample mean. This is an important distinction.

Confidence intervals convey more information to readers than *p*-values. Confidence intervals provide information regarding both the size and direction of the effect observed. When interpreting CIs, any value from the lower confidence bound up to and including the upper confidence bound could be the true value in the larger population of interest. Confidence intervals also allow readers to determine whether a finding is statistically significant by seeing whether the interval includes the null hypothesis value (eg, zero for a difference, one for a ratio). If the CI includes this null value, then statistical significance has not been achieved. Conversely, if the CI does not include the null value, then the results are statistically significant.

The width of a CI can be affected by several factors. Reduced variability in data from which the sample is drawn results in a narrower CI. Given a fixed SD, increasing the sample size or decreasing the confidence level (eg, going from 95% CI to 90% CI) will both result in a narrower CI. Although the CI is useful and provides the reader with more information compared with a *p*-value, it cannot control for errors in study design or improper selection of study subjects.

CONCLUSION

This chapter has provided information on foundational concepts/building blocks for understanding statistical findings. However, in the real world, several factors or variables often affect an outcome. In Chapter 9, we will expand on these topics to understand multivariate modeling and the translation of its findings to real-world settings.

REFERENCES

1. Casetta B, Videla AJ, Bardach A, et al. Association between cigarette smoking prevalence and income level: a systematic review and meta-analysis. *Nicotine Tob Res*. Published online September 27, 2016. https://doi.org/10.1093/ntr/ntw266
2. Papo Y, Harvey J, Williams D, et al. Building a telemedicine program to create a sustainable care delivery model for a rural hospital at risk for closure. *Telemed E-Health*. Published online February 20, 2025. https://doi.org/10.1089/tmj.2024.0488
3. Simpson AN, Harvey JB, DiLembo SM, et al. Population health indicators associated with a statewide telestroke program. *Telemed E-Health*. 2020;26(9):1126-1133. https://doi.org/10.1089/tmj.2019.0204
4. UCLA Statistical Consulting Group. What statistical analysis should I use? UCLA Institute for Digital Research and Education. https://stats.oarc.ucla.edu/other/mult-pkg/whatstat/. Accessed March 4, 2026.
5. Yuen B. Which statistical test? A flowchart for choosing statistical tests. University of Southampton. https://www.med.soton.ac.uk/resmethods/statisticalnotes/which_test_flow.htm. Accessed March 4, 2026.
6. Psoter KJ, Roudsari BS, Dighe MK, et al. Biostatistics primer for the radiologist. *Am J Roentgenol*. 2014;202(4):W365-W375. https://doi.org/10.2214/AJR.13.11657
7. Hazra A, Gogtay N. Biostatistics series module 9: survival analysis. *Indian J Dermatol*. 2017;62:251-257. https://doi.org/10.4103/ijd.IJD_201_17

ADDITIONAL READINGS

The following list of additional readings were selected from widely referenced entry-level statistics resources, relevant to healthcare research and evaluation. These readings are intended to reinforce key concepts, or "building blocks," that support a foundational understanding of statistics. In addition, these readings provide examples of statistical applications in healthcare management and administration. With a deeper understanding of statistical concepts, readers will be better equipped to interpret and apply statistical findings in real-world settings.

Bensken WP, Pieracci FM, Ho VP. Basic introduction to statistics in medicine, part 1: describing data. *Surg Infect (Larchmt)*. 2021. https://doi.org/10.1089/sur.2020.429

Canova S, Cartinovis DL, Ambrogi F. How to describe univariate data. *J Thorac Dis Stat Corner*. 2017. http://dx.doi.org/10.21037/jtd.2017.05.80

Cleff T. Univariate data analysis. In: *Exploratory Data Analysis in Business and Economics*. Cham, Switzerland: Springer International Publishing; 2014.

Denis DJ. *Applied Univariate, Bivariate, and Multivariate Statistics*. 2nd ed. Hoboken, NJ: Wiley; 2021.

Friedman LM, Furberg CD, DeMets D. *Fundamentals of Clinical Trials*. 4th ed. Cham, Switzerland: Springer International Publishing; 2010.

George A, Stead TS, Ganti L. What's the risk: differentiating risk ratios, odds ratios, and hazard ratios? *Cureus*. 2020;12(8):e10047. https://doi.org/10.7759/cureus.10047

Glanz SA. *Primer of Biostatistics*. 7th ed. New York: McGraw Hill; 2012.

Heumann C, Schomaker M, Shalabh MS. *Introduction to Statistics and Data Analysis: With Exercises, Solutions, and Applications in R*. 2nd ed. Cham, Switzerland: Springer; International Publishing; 2016.

Rosenthal DA, Kros JF. *Statistics for Health Care Management and Administration, Working with Excel*. 4th ed. Hoboken, NJ: Wiley; 2023.

Rovai AP. *Statistical Fundamentals: Using Microsoft Excel for Univariate and Bivariate Analysis*. Chesapeake, VA: Watertree Press, LLC; 2014.

Tessler M. Univariate analysis: variance, variables, data, and measurement. In: *Social Science Research in the Arab World and Beyond*. SpringerBriefs in Sociology. Cham, Switzerland: Springer International Publishing; 2023.

Van Belle G, Fisher LD, Heagerty PJ, Lumley T. *Biostatistics: A Methodology for the Health Sciences*. 2nd ed. Hoboken, NJ: Wiley; 2004.

Multivariable Analyses

9

Ralph Ward, PhD, and Annie N. Simpson, PhD

INTRODUCTION

In previous chapters, the fundamental concepts that underlie most healthcare outcomes studies were examined, including univariate statistical analyses. This chapter moves beyond these fundamentals to describe multivariable analyses—methods used to estimate the simultaneous effects of multiple explanatory variables (also termed covariates). While univariate analyses involve a single independent variable, the focus now shifts to estimating the effects of multiple independent variables on an outcome (or dependent) variable. For example, investigators studying factors related to lung cancer outcomes would likely want to account for more than the main exposure (smoking history) and might also include the simultaneous effects of age, sex and other demographic variables, comorbid conditions, other toxic exposures, and any family history of lung cancer. Note that specialized models with multiple outcomes are termed multivariate models, a term that should not be confused with the topic at hand: multivariable models.

While attempting to unravel these concurrent effects, investigators must contend with several new challenges not usually encountered in univariate methods. Potential explanatory variables are often strongly correlated, as seen with cigarette pack-year history and number of years smoked. When used in multivariable models, highly correlated variables could produce unstable or unreliable estimates. Additionally, some variables may interact with each other, as with simultaneous exposure to asbestos and tobacco smoke, which could lead to a substantially greater combined cancer risk than from exposure to either substance alone. Failure to account for such interactions could produce misleading conclusions. Other common challenges, discussed further below, include confounding, mediating, and moderating variables. In addressing such issues, the primary concern is to obtain estimates that have the smallest possible bias (systematic error) given the limitations of the dataset. Above all, it is important to remember that multivariable models built from observational data are rough maps rather than precise representations of reality.[1] These models can only account for the observed data and may be severely constrained by unknown or unmeasured factors. While they can help demonstrate that the strength of association exists between an explanatory variable and an outcome, much caution is warranted when attempting to claim causation—despite ongoing research in this area.

APPLICATIONS OF MULTIVARIABLE ANALYSES

Investigators usually apply multivariable methods to one of three distinct goals:

Descriptive Analyses

In this application, the research is designed to show which explanatory variables have the strongest associations with the outcome.

DOI: 10.37573/9781585287666.009

Predictive Analyses

The goal in this setting is to make predictions about a future outcome for a new patient or population based on findings from a population for whom the explanatory and outcome variables are already known. Predictive analyses may involve methods for splitting the data so that the model is developed by using a training dataset, after which its predictive performance is evaluated by using a separate validation dataset. The training model may also be validated using a new (external) population that was not included in the original dataset.

Causation Analyses

The goal is to make claims concerning whether an exposure or risk factor was responsible for causing the observed outcome. If the study was a randomized trial such that both known and unknown confounding factors were randomly distributed between the intervention and control arms, then claims for causation are usually credible. However, randomized trials are often very expensive to run and it may be unethical to randomize subjects to some exposures. Further, there is considerable interest in using retrospective real-world healthcare data drawn from electronic medical records or billing claims to approximate a randomized trial. This is an area of considerable research, but as emphasized above, it may be difficult to make claims for causation from observational data, and a great deal of care is needed to attempt to minimize possible sources of bias.

COMMON TERMINOLOGY

The following concepts are frequently encountered when exploring multivariable analysis techniques:

Regression

This statistical technique is designed to investigate (or model) the relationship between the dependent variable (also called the outcome, or Y) and one or more explanatory variables (X). A shorthand description for this model is "regress Y on X." Models with multiple explanatory variables are termed multivariable analyses. As noted, specialized models with more than one outcome are termed multivariate analyses.

Collinearity

If two independent covariates are strongly correlated, they are likely to have nearly identical associations with an outcome. Regression models may have difficulty distinguishing between the two when attempting to determine their separate effects, resulting in unstable or unreliable estimates with a large degree of uncertainty. For example, body mass index (BMI) and closely related variables, such as body fat percentage or waist circumference, are all strongly correlated and likely to have similar associations with many healthcare outcomes. Several options exist for addressing the problem, but most often it can be resolved by checking for correlation between explanatory variables and eliminating all but one from a closely related group. A closely related term is multicollinearity, in which there are more than two highly correlated variables.

Confounder

When risk factor A is associated with risk factor B and both are associated with the outcome (Y) but A and B are not on the same causal pathway for Y, then risk factor A's effect on Y may be distorted or confounded by B (**Figure 9-1a**). For example, exercise (A) is associated with weight loss (Y), and a healthy diet (B) is also associated with weight loss. Exercise and diet may also be associated with each other if subjects who exercise frequently are more likely to have healthy diets and vice versa. Diet is not on the casual path between exercise and weight loss, but improvements in both often occur simultaneously. A model's estimate of the impact of exercise on weight loss may be distorted (or confounded) from the true value if diet is not taken into account. One way to do this involves a stratified analysis, in which separate analyses are conducted for subjects with healthy and unhealthy diets. If the effects of exercise are substantially different between these groups, then diet can be identified as a confounding factor. When there are multiple confounders, multivariable analyses are the most effective way to simultaneously account for these and for other covariates of interest in order to produce an unbiased estimate of the exposure's true effect on the outcome.

Mediator

If two covariates (A and B) are on the same causal pathway with the outcome (Y), then the A's effect on Y may be mediated by B (**Figure 9-1c**). For example, exercise (A) may reduce the risk of subsequent falls (Y) through improved muscle strength (B) or improved balance (B); either of these might act as mediators between exercise and fall risk. If mediation is suspected, special statistical methods can be used to establish whether such relationships exist. If a mediator is confirmed to exist, the statistical results supporting this conclusion should be reported, along with an interpretation of the mediator's likely relationship with the independent variable and the outcome.

Moderator

If one covariate's effect (A) on the outcome is modified by a second covariate (B), then B may be a moderator (**Figure 9-1b**). For example, if drug (A) is more effective against disease (Y) among younger patients then its effects may be moderated by age. Note that A and B are not necessarily associated with each other, unlike the confounder relationship. A moderator can thus change the strength or direction of association but does not produce a distorted or false association. In regression analysis, an interaction term between the two independent variables (A*B) could be used to test for moderation. If a moderator is confirmed to exist, this term should be included in the analyses, and an interpretation of its effects should be provided. For example, the effects of A on Y could be provided for different levels of B.

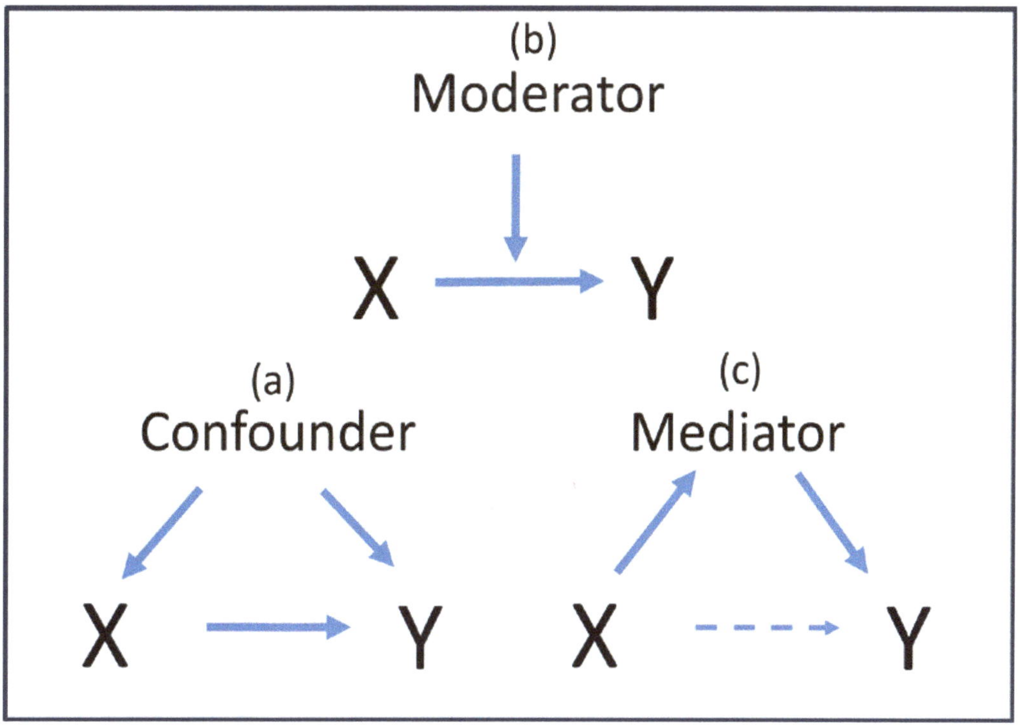

FIGURE 9-1. **Relationships between exposure (X) and outcome (Y) in the presence of confounding, moderation, and mediation. In (a), confounding exists when a separate factor associated with both X and Y can distort the apparent relationship between the two. Example: alcohol consumption (X) might be found to have a significant relationship with lung cancer (Y). However, this association is confounded by heavy smoking, which is associated with both alcohol consumption and lung cancer. The association between alcohol and lung cancer would disappear in a nonsmoking population. In (b), a moderator affects the strength of association between X and Y. Example: Age could moderate an exposure's effect, such that older subjects have a greater (or lower) response. In (c), a mediator falls on the causal pathway between X and Y. The dashed line between X and Y shows that a direct association is also possible. Example: Increased exercise (X) could reduce the risk of subsequent falls (Y) through several mediators (improved balance or muscle strength).**

DATA PREPARATION STEPS

This chapter's focus is on the application of multivariable analytic methods, but it is important not to overlook the crucial importance for the data preparation steps. In a large study drawn from complex healthcare databases with millions of patients, the actual analyses may be completed within a short time, but the data preparation steps will likely require several months of meticulous effort. An effective statistical analysis plan should include detailed steps for data preparation, and the study's success in attaining unbiased results depends as much on these preparatory steps as it does on the actual analyses. The data analyst and investigator should work closely to decide on approaches for handling missing, duplicated, or outlier values and should validate their work carefully to ensure that new errors are not inadvertently introduced. The following sections briefly describe some key data preparation steps.

Population, Exposure, and Outcomes Definitions

Precise definitions for the study's population, outcomes, exposures, and other covariates are needed to enable the analyst to extract the intended information without resorting to assumptions. When reading research papers, one indicator of methodical work is the care with which these elements are fully described. Experienced teams recognize that misunderstandings at this step could lead to a dataset with undetected deviations from the intended population. Examples to look for include the use of exact dates where appropriate, detailed listings of clinical codes or laboratory values used to define exposures or other variables (or an appropriate citation), and methods for determining death and cause of death.

Data Cleaning and Transformation

Observational datasets are likely to contain numerous errors, including duplicated, missing, or implausible values. Steps for addressing such areas should be established in advance. For example, a clinical team might establish thresholds for implausible values and decide whether they should be excluded or handled in some other manner. While there may be good reasons to exclude an outlier, caution is needed, because a seemingly implausible value may actually be valid and could be essential to correctly answering the study's questions.

Approaches for Missing Data

Large observational datasets usually have some degree of missing data, and methods for addressing this problem should be part of the statistical analysis plan. Because incorrect approaches to missing data could produce biased results, research papers should include full descriptions of the methods used to address the problem. Statistical software packages usually have default responses to missing values, and analysts must ensure that these are consistent with their planned approach. The common software default is complete case analysis, where any row with a missing value is simply ignored. However, this is only appropriate when values are missing completely at random, meaning the probability of missingness is purely owing to chance and is unrelated to any observed or unobserved factors. If values are missing at random (MAR), the probability of missingness is owing to other observed variables but not on the missing variable itself. For example, if older patients are less likely to respond to a follow-up survey, the probability of missing survey values is related to age but not to the survey itself. In this case, missing data methods that depend on the MAR assumption can be applied to produce unbiased inference; one common MAR method is multiple imputation. The most difficult missing data category is missing not at random (MNAR), in which the probability of missingness depends on the missing values themselves. For example, if severely depressed patients are less likely to report their symptoms in a mental health survey related to depression, then missingness is nonrandom. It may be very difficult or impossible to establish that MNAR conditions exist from the dataset alone, and the available methods to effectively address the issue are limited; one common approach involves sensitivity analyses.

Dataset Structure and Variable Types

The study's aims and design will also influence the choice of variable types and dataset structure. For example, as previously discussed in Chapter 3, a cross-sectional study involves a single snapshot in time for the population in which each subject usually has a single row of data. In contrast, a longitudinal study collects multiple observations for each subject over time so that each will have multiple rows of data. In either design, there could be clustered values that require appropriate statistical methods for analysis. For example, patient-level data could be clustered according to hospital or surgeon, while lung cancer nodule data would likely be clustered by patient.

Another important factor in data preparation is establishing variable types for the outcome, exposure, and explanatory variables. As discussed in Chapter 8, continuous (numeric) variables could include blood pressure or temperature. Nominal categorical variables could include blood type or gender, while ordinal categorical variables include pain level or cancer stage. Discrete (counts) variables might include numbers of visits or medications, and time-to-event measures could include time until recurrence, readmission, or death. The outcome variable's type will directly influence what types of analyses are possible; for example, logistic regression is often used for binary (yes/no) outcomes, Poisson regression for discrete outcomes, and survival methods such as Cox proportional hazards regression for time-to-event outcomes. Investigators may decide to group continuous values, such as age or BMI into categorical variables particularly if the research question involves specific widely accepted thresholds or groups. However, categorization can introduce unintended problems if not used thoughtfully. These can include a loss of statistical power owing to a loss of information. For example, a person aged 17 years and 11 months could be categorized as "pediatric," whereas someone just a month older would be considered an "adult" under a categorical age threshold of < 18 versus ≥ 18.

LINEAR MODELS

Deterministic and Statistical Models

Compare panels A and B in **Figure 9-2**, which represent a dataset of independent (X) and dependent variables (Y), respectively. The values in panel A on the left all exactly fall on the straight line plotted through them, whereas

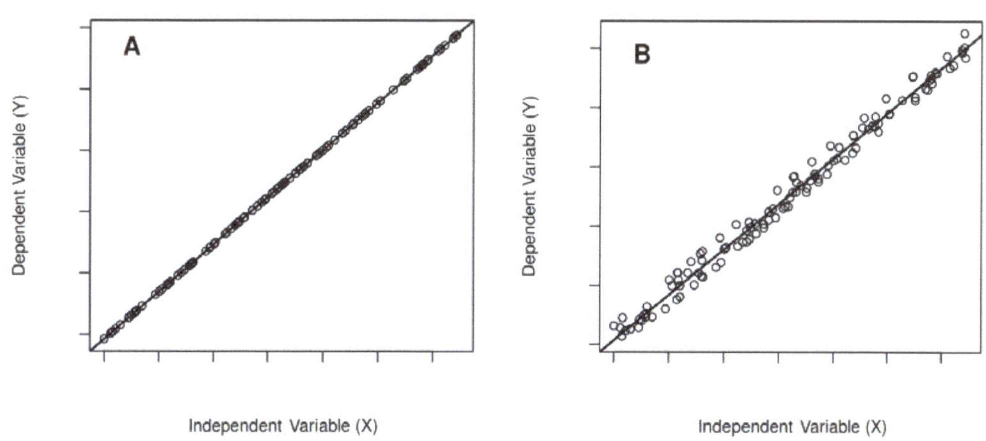

FIGURE 9-2. **Panel A represents a deterministic function, while panel B includes random error in the relationship between the independent (X) and dependent (Y) variables.**

those in panel B are scattered around the central line and often fall some distance from it. Panel A is an example of a deterministic function that could be represented by:

$$Y = \beta_0 + \beta_1 X$$

This is the equation for a straight line, where the y-axis intercept is defined by β_0 and the slope of the line by β_1. This is a deterministic relationship, because only one value of Y is possible for each value of X. Panel B could be represented by:

$$Y = \beta_0 + \beta_1 X + \varepsilon$$

The new term (ε) represents the random error that is usually observed in datasets captured from real-world processes and accounts for the random distribution in values of Y that may occur for a single value of X. For example, if X represents body weight, subjects with the same weight may have different values of blood pressure (Y), although blood pressure would generally be expected to increase with weight. The straight line through the scattered data in panel B represents the results of a statistical model, in which estimates were derived for parameters β_0 and β_1 based on a sample of real-world data. This is considered to be a linear model, because the unknown parameters (β_0 and β_1) are constants or have linear relationships with the outcome Y.

Ordinary Least Squares Regression

Ordinary least squares (OLS) regression is one method for estimating a solution for the fitted line shown in **Figure 9-3**, where a vertical

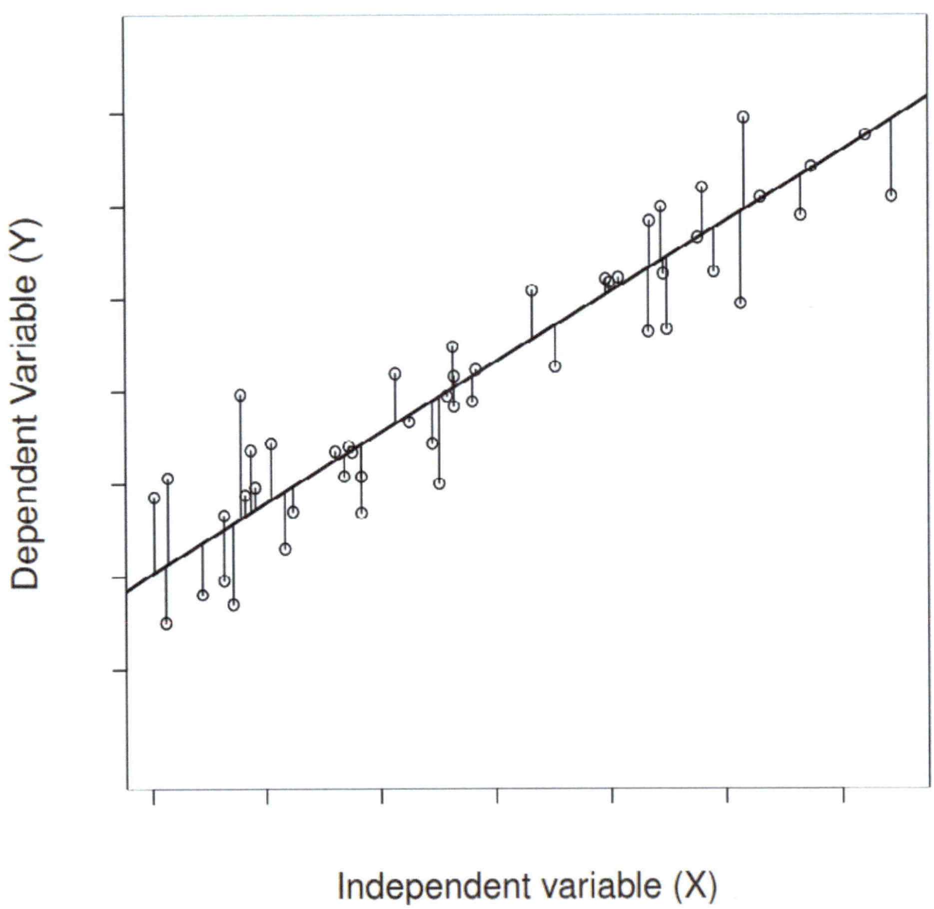

FIGURE 9-3. **Illustration of residuals, the vertical distance between the fitted and observed values of Y.**

line has been added between each observed (actual) value of Y and the corresponding estimated value of Y (on the fitted line). Graphically, this collection of vertical distances is called the residuals. Each residual is a measure of the model's error for that single data point. As in the previous section, the objective in OLS is to estimate the model's parameters, where the y-axis intercept is defined by β_0 and the slope of the line by β_1. In an OLS solution, the values for β_0 and β_1 will minimize the sum of the squared residuals:

$$\sum_{i=1}^{N} \varepsilon_i^2$$

where N is the number of observations in the sample. Conceptually, OLS is equivalent to the following steps:

1. Calculate the distance (residual) between each observation and a candidate solution for the fitted line.
2. Square each residual such that the positive and negative residuals do not cancel and find the sum of squares.
3. Pick the candidate line through the observed data that best minimizes the sum of the squared residuals.

Note that the OLS solution depends on the model's assumed structure and will produce parameter estimates that satisfy its objective function. In this example, a straight line (linear model) was a good fit for the data, but if the relationship between X and Y were not linear, the underlying model would be wrong, and an OLS solution will not likely produce reasonable estimates. In **Figure 9-4**, the

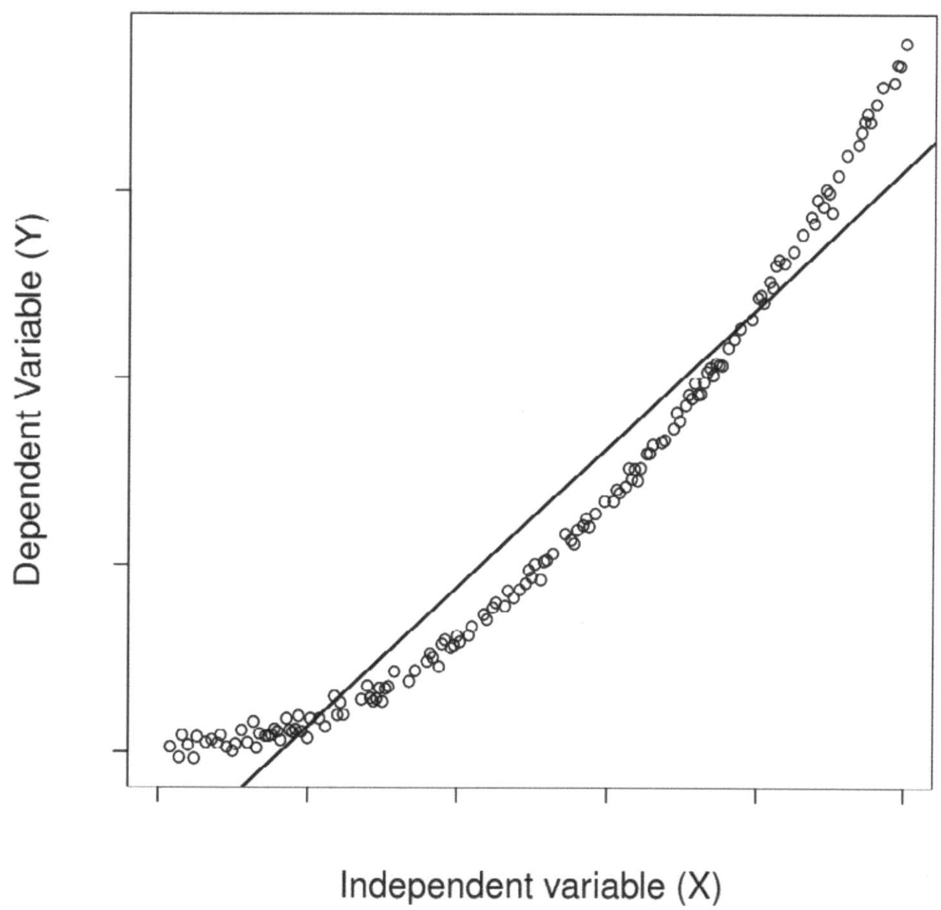

FIGURE 9-4. **The OLS solution from a linear model is a straight line while the observed data have a nonlinear association. Errors between observed and fitted values become particularly large at the smaller and larger values of X.**

OLS solution from a linear model is a straight line while the observed data have a nonlinear association. Errors between observed and fitted values become particularly large at the smaller and larger values of X. See Draper and Smith for more detailed descriptions of OLS analyses.[2]

Ordinary Least Squares Example

Simulated dataset for randomized drug trial. Examples in the remainder of this chapter will make use of a simulated dataset based on a randomized drug trial in which patients either received a new drug or were treated with an existing standard treatment (TRT). **Table 9-1** contains a summary of the dataset's variables. The outcome or dependent variable (Y) is a continuous measure of the new drug's effectiveness based on serum viral load (VL) levels. Explanatory or independent variables (Xs) that could conceivably influence patient outcomes include the baseline viral load (BVL), age, and a binary variable to indicate use of illicit intravenous (IV) drugs. The BVL recorded at the beginning of the study is intended to control for disease severity, because those with a higher initial VL might have a different treatment response. Patient age was collected as a continuous variable but then transformed into a series of binary (or dichotomous) variables. For the age 30–44 group, patients were assigned a value of either 1 (if they fell in that age range) or 0 (if they were either older or younger). A similar variable was created for those older than 44. In the model, these two age groups were compared with the reference age group of those younger than 30. Patients who were younger than 30 were identified as those coded with a 0 for the other two age categories. Accordingly, the reference age category does not appear as a unique variable in the equations; it is the omitted variable. Finally, an interaction term was used to assess whether the new drug works significantly differently for patients with either very high or very low BVLs.

Model 1: Simple treatment effect. The first basic model involves only the variables TRT, BVL, and VL. Recall that VL and BVL are continuous variables, while TRT is binary, meaning it is set at 1 if the subject received the new drug and 0 otherwise. The following equation describes the model, where OLS regression will be used to estimate β_0, β_1, and β_2:

$$VL = \beta_0 + \beta_1 TRT + \beta_2 BVL + \varepsilon$$

Recall that β_0 is the model's estimate for the intercept; this is the expected value of VL when TRT and BVL are both 0. Panel A

TABLE 9-1. Variables Used to Model a Patient's Drop in Viral Load with New Drug Therapy

Variable Type	Variable Name	Description
Outcome variable	Viral load (VL)	Patient's viral load at the conclusion of the study
Treatment variable	TRT = 1 patient received new drug TRT = 0 patients received standard care	Dichotomous variable indicating whether the patient received the new drug
Patient characteristics	Baseline viral load (BVL)	Measure of the patient's viral load at the beginning of the study
	IV drug user	Dichotomous variable indicating whether the patient is an IV drug user
	Age categories	
	< 30	Reference (ie, omitted) age category
	30–44	Dichotomous variable indicating whether the patient is between ages 30 and 44
	Age 45+	Dichotomous variable indicating whether the patient is age 45 or older
Interaction term	TRT * BVL	Product of the new drug and baseline viral load variables

IV = intravenous; TRT = treatment.

in **Figure 9-5** shows the fitted lines from this model for subjects with or without the new drug. The top line gives the result for TRT = 0, indicating only standard care was provided, while the bottom line represents TRT = 1, treatment with the new drug. The vertical distance between the two lines is β_1 and reflects the new drug's effectiveness. The line for TRT = 1 is lower, because the estimate for β_1 was negative, indicating a beneficial (lower) final viral load. Note that the two treatment lines are parallel as expected, because the model did not account for any change in treatment effect with changing BVL.

Model 2: Interaction term added. However, the new drug may be more effective for people with a higher BVL than for those with low BVLs. An interaction term will be used to model this possibility, which involves the TRT and BVL terms multiplied by one another. Thus, the new model specification is:

$$VL = \beta_0 + \beta_1 TRT + \beta_2 BVL + \beta_3 TRT * BVL + \varepsilon$$

Here, β_1 reflects the effect of the new drug regardless of BVL and β_3 measures the effect of the new drug as BVL changes. Thus, a negative estimate for β_3 can be interpreted to mean that the effect of the new drug on the outcome is more beneficial as BVL increases, because a larger drop in final viral load would be produced. Panel B in Figure 9-5 displays the model output. As before, the top line represents TRT = 0 (standard care level provided), and the bottom line represents TRT = 1 (new drug treatment). However, although panels A and B look similar at the lowest values for BVL, the lines are no longer parallel owing to the interaction term, indicating that the new drug's estimated effect is greater as BVL increases.

Model 3: Full model. In the final model, the influence of other important patient characteristics will be added, including whether the subject is an IV drug user, entered as a binary (equal to 0 if no, 1 if yes), and the two age group variables (age 30–44 and age 45+). The variable for the youngest group (age < 30) is omitted from the model, because it serves as the reference group; note that this group is already represented in the data when the other two groups' dummy variables are both set to 0. The final model is thus:

$$VL = \beta_0 + \beta_1 TRT + \beta_2 BVL + \beta_3 TRT * BVL + \beta_4 IV + \beta_5 age30\_44 + \beta_6 age45 + \varepsilon$$

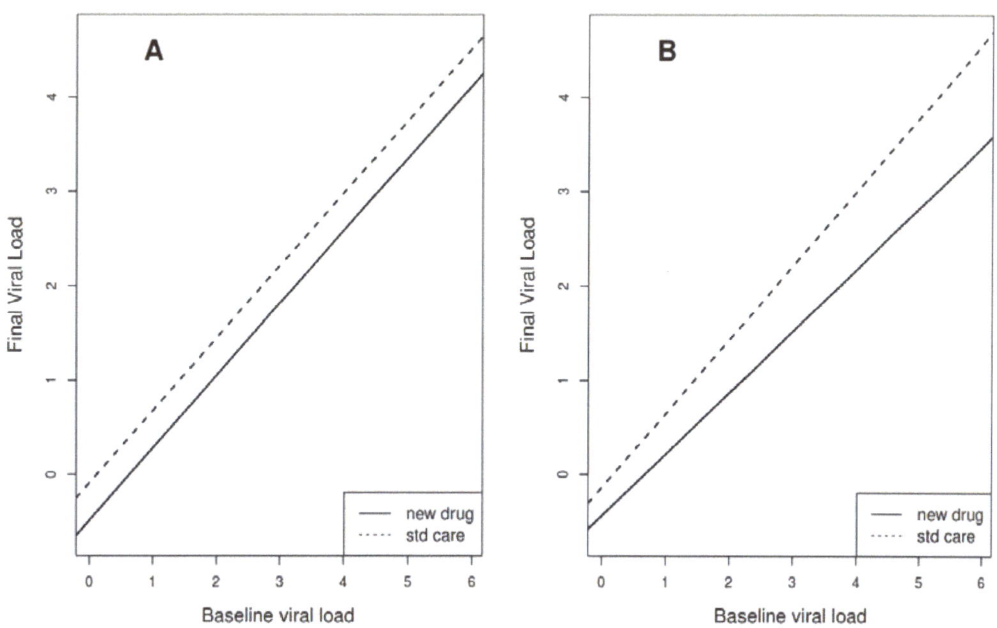

FIGURE 9-5. **Comparison of scenarios without (A) and with (B) an interaction between screening arm and baseline viral load.**

Table 9-2 gives the model's OLS parameter estimates, their standard errors, and *p*-values. Recall that the outcome and baseline viral load are both continuous variables, while the other explanatory variables are all binary categorical variables. Parameter estimates for binary variables show the estimated change in the outcome (final viral load) when the binary variable changes from 0 to 1, again assuming all other variables are held constant. To get an overall understanding of the new drug's effect, the combined effects of the TRT and TRT*BVL must be taken into account, because the interaction term was highly significant ($p < 0.0001$). Assuming that BVL = 5.0 and TRT = 1, the overall treatment effect (or vertical distance between the treatment lines) becomes:

$$VL = \beta_1 TRT + \beta_3 TRT * BVL = -0.40 * 1 - 0.099 * 5.0 * 1 = -0.895$$

The model estimates that patients with the new drug and baseline viral loads of 5.0 would have final viral loads approximately 0.9 units lower compared to similar patients without the new drug. Conversely, when BVL = 0 (no baseline viral load), the interaction term becomes zero in the above equation, and the treatment effect is now less than half as large, with final VL –0.4 units lower compared with similar patients with standard care. The parameter estimate for the continuous variable BVL (0.77) indicates the expected magnitude of change in the outcome for a 1-unit change in BVL, assuming all other variables are held constant during that change. Thus, the final viral level is estimated to grow in direct proportion with the BVL, but at a less than one-to-one relationship. Note that the estimate for IV (0.0076) was positive, suggesting that IV drug use possibly contributed to higher final viral loads. However, this result was not statistically significant ($p = 0.28$) and does not support making firm claims about IV drug use. Similarly, the estimates for the two older age groups had negative estimates, indicating that older patients may have been more likely to have lower final VLs compared with the youngest group, but again these results were not statistically significant.

Goodness of Fit and Hypothesis Tests

Several other areas are worth exploring from the model results in Table 9-2. First, the R-squared statistic provides a "goodness of fit" for the model and is the proportion of the dependent variable's variance that can be explained by the independent variables. Possible values for R-squared range between 0 and 1, where higher values indicate a better model in which the sum of squared residuals is small. One drawback of R-squared is that it always increases as additional variables are added to the model, even if they have no association with the outcome. The

TABLE 9-2. OLS Regression Modeling a Patient's Drop in Viral Load with New Drug Therapy

Variable	Definition	Estimate	Standard Error	*p*-Value
Intercept		–0.1058	0.0117	< 0.0001
TRT	Receipt of new drug	–0.4032	0.0138	< 0.0001
BVL	Baseline viral load	0.7690	0.0028	< 0.0001
IV	Intravenous drug use	0.0076	0.0071	0.28
Age 30–44	Reference group: age < 30	–0.0017	0.0083	0.84
Age 45+		–0.0135	0.0084	0.11
TRT*BVL	Interaction term	–0.0991	0.0039	< 0.0001
Multiple R-squared: 0.9773				
Adjusted R-squared: 0.9767				

adjusted R-squared statistic was developed in response to this problem and includes a penalization factor that reduces the overall result in proportion to the total number of predictor variables. The values for R-squared and adjusted R-squared in Table 9-2 indicate that the model is a good fit for the simulated data and that the penalty for the relatively small number of predictors did not substantially affect this conclusion.

The *p*-values in Table 9-2 illustrate that hypothesis tests are usually performed to assess whether the parameter estimates are statistically significant. The following steps outline how a hypothesis test is conducted:

1. Researchers specify a null hypothesis (H_0) of no effect, commonly set up as follows: Dependent variable (X) has no effect on the independent variable (Y)

$$H_0: \beta = 0$$

2. The alternative hypothesis (H_A) specifies a potential relationship between X and Y. It most commonly takes the form of a two-tailed test, meaning that X has either a positive or negative effect on Y, but one-tailed tests that specify the most likely direction of the proposed relationship are also possible:

   $H_A: \beta \neq 0$ (two-tailed test)

   $H_A: \beta > 0$ (one-tailed test for positive effect)

   $H_A: \beta < 0$ (one-tailed test for negative effect)

3. The *t* statistic is then easy to calculate in statistical software or using the following formula:

$$t = \frac{\hat{\beta}}{SE(\hat{\beta})}$$

   where $\hat{\beta}$ is the parameter estimate and $SE(\hat{\beta})$ is its standard error. The "hat" symbol indicates that this is an estimate for the true population parameter (β), an estimate that was based on the specific sample. The *p*-value is then derived from *t*-distribution tables or statistical software with the following inputs: the *t*-statistic; the degrees of freedom $n-p$, where n is the sample size and p is the number of explanatory variables; and the alternative hypothesis (one- or two-tailed test).

4. The *p*-value is then interpreted based on a prespecified margin for statistical significance, most commonly $p = 0.05$. A smaller *p*-value ($p < 0.05$) provides strong evidence in support of the alternative hypothesis, indicating that $\hat{\beta}$ is different from 0. In such cases, $\hat{\beta}$ is considered statistically significant and the null hypothesis is rejected based on this evidence. The *p*-value can be interpreted as the probability of observing this result (or something even more extreme) given that the null hypothesis is true. A large *p*-value ($p > 0.05$) means that there is not sufficient evidence to reject the null hypothesis and that $\hat{\beta}$ is not considered to be statistically significant. This does not imply that the null hypothesis is true; it only indicates there was not enough evidence to reject it. Another study with a larger population might yield different results.

Assumptions Behind Ordinary Least Squares Regression

When conducting analyses or reading about another investigator's work involving an OLS model, it is important to keep several important assumptions in mind. These should be verified as part of the modeling process:

1. The observations are independent of each other, meaning the information from one observation does not reveal anything about another. Independence would be violated if there were repeated observations from the same patient or if observations were clustered such that patients within a cluster might have similar responses (by hospital for example).
2. The outcome *Y* has a linear relationship with the independent variables in the model. This linear relationship could be verified by plotting each variable against Y.
3. The variance of residuals is constant across all values of *X*, especially for small samples. This condition is called homoscedasticity. For example, this assumption might be violated if there were more

variation in cancer outcomes among the elderly compared with younger patients.

4. The residual terms should have a normal distribution, with a mean value of 0.
5. None of the independent variables are correlated with the error term, meaning no endogeneity exists. This is consistent with the idea that the error term represents random error that is not associated with any observed data.
6. None of the independent variables are perfectly correlated with another. As discussed earlier, this problem is termed collinearity, in which the model may be unable to distinguish one variable from the other as they describe the same information.

MODELS FOR NONLINEAR RELATIONSHIPS

Recall that a linear model was defined earlier as one in which the unknown parameters were either constant or had linear relationships with a continuous outcome. The discussion now moves to models in which the relationship between an outcome and parameters is given by some type of nonlinear function. The choice of function usually depends on the outcome's distribution, and outcomes may be continuous, discrete, or categorical. The focus in this section is on logistic regression, which originates from a broader group of closely related statistical models known as generalized linear models. These are based on the exponential family of distributions; examples from this family include:

1. Normal (or Gaussian) distribution: used to model outcomes that approximate the familiar symmetric bell-shaped distribution.
2. Binomial distribution: used to model discrete outcomes. The next section demonstrates how a special case of the binomial distribution, known as the Bernoulli distribution, serves as the basis for logistic regression.
3. Poisson distribution: used to model discrete counts of outcomes.
4. Gamma distribution: used to model skewed, continuous outcomes.
5. Negative binomial distribution: sometimes used instead of the Poisson distribution for discrete count outcomes when it provides a better fit for the observed data.

Return to Randomized Drug Trial Data

A simulated dataset involving a randomized drug trial was used earlier to help illustrate the OLS regression method, where the outcome was a continuous measure of serum viral load. For the logistic regression model, a binary (yes/no) or dichotomous outcome is needed to indicate whether the VL is detectable. Continuous values that are above a detectability threshold will be labeled as "positive" or "yes" values, whereas the remainder will be "negative" or "no" values. The same explanatory variables will be used as before in the OLS models.

OLS for Binary Outcomes?

It is important to understand that the OLS approach for linear models could be used with a binary dependent variable; no statistical package will object to such a model. However, several problems would result as shown in **Figure 9-6**, which gives a comparison between linear and nonlinear solutions for the drug trial data. Recall that the binary outcome indicates whether the final VL is below the detectable limit (yes/no). The outcome values are limited to 1 or 0 (or yes and no), and the OLS solution (as depicted by the heavy straight line) attempts to provide a linear solution for this relationship. The logistic model solution is given by the curved (nonlinear) line, and horizontal probability lines (at 0%, 50% and 100%) indicate that logistic models deal in smooth probability functions that asymptotically approach 0% and 100% (more on this later). Note that the observed binary outcomes on the yes line are grouped to the left (lower baseline viral load), and outcomes on the no line are associated with higher baseline viral load. The OLS solution can take any value along the y-axis since the OLS model can yield impossible estimates greater than 1 or less than 0. Next, an OLS model assumes a linear relationship exists even though the marginal effect of a change in an independent variable

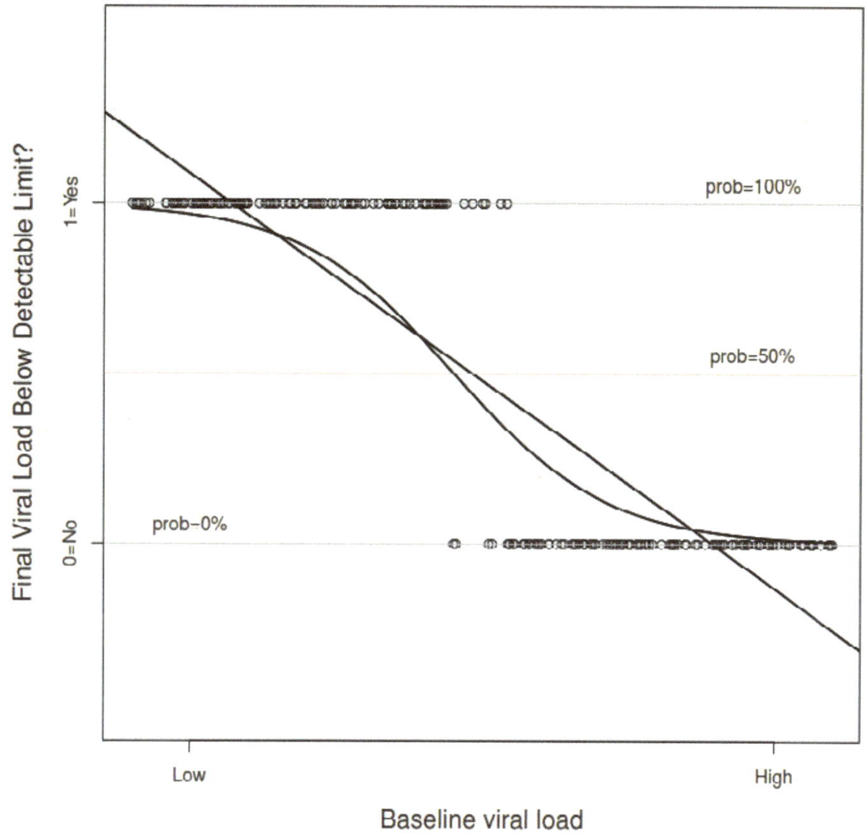

FIGURE 9-6. **Comparison between linear and nonlinear solutions for the drug trial data.**

generally attenuates at extremely high or low values of that independent variable (as shown by the curved line in Figure 9-6). Finally, the OLS model will violate the homoscedasticity assumption (ie, error terms with nonconstant variance). As we will see, the logistic model solves these problems by assuming a nonlinear relationship between the binary outcome and the dependent variables.

Logistic Regression

Logistic regression is part of a family of generalized linear models, in which the nonlinear outcome is transformed to take on a linear form. As indicated earlier, the binomial distribution is the basis for logistic regression. This distribution predicts the number of successful outcomes for a given number of attempts (flipping a coin) based on the probability of success for each coin flip, which is called p. When restricted to a single attempt (binary outcome), this reduces to the Bernoulli distribution, for which the probability of success is p and the probability of failure is $1-p$. The ratio of success and failure probabilities $p/(1-p)$ is known as the odds of success. Logistic regression deals with the natural logarithm of the odds, called the log-odds or logit (p). As Figure 9-6 shows, p is nonlinear when plotted against the independent variable, whereas the logit has a linear relationship. In **Figure 9-7**, this is evident in the plot of the baseline viral load against the log-odds for undetectable viral load. Owing to this linear relationship, the same linear equation for the explanatory variables that was used for OLS models can be used but altered to include the binary outcome probability transformed by the logit function:

$$log\left(\frac{p}{(1-p)}\right) = \beta_0 + \beta_1 TRT + \beta_2 BVL + \beta_3 TRT *$$
$$BVL + \beta_4 IV + \beta_5 age30_{44} + \beta_6 age45$$

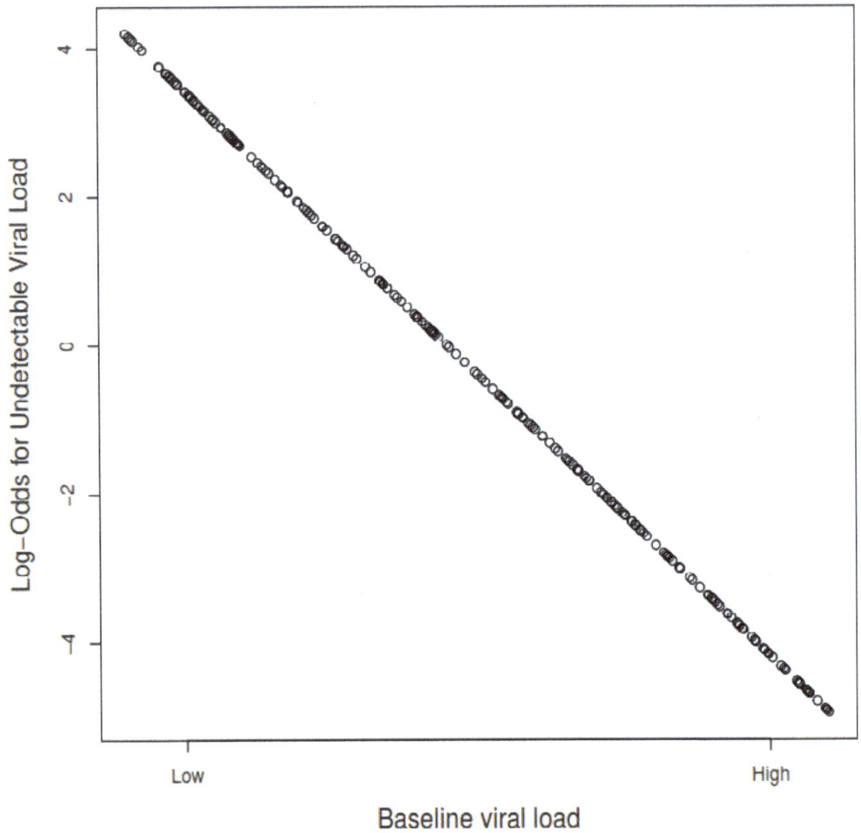

FIGURE 9-7. **Plot of the baseline viral load against the log-odds for undetectable viral load.**

where p is the probability of an undetectable viral load at the end of the study. A shorthand version of the above equation is:

$$log\left(\frac{p}{(1-p)}\right) = \beta' X$$

where β' represents the unknown parameters $(\beta_0, \beta_1, \beta_2, \beta_3, \beta_4, \beta_5, \beta_6)$, X is the data for the observed independent variables, and the apostrophe is shorthand matrix notation that indicates in this case that the corresponding terms of β' and X are multiplied by each other and then summed to give the original equation. To obtain the individual outcome probabilities for each patient in the dataset, the above equation is solved for p:

$$p = \frac{1}{(1+\exp(-\beta' X))}$$

This equation could also be used to make predictions about new patients by using the parameter estimates $(\hat{\beta})$ from a model developed from an existing group of patients with known outcomes and the observed values (X) for the new patients. A threshold must be chosen for the predicted outcome probability to define where the binary outcome should occur. While 50% might be a reasonable choice, lower thresholds may be appropriate for less common outcomes.

Solution by Maximum Likelihood Estimation

Maximum likelihood estimation (MLE) is a standard method for estimating nonlinear model parameters. Note that MLE could have been used in lieu of OLS for the linear model example and would have produced identical results, although the reverse is not true as shown above: the OLS method is limited to linear regression models. While an explanation of MLE theory is beyond this chapter's scope, the overall approach is to find a set of parameters that makes the observed data the most probable result given the defined model. The MLE equations will vary depending on the underlying distribution and design features, and in many cases (including logistic regression) there are no closed-form solutions. Specialized statistical software that uses iterative numerical techniques is typically needed to determine parameter estimates. For more information on generalized linear models, refer to Agresti,[3] Dobson,[4] or Myers et al.[5]

Interpretation of Results from Example Logistic Model

Table 9-3 gives the results from a logistic regression model for the simulated dataset involving a randomized drug trial. The columns labeled "Estimate" and "Std. Error" are the parameter estimates ($\hat{\beta}$) and their respective standard errors. Logistic model results are usually given in terms of odds ratios (OR), which can be calculated from the model's equation by forming the ratio of two comparison patients where there is a difference in only one term (age for example). The goal is to compute how much the odds of the outcome change when the second patient is compared with the first. Note that there must always be a comparison (or reference) patient in order to form an odds ratio. In Table 9-3, the column labeled "Level" often helps to define the reference patient. For example, in the treatment variable (yes vs. no) the reference level is a patient with "no" treatment; for age group, the reference is given in the first column. If the variable is continuous (baseline VL), unless otherwise indicated, the OR is defined as the effect from adding a single additional unit (of viral load in this case). To illustrate, the logistic model will be used with the example data to compute the OR for a patient aged 45 against a reference patient aged 25. Starting with the log-odds equations for each:

$$\text{Patient \#1: log-odds}(VL_1) = \beta_0 + \beta_1 TRT + \beta_2 BVL + \beta_3 TRT * BVL + \beta_4 IV + \beta_6 age45$$

$$\text{Patient \#2: log-odds}(VL_2) = \beta_0 + \beta_1 TRT + \beta_2 BVL + \beta_3 TRT * BVL + \beta_4 IV$$

The second patient's equation is identical except the age term dropped out, because he or she is age 25 such that the binary variables *age30_44* and *age45* are both 0 and the terms drop out. Next, the ratio of the two is formed and both sides are exponentiated such that the left side is the ratio of the odds for each patient:

$$OR = \frac{odds(VL_1)}{odds(VL_2)} = \frac{\exp\begin{pmatrix}\beta_0 + \beta_1 TRT + \\ \beta_2 BVL + \beta_3 TRT \\ *BVL + \beta_4 IV \\ +\beta_6 age45\end{pmatrix}}{\exp\begin{pmatrix}\beta_0 + \beta_1 TRT \\ +\beta_2 BVL + \beta_3 TRT \\ *BVL + \beta_4 IV\end{pmatrix}}$$

Recall that the two patients are identical in all terms except age, such that values for TRT, BVL, and IV are the same in the numerator and denominator. Because these are exponentials, the identical terms in the denominator can be subtracted from those in the numerator.

TABLE 9-3. Logistic Regression Model for Undetectable Final Viral Levels

Variable	Level	Estimate	Std. Error	Odds Ratio (OR) (95% Confidence Interval)	*p*-Value
Treatment	Yes vs. no	0.456	0.148	1.58 (1.18, 2.11)	0.002
Baseline viral load		−0.133	0.061	0.88 (0.78, 0.99)	0.03
IV user	Yes vs. no	−0.277	0.173	0.76 (0.54, 1.06)	0.11
Age group reference = age 18–29	Age 30–44	0.217	0.14	1.24 (0.94, 1.63)	0.12
	Age 45 and greater	0.323	0.184	1.38 (0.96, 1.98)	0.08

Because the binary variable age 45 is 1 for patient #1, this simplifies to:

$$OR = \frac{odds(VL_1)}{odds(VL_2)} = \exp(\beta_6)$$

where OR stands for odds ratio. From Table 9-3, the value for β_6 (age 45 or greater) is 0.323, which when exponentiated is 1.38. This odds ratio could be interpreted as, "A subject aged 45 has 38% greater odds of undetectable VL compared with a subject aged 25." Note that this is described as "38% greater odds" and not "38% greater risk"; more on this in the next section. Because the OR involves a multiplicative relationship, this result could have also been interpreted as the older subject having odds that were "nearly 1.4 times greater than for a subject aged 25." The 95% confidence intervals in Table 9-3 are calculated from the estimate and its standard error (see Chapter 8); recall that if this randomized trial were repeated many times, then 95% of the time the true population parameter would fall within the confidence limit. The *p*-value is also directly related to the parameter estimate and its standard error; these estimates generally follow a standard normal distribution, where the Z statistic is the ratio of the parameter estimate and its standard error.

Odds Ratios Versus Risk Ratios

As discussed, results from logistic regression are usually discussed in terms of odds ratios owing to the model's log-odds (or logit) link. Refer to Chapter 3 for a comparison of odds ratios and risk ratios, which result from other types of analyses. It is worth highlighting again that when the outcome is relatively common, the odds ratio may substantially overestimate the risk ratio. In such cases, logistic regression may not be the most appropriate method, and an alternative approach, such as Poisson regression, may be more suitable.

ADVANCED TOPICS

The previous sections gave brief introductions to the OLS and MLE methods for estimating parameters for simple linear and nonlinear regression models. These methods form the basis for a number of more advanced methods that are needed when the dataset's structure or the research questions dictate more sophisticated approaches. The following sections give a brief introduction to some of these with typical applications. Each topic branches to many additional types of specialized models, and references are provided for those needing more information.

Clustered Data

Clustered data involves observations that are not independent, as they are grouped in some manner such that a correlation exists between related rows. For example, health outcomes data frequently involve repeated measurements taken over time, such that each patient has multiple observations (or rows) that can cover many days, months, or years. These are often referred to as longitudinal data. Observations can also be clustered by other factors, such as location (eg, by hospital, geographic region). If such clustering is not accounted for during the analysis, the population's true variability may be underestimated. For example, 10 blood pressure measurements recorded from one patient within a short timeframe are likely to be highly correlated compared with 10 measurements recorded from 10 different subjects. Failing to account for this correlation could lead to incorrect conclusions that might involve inflated type I errors and confidence intervals that are too narrow. There are a wide range of approaches designed to handle clustered data, including linear mixed models (LMM) and generalized linear mixed models (GLMM); these are extensions of linear models (LM) and generalized linear models (GLM) discussed earlier. In mixed models, random effects are estimated to help account for the correlation within clusters. Random effects are a separate class of parameters estimated by the mixed models in addition to the familiar fixed effects that are part of basic LMs and GLMs. Random effects can be random intercepts or random slopes and allow the model to estimate separate solutions for each patient (or other cluster groups) such that the fixed effect estimates give a better estimate for the population's true variability. Owing to their greater complexity, mixed models can be more computationally intense, particularly for large datasets, and problems with convergence can occur. Analysts may need to attempt different random effect covariance structures or different numerical estimation techniques to obtain useful results. Another very useful option for clustered data is generalized estimating equations (GEE) models. This approach does not estimate random effects and thus can only make estimates at the population level. Generalized estimating equation models account for clustered observations through a working correlation matrix that has an assumed covariance structure. One distinct advantage for GEE models is that they provide robust standard errors for fixed-effect estimates that are valid even when the working correlation matrix structure is mis-specified. For more information on GLMM and GEE models, refer to Diggle et al.[6] and Hardin et al.,[7] respectively.

Time-to-Event Outcomes

Healthcare outcomes researchers are frequently interested in assessing outcomes based on how long it took for an event to occur rather than whether it simply occurred at all. Such studies are challenged by the fact that some subjects may be lost to follow-up without experiencing an event. For example, cancer studies are often designed to determine whether a new treatment might extend the time to relapse or death. These questions involve time-to-event (or survival) analyses, and two of the most common approaches in this field will be described: Kaplan-Meier curves and proportional hazards models. The time-to-event datasets used in both approaches include two types of dependent variables. The first is a censoring variable to indicate the subject's current status, which could include whether the event of interest occurred at that point (eg, lung cancer relapse or death), or that a different event related to a competing risk occurred (death owing to a nonlung cancer reason), or that no event had occurred by the end of the study (eg, the subject was censored). The second dependent variable is used to give the time of each observation such that combination of the two gives us a full description of each subject's time-to-event outcome.

Kaplan-Meier Curves

The survival function $S(t)$ describes a subject's probability of surviving past time t, and Kaplan-Meier (KM) curves are typically used to compare estimated survival functions between two groups by plotting each group's survival over time, such that a stair-step vertical drop is shown for each event to indicate the overall proportion still surviving. Tick marks are also included at censoring points (without a drop in survival) to show where subjects who never experienced events were last observed. Several statistical methods could be used to compare KM curves; for example, the log-rank test is often used to test for differences between survival curves. While KM curves support comparing survival between groups stratified by a single variable of interest, they do not allow simultaneous adjustment for other covariates, including potential confounders or interactions. A regression-based approach is needed to be able to incorporate those steps.

Cox Proportional Hazards Regression

As in the multivariable models reviewed in previous sections, Cox proportional hazards (CPH) models can be adjusted for other covariates that are potentially related to the outcome. Unlike previous designs, however, CPH models estimate the hazard rate $h(t)$ and also incorporate a baseline hazard rate. The hazard rate is the instantaneous risk that an event might occur, given the subject has survived to that point. Hazard ratios (HR) and their confidence intervals are used to compare the hazard rates for two groups based on the parameter estimates from CPH models. While ORs compare the odds of an event ever occurring during the study, the HR compares the instantaneous risks for the event at a specific time. Cox proportional hazard models depend on an assumption that when relative hazards are compared between two risk groups, this comparison remains the same (proportional) over time. This may be a poor assumption, and investigators should report how they verified it was valid. For more information on analysis of time to event outcomes, refer to Klein et al.[8]

Zero-Inflated Data

Many healthcare studies involve count outcomes that are not appropriate for OLS analysis, because they are not normally distributed. Generalized linear models under the Poisson or negative binomial distributions are possible options depending on the outcome's characteristics. For the Poisson distribution, the mean and variance should be approximately equal;

in overdispersed cases where the variance is greater than the mean, the negative binomial distribution may be appropriate. However, counts outcomes often involve an excess number of zeros such that neither distribution is appropriate. This situation is common in studies of healthcare costs, where subjects can have zero costs in many months but very large costs in others. Similarly, inpatient admissions and emergency department utilization may involve zero-inflation. Specialized methods are needed to analyze zero-inflated data that incorporate separate assumptions for the source of zero and nonzero values. Common approaches involve two-part models, where the first model is used to estimate the probability of a zero outcome and the second estimates the probability of a nonzero outcome. Logistic regression is a common option for the first model, whereas the second could involve Poisson or negative binomial distributions. These two-part models are referred to as zero-inflated Poisson (ZIP) and zero-inflated negative binomial (ZINB) models, respectively. In both models, it is important to recognize that a zero can arise from two situations: (1) structural zeros occur when a subject cannot have the outcome. For example, those without access to healthcare will not have healthcare costs or utilization. (2) *Random zeros* can occur among patients who are at risk for the outcome; those with healthcare access will have some months without any claims. From the data alone, it may not be possible to distinguish between structural and random zeros, although an important alternative design known as two-part hurdle models is based on the assumption that all zeros are structural in nature. For more information on analysis of zero-inflated data, refer to Lambert[9] and Cameron et al.[10]

Penalized Regression

Recall that in OLS regression, the goal was to minimize the sum of the squared residuals, where the fitted parameter estimate for a sample of N subjects could be represented by:

$$\hat{\beta} = \underset{\beta}{\text{argmin}} \frac{1}{N} \sum_{i=1}^{N} (Y_i - \beta' X_i)^2$$

For large datasets involving many hundreds or thousands of covariates, the OLS process will produce parameter estimates for every covariate included in the model, including those with little or no association with the outcome of interest. This could lead to overfitting, a situation in which the model's prediction accuracy suffers, because the model attempts to account for every available feature, even those due to random noise. One approach to reduce overfitting is to add a penalty term that accounts for increased model complexity. These penalties can work to reduce or even eliminate less important terms from the model. For example, ridge regression adds a penalty term to the above equation that is based on the squared parameters:

$$\widehat{\beta_R} = \underset{\beta}{\text{argmin}} \frac{1}{N} \sum_{i=1}^{N} (Y_i - \beta' X_i)^2 + \lambda \sum_{j=1}^{d} \beta_j^2$$

where λ is known as a tuning parameter that controls the size of the penalty term. Ridge regression generally shrinks parameter estimates for less important covariates but does not entirely eliminate them. Another important option is LASSO penalized regression, which stands for Least Absolute Shrinkage and Selection Operator. Here, the penalty term involves the sum of parameters:

$$\widehat{\beta_L} = \underset{\beta}{\text{argmin}} \frac{1}{N} \sum_{i=1}^{N} (Y_i - \beta' X_i)^2 + \lambda \sum_{j=1}^{d} |\beta_j|$$

In contrast with Ridge regression, LASSO regression performs a variable selection role, because it will eliminate less important covariates by shrinking the parameter estimate to 0 if λ is large enough. However, for correlated variables, one variable may be randomly selected to be retained from the group while the others are eliminated. In contrast, Ridge regression would likely shrink all related variables by the same degree. Next, the Elastic Net design includes a weighted combination of the LASSO and Ridge penalties:

$$\widehat{\beta_E} = \underset{\beta}{\text{argmin}} \frac{1}{N} \sum_{i=1}^{N} (Y_i - \beta' X_i)^2 + \alpha \sum_{j=1}^{d} \beta_j^2 + (1-\alpha) \sum_{j=1}^{d} |\beta_j|$$

where α is the tuning parameter that controls which penalty term predominates in the model. Elastic Net is designed to incorporate strengths from both LASSO and Ridge models and is often the top choice when the three models' predictive performance is compared using techniques such as cross-validation. For more information on penalized regression, refer to Zou and Hastie.[11]

Bayesian Methods

Every model described thus far in this chapter comes from a branch of statistics known as frequentist statistics, but readers are likely to also see studies that involve Bayesian methods, and it is important to understand some basic distinctions between the two approaches.

As described in previous chapters, the frequentist approach includes a focus on hypotheses testing, where a null hypothesis is assumed to be true. Data are next sampled from the population of interest and tested against the null hypothesis to determine the probability (*p* value) for how unlikely these results are under the null hypothesis. This probability is an indication of how likely it is to obtain another result from a new random sample of the population that is at least as extreme as the current result if the null hypothesis were true. If this probability is very low, the null hypothesis is rejected, and this is considered evidence in favor of the alternate hypothesis. The *p*-value does not allow us to firmly conclude that that either hypothesis is correct or incorrect, only that the current sample provided evidence about the null hypothesis, although such results could be due to random chance. As seen in discussion of the OLS and MLE models, frequentist hypothesis tests are an integral part for testing whether a model's parameter estimates are statistically significant, usually under a null hypothesis of $\beta = 0$. Confidence intervals are also used to help give a better understanding for a result's importance. As discussed in earlier chapters, recall that, for a 95% confidence interval, if the same analysis were repeated many times with independent random samples, then 95% of the time, the confidence interval would contain the true population value. Note this is *not* the same thing as saying that there is a 95% probability that the true value lies within the confidence interval. Such a statement would be incorrect and is a key example of why frequentist concepts are confusing to many readers.

The Bayesian approach is named after Rev. Thomas Bayes (1701–1761), who is credited with Bayes' theorem:

$$p(\theta \mid Data) = \frac{p(Data \mid \theta)p(\theta)}{p(Data)}$$

where θ is the parameter or hypothesis to be estimated from the data. The term on the left is called the posterior probability and is the probability of the parameter θ given the data. For example, if estimating the probability of having a given disease given that a screening test was positive, the posterior probability would become $p(disease \mid test+)$. On the right side, the numerator term $p(Data \mid \theta)$ would become $p(test+ \mid disease)$, or the probability of a positive test given the patient has the disease. The denominator would become $p(test+)$, or the overall probability of a positive test in the population. The ratio of these two terms is the relative probability of a positive test among those with the disease compared with those in the full population. The posterior probability is obtained when this ratio is multiplied by $p(\theta)$, or p(disease) in the example, which is the disease prevalence in the overall population. In Bayesian statistics, $p(\theta)$ is called the prior probability, which can reflect any prior beliefs about the parameter in question. Values selected for the prior can strongly influence the posterior probability. The elements of Bayes' theorem can also be applied to models, where the analyst makes assumptions about the distribution of the prior probability. It can be difficult to obtain closed-form solutions for the posterior probability distribution, and iterative numerical methods, such as Markov Chain Monte Carlo (MCMC) sampling, are typically used to estimate them.

When frequentist and Bayesian statistics are compared, several key distinctions arise. In the frequentist approach, the *p*-value involves a probability for whether the current data support the null hypothesis, and the confidence interval is interpreted in terms of many repeated samples. In the Bayesian approach, these concepts are reversed; here, the posterior probability involves the probability of the hypothesis given the data, and there is a 95% probability that the parameter estimate falls within the 95% credible interval (used in place of confidence intervals). Whereas interpretation of Bayesian concepts often makes more intuitive sense to readers, it is also important to understand important distinctions, particularly the role of the analyst's beliefs about the prior probability distribution. For more in-depth information about Bayesian analyses, refer to Lesaffre and Lawson[12] or Sivia.[13]

Machine Learning Algorithms

All discussion on multivariable analyses thus far has involved statistical models, which are typically used to help explore and possibly explain associations between exposures, covariates, and outcomes. Some models are also used to make predictions about new subjects given what was learned about an existing population. Machine learning algorithms are a related field, and it can be difficult to define consistent distinctions between the two. An algorithm in this context is an automatic procedure for processing a dataset, usually with the goal of being able to make accurate predictions. There is usually less focus on testing hypotheses or attempting to determine what factors could explain the outcome. For example, the random forest (RF) algorithm uses a collection of decision trees that form a "forest," each automatically generated from the data.[15] Each tree is grown from a bootstrapped version of the data, meaning the data are sampled with replacement; part of the data used in each tree is also set aside (or bagged) to be used to validate the forest's performance. At each decision point (branch) in a tree, the algorithm selects one variable from a randomly selected group; this choice is based on which variable is best at splitting the data against the outcome. This branching process is automatically repeated until a tree is grown to a prespecified size. Because the trees are created based on an identified outcome, RF is termed a supervised method, whereas machine learning methods that look for patterns in data without regard for an outcome are termed unsupervised. Once the forest is created, the trees can "vote" on each case in the bagged data for whether that subject had the outcome or not. The sum of votes (or in some cases the average of votes depending on the specific application) is used to assign a predicted outcome. This result can be compared with the actual outcomes to determine prediction performance in the held-out validation data. The RF algorithm can be extremely effective as a prediction algorithm and (like penalized regression models) is a useful tool for determining variable importance. Random forest is only one example from a multitude of decision tree algorithms, which in turn is only one of many classes of machine learning algorithms. Of particular note are neural networks, which form the basis for recent important advances in artificial intelligence tools, including image recognition and large language models. For more information on machine learning methods, refer to Hastie et al.[14]

CONCLUSION

In this chapter, the foundations of multivariable analysis were explored, including the use of OLS and nonlinear regression techniques to estimate the simultaneous effects of multiple independent variables on a dependent variable. While these fundamental approaches may be sufficient for many simple analyses, several examples of advanced topics were briefly introduced, including methods involving time-to-event (survival) analysis, clustered (or longitudinal) data, zero-inflated data, penalized regression, Bayesian statistics, and machine learning algorithms. These tools provide a robust framework for analyzing complex datasets, and each in turn lays the groundwork for a wide range of even more specialized methods.

REFERENCES

1. Spiegelhalter D. *The Art of Statistics: How to Learn from Data.* New York: Hachette Book Group; 2021.
2. Draper NR, Smith H. *Applied Regression Analysis*. 3rd ed. New York: John Wiley & Sons; 1998.
3. Agresti A. *Categorical Data Analysis*. 2nd ed. New York: John Wiley & Sons; 2002.
4. Dobson A. *An Introduction to Generalized Linear Models*. London: Chapman & Hall; 1990.
5. Myers RH, Montgomery DC, Vining GG. *Generalized Linear Models with Applications in*

Engineering and the Sciences. New York: John Wiley & Sons; 2002.

6. Diggle PJ, Liang K-Y, Zeger SL. *Analysis of Longitudinal Data*. Oxford: Clarendon Press; 1994.
7. Hardin JW, Hilbe JM. *Generalized Estimating Equations*. Boca Raton, FL: Chapman & Hall/ CRC; 2003.
8. Klein JP, Moeschberger ML. *Survival Analysis Techniques for Censored and Truncated Data*. 2nd ed. New York: Springer; 2003.
9. Lambert D. Zero-inflated Poisson regression with an application to defects in manufacturing. *Technometrics*. 1992;34:1-14.
10. Cameron AC, Trivedi PK. *Regression Analysis of Count Data*. Cambridge: Cambridge University Press; 1998.
11. Zou H, Hastie T. Regularization and variable selection via the elastic net. *J Royal Statistical Society, Series B*. 2005;67:301-320.
12. Lesaffre E, Lawson AB. *Bayesian Biostatistics*. Chichester, UK: John Wiley & Sons; 2012.
13. Sivia DS. *Data Analysis: A Bayesian Tutorial*. 2nd ed. Oxford: Oxford University Press; 2006.
14. Hastie T, Tibshirani R, Friedman J. *The Elements of Statistical Learning: Data Mining, Inference, and Prediction*. New York: Springer; 2009.
15. Random Forest: Breiman L. (2001) Random Forests. *Machine Learning* 45, 5-32.

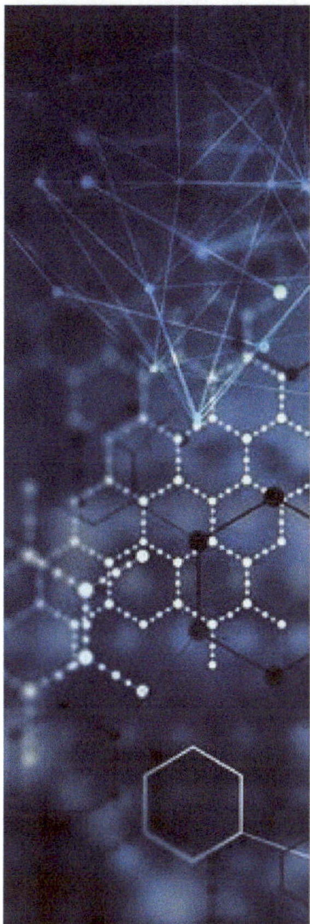

SECTION THREE

Real-World Evidence

DOI: 10.37573/9781585287666.TITLE

Introduction to Real-World Evidence

10

Kit N. Simpson, DrPH, MPH

INTRODUCTION

The growth of health economics and outcomes research (HEOR) is reflected in advancements in research designs, analytical approaches, and use of observational data for examining treatment outcomes that patients and providers care about. Indeed, a large HEOR consulting and data vendor industry has emerged over the past decade. The increasing availability of billing and electronic health record (EHR) data has led to exponential growth in the use of quasi-experimental study designs that use archival data for postlaunch medication studies by pharmaceutical companies, program evaluations by demonstration project funders, and quality improvement research to assess the effectiveness and cost of new programs. Real-world evidence (RWE) using real-world data (RWD) is now routinely used to assess the effectiveness of interventions under actual practice conditions, once efficacy has been assessed in randomized controlled trials (RCTs). The practice grew exponentially after the 21st Century Cures Act (2016) specified that the US Food and Drug Administration (FDA) should develop a program to evaluate the potential use of RWE for assessing effectiveness.[1]

The increasing availability of large amounts of RWD spurred the development of study designs and statistical methods capable of minimizing selection bias, which is ubiquitous in observational studies and a constant barrier to the unbiased use of stored data. Thus, deriving RWE from RWD only became possible once researchers started developing, testing, and documenting the performance of innovative research designs, such as propensity score matching, inverse-probability weighting, use of instrumental variables, difference-in-differences, and interrupted time series study designs (discussed in detail in Chapter 4).

The largest sources of RWD include archival data from EHRs and billing data from insurance claims. Other RWD sources include disease or population-specific patient registry data. These data have strengths and weaknesses that vary across data vendors and over time as payment regulations change and EHR systems are modified. In general, insurance billing data presents as a list of variables with very sparse explanations, while detailed EHR documentation is often only available to the information technology data managers who extract the data for research purposes. Chapter 11 compares the strengths and weaknesses of each and discusses the uses and usefulness of the major data sources.

REGULATORY SUPPORT FOR RWE EVOLUTION

The FDA created a "Framework for FDA's Real-world Evidence Program" in 2018 with guidance on the use of RWD in generating evidence and how best to evaluate that evidence in regulatory decisions.[2] They defined RWD as "the data relating to patient health status and/or the delivery of health care routinely collected from a variety of sources," and RWE is the "clinical evidence regarding a medical product's use and potential benefits or risks derived from analysis of RWD." The National Institutes of Health (NIH) define RWE as clinical evidence regarding the usage and potential

DOI: 10.37573/9781585287666.010

benefits or risks of a medical product derived from analysis of RWD, and its National Center for Advancing Translational Science provides a toolkit emphasizing the importance of including "patients voices" when designing RWE studies.[3] Support and guidance from the FDA and NIH facilitated the orderly scientific development and testing of new study designs, data sources, and analytic methods. A great source of additional information is available at the FDA's Center for Biologics Evaluation and Research and Center for Drug Evaluation and Research Real-World Evidence.[4] International organizations are also excellent sources of guidance, in particular the International Council for Harmonisation and the National Institute for Health and Care Excellence (NICE) in the United Kingdom.[5]

Consulting groups, academic researchers, and data vendors are also sources of examples and innovations in RWD/RWE. A 2025 search of the Internet for "resources for RWE" showed 14 data vendors or consulting firms and three YouTube videos for RWD/RWE on the first page. This indicates a rapidly changing scientific and commercial field with many stakeholders, indicating the need to use multiple peer-reviewed sources for information to inform study design and evidence interpretation in this area.

USES AND USEFULNESS OF REAL-WORLD EVIDENCE

Amit Dang recently published a primer on RWE that outlines some important points for readers to consider, mainly that (1) RWE is medical evidence generated during routine patient visits; (2) there are multiple sources of RWE data generated from EHRs, pharmacy records, medical insurance claims, patient registries, and social media; and (3) different regulatory bodies have provided guidelines for generating RWE.[6] He goes on to discuss RWD collection and the importance of using RWD to examine the efficacy and safety of new drugs. While such data have been in use for many years, they have often been reported to authorities on a voluntary basis. Real-world data from routine clinical sources may be much better at identifying small, but important, risks that can only be found in large datasets. He also points out that the new wearable devices, sensors, and social media platforms may be important sources of data for identifying subtle treatment effects in large populations. In 2025, this area of inquiry is not yet well developed, but it holds great promise for future research. He reviews the different study designs that are useful for RWE studies and discusses areas where RWE may be supplemental to clinical trial efficacy measures in informing practice and especially risks to patients. Finally, he provides a table of RWE studies that have been used for licensure approvals and discusses the stakeholders to consider in RWE studies. The latter list is insightful, because it includes both medical device companies with interests in licensure and market expansion and patients/family members concerned with access to new and/or affordable treatments.

The potential "tokenization" of patient data, where patients lose control of their own data when it is sold to vendors, is an important issue.[6] Other important considerations are the equity and ethics related to doing studies in poorer countries where economic access to the drugs examined may be limited. He describes the roles of payers and regulators in raising barriers to access and the impacts of new drugs' cost of care. The paper also provides a well-rounded discussion of agencies, such as NICE and the FDA, and their roles in RWE research. This primer is recommended as a valuable resource for both students and new researchers contemplating RWE studies.

Recent studies have highlighted the role that RWE can play in improving care for specific diseases or populations, especially in the field of orphan drugs for rare diseases. During an 18-month period ending June 2021, three of the 30 neuroscience-related new drug or biologically similar applications approved by the FDA included RWE as evidence of efficacy or effectiveness.[7] All three approvals were for drugs to treat rare diseases, specifically Zolgensma for the treatment of pediatric patients younger than 2 years with spinal muscular atrophy, Risdiplam for the treatment of spinal muscular atrophy, and Viltolarsen for patients with Duchenne muscular dystrophy

(DMD) and a specific gene mutation.[8-10] The studies used existing patient registries for endpoints easily determined therein, such as survival, time to death, permanent intubation/tracheostomy, or functional measures, such as a 6-minute walk.[10-12] What stands out about these studies is that RWD successfully generated evidence for efficacy and effectiveness to support the FDA approval of the three medications.

One key finding from this study is that the definitions for RWD and RWE are not consistent across studies, a major impediment to their use. In May 2024, the NIH and FDA collaborated to release a request for information (RFI) to solicit public feedback on a draft glossary of terms related to use of RWD and RWE in clinical research.[13] The goal of the RFI was to improve communication and understanding within the research community by establishing a common vocabulary.

Other examples of collaborations to advance the use of RWD and RWE include the international I-O Optimize initiative, which was established to foster real-world insights into thoracic cancer. Other special data sources are Pediatric Neuromuscular Clinical Research Network database,[14] the Real-World Evidence Collaborative at the Margolis Institute at Duke University, and the Real-World Evidence Collaborative at the International Society for Pharmacoepidemiology.[14-17] These organizations will help to refine and to clarify the use of RWD for RWE over time. In the meantime, it is up to the individual student/researcher to judge the data and evidence in an informed but cautious manner. Chapter 11 describes specific types of RWD and provides examples of their strengths and weaknesses, and Chapter 12 dives into the issues to consider when planning, performing, and using this type of data for research.

REFERENCES

1. H.R.34 - 21st Century Cures Act114th Congress (2015-2016). https://www.congress.gov/bill/114th-congress/house-bill/34. Accessed March 4, 2026.
2. U.S. Food & Drug Administration. *Framework for FDA's Real-World Evidence Program.* 2018. https://www.fda.gov/media/120060/download?attachment. Accessed February 9, 2026.
3. NIH National Center for Advancing Translational Science (NCATS) Toolkit. Toolkit for patient-focused therapy development (NCATS Toolkit). https://toolkit.ncats.nih.gov/about/. Accessed February 9, 2026.
4. Center for Biologics Evaluation and Research & Center for Drug Evaluation and Research Real-World Evidence. *CBER and CDER RWE Program.* https://www.fda.gov/science-research/real-world-evidence/center-biologics-evaluation-and-research-center-drug-evaluation-and-research-real-world-evidence. Accessed March 16, 2026.
5. NICE real-world evidence framework. Corporate document. Reference number: ECD9. Published June 23, 2022. https://www.nice.org.uk/corporate/ecd9/chapter/introduction-to-real-world-evidence-in-nice-decision-making. Accessed February 9, 2026.
6. Dang A. Real-world evidence: a primer. *Pharmaceut Med.* 2023;37(1):25-36. https://doi.org/10.1007/s40290-022-00456-6
7. Bloomfield-Clagett B, Rahman M, Smith K, Concato J. Use of real-world evidence in neuroscience-related new drug and biologics license applications for novel therapeutics. *Clin Pharmacol Ther.* 2023;114(5):1002-1005. https://doi.org/10.1002/cpt.3018
8. Center for Biologics and Evaluation Research (CBER). Zolgensma (Onasemnogene abeparvovec) product approval package: US Food and Drug Administration (FDA). Updated August 10, 2022. https://www.fda.gov/vaccines-blood-biologics/zolgensma. Accessed March 4, 2026.
9. Center for Drug Evaluation and Research (CDER). Evrysdi (risdiplam) product approval package: US Food and Drug Administration (FDA). https://www.accessdata.fda.gov/scripts/cder/daf/index.cfm?event=overview.process&varApplNo=213535. Accessed March 4, 2026.
10. Center for Drug Evaluation and Research (CDER). Viltepso (viltolarsen) product approval package: US Food and Drug Administration (FDA). https://www.accessdata.fda.gov/scripts/cder/daf/index.cfm?event=overview.process&varApplNo=212154. Accessed March 4, 2026.
11. Cooperative International Neuromuscular Research Group Natural History Database. https://cinrgresearch.org/. Accessed March 4, 2026.

12. NeuroNEXT database. https://neuronext.org/. Accessed March 4, 2026.
13. National Institutes of Health. Request for Information: FDA-NIH resource on terminology for clinical research notice number: NOT-OD-24-112. https://grants.nih.gov/grants/guide/notice-files/NOT-OD-24-112.html. Accessed March 4, 2026.
14. Pediatric Neuromuscular Clinical Research Network database. https://neuromuscularstudygroup.org/resources/. Accessed March 4, 2026.
15. Johnsen SP, Baas P, Sørensen JB, et al. Advancing real-world research in thoracic malignancies: learnings from the international I-O Optimise initiative. *Future Oncol.* 2025;21(7):867-878. https://doi.org/10.1080/14796694.2025.2466416
16. The Real-World Evidence Collaborative at the Margolis Institute at Duke University. https://healthpolicy.duke.edu/projects/real-world-evidence-collaborative. Accessed February 9, 2026.
17. The Real-World Evidence Collaborative. International Society for Pharmacoepidemiology. https://www.pharmacoepi.org/communities/sigs/rwe-collaborative/. Accessed March 4, 2026.

11 Data Available and Data Issues for Real-World Studies

Kit N. Simpson, DrPH, MPH

The 21st Century Cures Act passed by Congress in 2016 had a huge effect on the use of real-world data (RWD) in US research and the approaches used by US health systems to improve care. One of the goals of the act was to facilitate research collaboration and data sharing to better use large, new archival data resources (electronic health records [EHRs], billing records, and patient registry data) to measure the effectiveness of new therapies and to improve diffusion of medical innovations and access to treatments for patients.[1] It also charged the US Food and Drug Administration (FDA) with developing mechanisms for using real-world evidence (RWE) for informing treatment, program, or policy decisions by using RWD to augment efficacy information from clinical trials with effectiveness information from routine practice settings.

Health services researchers have been using RWD for decades to examine access to quality of care, treatment adherence, and variations in everyday practice settings. However, before 2016, such data were rarely used to inform new drug approvals. The act changed the perceived value of RWD and fostered the rapid development of quasi-experimental research designs. The National Institutes of Health (NIH) and the Agency for Healthcare Research and Quality (AHRQ) grant applications using RWD were increasingly funded to examine differences between efficacy and effectiveness, geographic variations in access, and quality improvements. At the same time, universities experienced an increased demand for training of PhD students and clinical researchers in the appropriate use of RWD and quasi-experimental designs.

Now, nearly a decade after the act passed, RWD resources are much more plentiful. However, they are often more expensive to access, because commercial vendors have entered the market and government agencies have increased charges or changed access from physical data licensures to cloud-based "seat licensure" payments.

The current market for RWD is in flux, which makes it hard to describe succinctly in a textbook. The proliferation of commercial vendors who sell or license the use of RWD and the proposed changes by the Centers for Medicare & Medicaid Services (CMS) in ways to access their data means that the situation in 1 month may change a few months later. It is still essential for data users to understand the basics of how these data are derived and structured.

This chapter first describes the three types of data submission forms that are used to structure and submit archival billing data and provides structured comparisons of different datasets. Examples of RWD extracted from EHRs and patient registry data help to better illustrate these points.

OVERVIEW OF RWD SOURCES AND DATA CHARACTERISTICS

Real-world data from various sources is used to complement findings from clinical trials and helps to inform treatment decisions, assess safety and effectiveness, and support regulatory decisions. They are used to measure health-system performance and examine

DOI: 10.37573/9781585287666.011

provider responses to reimbursement, regulation, or policy changes. Common data sources include EHRs, claims databases, patient registries, and digital health technologies. **Table 11-1** contains some examples but not a comprehensive listing, because data sources, vendors, and access rules change often. Thus, a comprehensive list would quickly become outdated. The fact that a research project is often limited to a subset of RWD that is available to a given researcher or institution is an important point and one that often catches novice researchers by surprise.

MEDICAL SERVICE BILLING DATA

Medical service billing data were the first types of data available to all researchers for RWE studies.[2] The AHRQ's Healthcare Cost and Utilization Project (HCUP) was a catalyst for studies using billing data to examine access, quality, and outcomes of care under real practice conditions, making this type of data easily available for researchers across the United States. These data sources were undervalued until the advent of the HCUP, a federal and state partnership. Once accessing billing data became easily available, publications using RWD blossomed and provided important insights into how to improve healthcare policy and processes. The importance of billing data for examining RWE lies in the fact that the medical bills (whether paid by an insurer, patients, or resulting in a "bad debt" write off) are the footprints of the medical care process and contain essential information useful for research, policy, and program evaluation and quality improvement.

Medical bills have patient demographic, diagnosis, procedure, provider type, resource use measures, and charge data. Electronic payment records have (mostly) all of these plus the actual payment amount, patient share of payment, payment denials, and insurance type. Thus, these data are a gold mine for investigators who wish to pose questions about access, cost, and quality of current medical practice, as well as specific examinations of new drugs, procedures, population health indicators, and budget impacts.

It is important to remember that billing data are "garbage data"—records that are residuals of the billing and payment process, not designed to capture detailed medical symptoms and outcomes. For that reason, they can be difficult to work with and may not be able to answer important questions about details of care, severity, or symptoms. Furthermore, billing data often have rudimentary data dictionaries, which is a limitation to most studies using this type of RWD.

TABLE 11-1. Examples of Archival Billing Dataset Characteristics

Dataset Name	Abbreviation and Data Form(s)	Population	Years (lag time)	Source
National inpatient sample	HCUP NIS (UB04 data)	20% sample of inpatient admissions for about 46 states	1988–2024 (18 months)	AHRQ
State inpatient data	HCUP SID (UB04 data)	All inpatient admission for a state for a calendar year	Varies by state (18 months)	AHRQ or individual state agencies
MarketScan® Commercial Data	MSC (UB04, CPT, SDF data)	All bills for enrolled patients from a changing cohort of large insurers	Data from 2013 to present (6 months)	Merative MarketScan Databases®, Merative, Ann Arbor, MI
Medicare 5% limited dataset	Medicare 5% LDS (UB04, CPT)	All bills for a 5% sample (18 months)	Data linkable by patient from 2015 and onwards	CMS

AHRQ = Agency for Healthcare Research and Quality; CMS = Centers for Medicare & Medicaid Services; HCUP NIS = Healthcare Cost and Utilization Project National Inpatient Sample; HCUP SID = Healthcare Cost and Utilization Project State Inpatient Databases; LDS = limited dataset.

DESCRIPTION OF DATA FORMS USED FOR STRUCTURING MEDICAL SERVICE BILLING DATA

It is vitally important to understand the data submission forms used to structure the data at the source (hospital, surgery center, inpatient rehabilitation hospital, skilled nursing facility, medical office, laboratory, outpatient service center, hospice, or pharmacy). Originally submitted on paper, they are now transmitted electronically with rare exceptions. There are three main forms: the UB04, the CMS 1500, and the Standard Drug Form. Examples of these forms are provided in **Figure 11-1**. The forms, format, and type of data collected were developed for and used in specific settings by providers. Information is not standardized across forms.

The UB04 form (also called the CMS 1450) meets billing requirements specified in the Uniform Budget Act of 2004.[3] It became the official billing form for the CMS in 2007 and is used by institutional providers, such as hospitals, nursing facilities, outpatient surgery centers, and other facilities. It contains multiple ICD-10 diagnosis and procedure codes, diagnosis-related groups (DRGs) for hospital admissions only, and patient age, sex, race, insurer, resource use, admission source, and discharge destination codes.

The CMS 1500 form is used for provider billing and is also known as "Part B billing." It is submitted by physicians, laboratories, imaging centers, infusion providers, and others who provide professional services to patients. This form has space for four ICD-10 diagnosis codes and requires procedures to be coded using CPT codes. Thus, hospital surgery may generate two forms: a UB04 form billing for the facility's use using ICD-10 procedure codes and surgeon/anesthesiology professional services bills using CPT procedure codes. The use of different procedure coding is one of the issues that can complicate the use of these data for research.

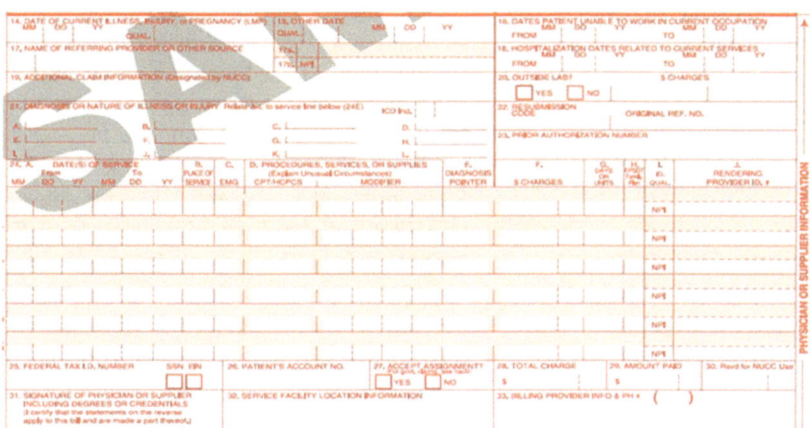

The **UB04** (**CMS 1450**) is a facility **claim form** used by hospitals, nursing facilities, inpatient, and other facility providers. On the other hand, the **HCFA-1500** (**CMS 1500**) is a provider **claim form** filed by individual doctors and practices, nurses, and professionals, including therapists, laboratories and outpatient clinics. **Prescription Claim** is submitted by outpatient and retail pharmacies.

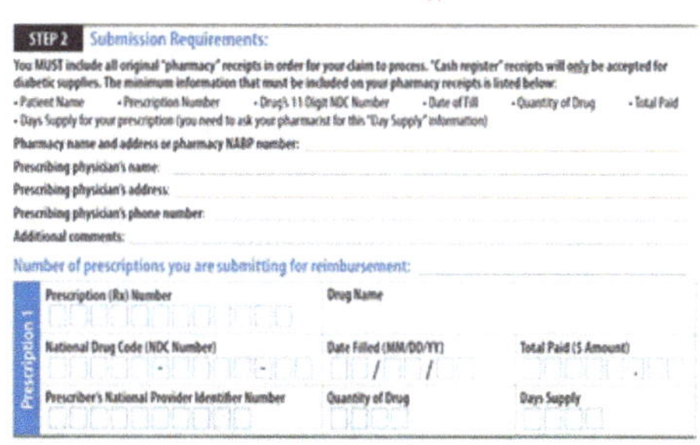

STEP 2 Submission Requirements:

You MUST include all original "pharmacy" receipts in order for your claim to process. "Cash register" receipts will only be accepted for diabetic supplies. The minimum information that must be included on your pharmacy receipts is listed below:

- Patient Name • Prescription Number • Drug's 11 Digit NDC Number • Date of Fill • Quantity of Drug • Total Paid
- Days Supply for your prescription (you need to ask your pharmacist for this "Day Supply" information)

Pharmacy name and address or pharmacy NABP number:

Prescribing physician's name:

Prescribing physician's address:

Prescribing physician's phone number:

Additional comments:

Number of prescriptions you are submitting for reimbursement:

Prescription 1

Prescription (Rx) Number | Drug Name

National Drug Code (NDC Number) | Date Filled (MM/DD/YY) | Total Paid ($ Amount)

Prescriber's National Provider Identifier Number | Quantity of Drug | Days Supply

FIGURE 11-1. **Examples of formats used for submitting UB04, CPT, and prescription billing data.**

The Standard Drug Form (SDF) is used by retail or outpatient pharmacies that fill prescriptions. It contains 11-digit National Drug Codes (NDCs), which are issued by the FDA for approved medications. National Drug Codes are complex to use in research, because each combination of the drug compound, manufacturer, dose, and formulation has its own NDC. Codes are also discontinued over time as patents expire, generic versions proliferate, and new drug combinations are approved. Thus, a researcher may need to use between 20 and 1,000 NDCs to capture bills for just one type of medication. In a recent study of two new injectable weight-loss drugs (semaglutide and tirzepatide), 33 different NDCs were needed to extract the prescription bills. For older drugs and drugs that have generic versions, the number of NDCs needed for extraction are much higher. It is important to note that drugs that require infusion, such as drugs for cancer treatments, may be billed by using CPT coding with specific codes issued by CMS.

In summary, to work successfully with archival billing data for RWE studies, one must consider several issues related to the selection of data sources and definition of study measures. Key takeaways include:

1. What are the diagnosis codes required to identify the study population?
2. Will those data be structured by a UB04, CPT, or SDF or by multiples of the three types?
3. How are all the individual bills going to be combined and operationalized into variables that measure disease severity, treatment(s) received, and patient outcome?
4. These datasets are big (often terabytes), and their handling and storage are protected under data use agreements; thus, where can these data be safely stored?
5. Is there a computer workstation available that can handle big data?
6. Given the complexity of generating an analytical dataset from these data, how will systematic quality control procedures be performed on the programming?
7. What study design and statistical approach is best to minimize biased results?

BRIEF DESCRIPTION OF THE HCUP AND ALL-PAYER STATE-SPECIFIC DATASETS

These three datasets were selected, because they are among the earliest RWD sets used for RWE studies and can serve as examples of specific data types. The National Inpatient Sample (NIS) for the Healthcare Cost and Utilization Project uses state data reported on the UB04 form used by healthcare institutions. The NIS is a 20% national sample of data from individual states that are members of the partnership. State membership varies by year; there were eight states represented in 1988 and 49 in 2024. Before purchasing the NIS or other HCUP databases, researchers are required to complete a training session, and their access is then limited by a data use agreement (DUA) specific to their project approved. The HCUP family of datasets includes the inpatient sample, emergency department (ED) sample, outpatient surgery sample, a sample of pediatric events, and a special sample of data that is linked so that hospital readmissions can be examined. The HCUP also contains state-specific data consisting of all inpatient, ED visits, or outpatient surgery records for a year for the state, data that can also be accessed through individual state agencies. The HCUP State Inpatient Databases (SID) are delivered to AHRQ and standardized by using the HCUP variable names. The datasets for specific states have DUAs that set limits to each state's data use based on that state's legislation. Thus, some HCUP SID data contain encrypted linkage variables that allow examination of utilization by specific patient groups and/or identification of readmissions, and some states' SID data also have hospital identifiers that can be linked with the American Hospital Association survey datasets. Furthermore, the cost of licensing these data varies greatly across states. One important point for using HCUP data within the limitations of the DUA is that no results may be reported for categories of variables with fewer than 11 patients in each category. This is strictly enforced by AHRQ checking published studies owing to the critical nature of the data for protection of patient anonymity. The HCUP website has well-documented data dictionaries and lists and contact information for the state partners who contribute all-payer discharge data to AHRQ.

COMPARISON OF FOUR DATA SOURCES: EXAMPLE OF TELEHEALTH VISITS

Publicly available licensed data are increasingly being used in telehealth studies; however, their usefulness for measuring telehealth utilization varies. Such data are expensive to license, and sometimes details that are important for telehealth studies (or other studies that require CPT or Healthcare Common Procedure Coding System [HCPCS] codes) may not be part of their documentation. Thus, investigators are left to learn by trial and error, and expensive licensing mistakes are not unusual. A recent analysis by this author used CMS 1500-formatted outpatient data from 2022 to describe the characteristics important for telehealth measurement for licensed data that rely on ICD-10, CPT, HCPCS, and NDCs for structuring events.

The four data sources compared in this analysis were MarketScan® Commercial, Medicare and Medicaid data from the Merative family of datasets, and the Medicare limited dataset 5% sample from CMS. However, there are many other commercial and public sources of CMS 1500 (Part B data) that could be used for similar studies.

The first step in a study like this was to construct an electronic phenotype to be used for data extraction. SAS version 9.4 (SAS Institute, Cary, NC) was used to extract the data, because the datasets were stored in an SAS format. However, other statistical or data manipulation programs would also work. The phenotype extraction code is shown in **Figure 11-2**. Three types of variables were used for extraction: CPT codes specific for telehealth visit billing; CPT Modifier codes that were added to billing codes for other types of visits to indicate that the visit was delivered via telehealth; and a location of service code, which indicated that the bill was for a telehealth service.

The same analyses were performed for all four datasets to compare volume, national reach, potential missingness owing to data structure, and population rates of telehealth use by state (except for Medicaid data, which does not have geographic identifiers) and to show the following:

1. Frequencies of events and the descriptive statistics for beneficiaries generating the events
2. Underascertainment bias in databases that contain only one Modifier code
3. Heat maps of state rates of telehealth use per 100 beneficiaries for 2022 for two age groups
4. Most common primary diagnoses for telehealth visits/consults

Medicare LDS 5% Sample Age > 64 for Year 2022

We used the following CPT, HCPCS Modifier, and Place of service codes. (All data set extractions used a similar approach.)

```
IF ProcedureCode1 in:
('99421','99422','99423','99441','99442','99443','99446','99447','99448','99449','99451','99452','G0406','G0407','
G0408','G0425','G0426','G0427','G0459','G0508','G0509','G2010','G2012','G2061 ','G2062','G2063','G2250','G2
251','G2252') then Telehealth=1;

IF ProcedureCodeModifier1 in: ('G0','GT','GQ','95','93') then Telehealth=1;

IF ProcedureCodeModifier2 in: ('G0','GT','GQ','95','93') then Telehealth=1;

If Placeofservice=2 then Telehealth=1;
```

FIGURE 11-2. **SAS program used to extract telehealth visits from data.**

The telehealth electronic phenotype was applied to all four datasets for 2022, yielding just over 27 million telehealth visits/consults. These data represent billed telehealth utilization by nearly 35 million beneficiaries from all 50 states. The mean use of telehealth in 2022 for insured patients was 78 visits per 100 individuals. For commercially insured patients, state telehealth use rates ranged from 25 to 242 annual visits per 100 people younger than age 65 (**Figure 11-3**). In contrast, telehealth use rates ranged from 21 to 122 telehealth visits per 100 Medicare beneficiaries age 65 and older.

Table 11-2 shows that the Medicare 5% sample was superior to the MarketScan® datasets in this particular type of analysis. It had the advantages of including all Modifier codes, variables on race, dual Medicare/Medicaid eligibility status, date of death, state of patient residence, counties, charges, payments, coinsurance, and deductibles. Furthermore, the Medicare 5% sample would be linked to social determinants of health and rurality data.

The MarketScan® datasets also have a number of advantages. They contain prescription records and calculate inpatient physician payment amounts from Part B bills, providing a variable that shows this amount on the relevant hospital admission record. This is a great help in estimating total hospitalization costs. It is important to note that each dataset has advantages and drawbacks that may or may not be important for a specific analysis. The dataset should be based on the research question posed.

EXAMPLE STUDIES USING RWD IN RWE STUDIES

State Discharge Data

State all-payer databases, or HCUP SID, and state ED databases data are especially useful for program evaluation studies. For example, Curfman and colleagues used the ED and Hospital UB04 records for program participants

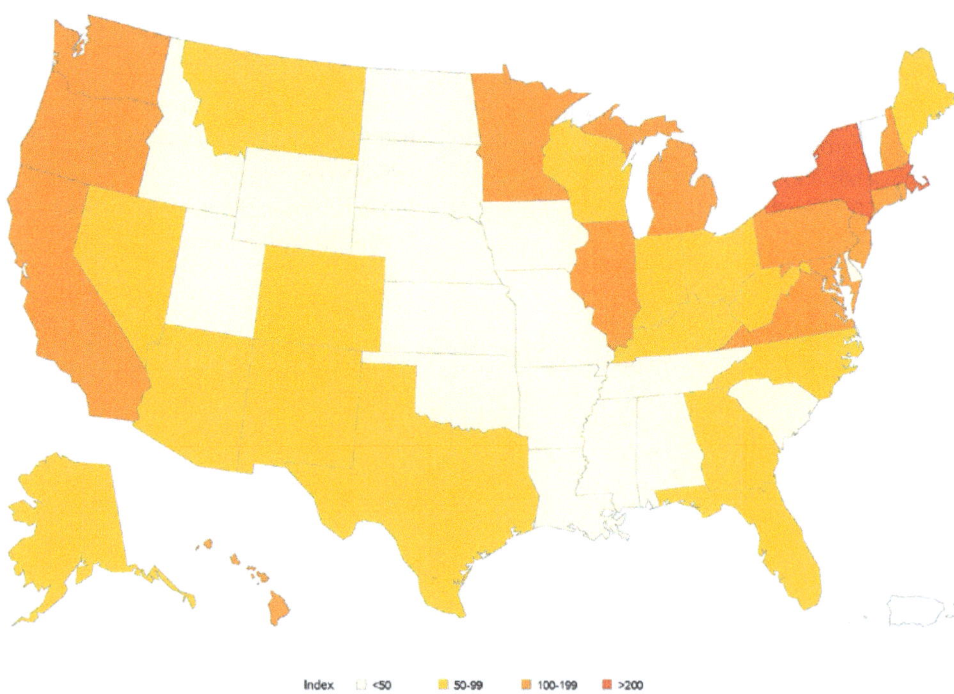

FIGURE 11-3. Example of telehealth heat map showing population rates for US states based on beneficiary data included in 2022 data sample (rates for other years and samples may differ).

TABLE 11-2. Comparisons: Number of Events in 2022, Telehealth Coding, Population Size, and Potential for Selection Bias

	MarketScan® Commercial	MarketScan® Medicare	Medicare LDS 5% Sample	MarketScan® Medicaid
Total events	15,903,345	862,628	1,494,479	8,835,391
Beneficiaries in this dataset	19,136,928	1,371,935	3,414,596	11,016,757
Type of coding used in extract:				
CPT	5.0%	11.8%	9.3%	2.4%
Modifier 1	37.5%	57.9%	64.6%	60.2%
Modifier 2	NA	NA	4.0%	NA
Place of service	57.5%	30.3%	22.2%	37.4%
Representative of state or US population	Uncertain, overall US representation, data are from commercially insured convenience sample from all states	Uncertain, overall US representation, data are from Medicare patients with supplemental commercial insurance convenience sample from all states	Representative, 5% sample of Medicare patients from all states	Uncertain, data from Medicaid patients from 10 representative, unknown states

LDS = limited dataset.

in Missouri to evaluate the effectiveness of the implementation of a "Wraparound Virtual Care" program for children with medical complexity. Data were accessed through the Hospital Industry Data Institute, which is the custodian of the Missouri ED and hospital all-payer data.[3] This retrospective pre-post analysis of data contained inpatient, outpatient, and ED utilization and charge records from before implementation and during the 2 years of the program. Eighty ($n=80$) children were included in the evaluation, and 75 had sufficient data for analysis. This is a very good level of linkage between program data and archival billing records. One of the most common problems in the use of billing data for program evaluation is that the "match" rate between program records and billing data is rarely perfect. Thus, a 94% match rate, as seen in the Curfman study, should be considered very good. The authors compared medical care utilization measures for the 12 months before enrollment to measures for the 24 months in the program. They observed that patients had a 35.3% reduction in hospitalizations ($p=0.027$), a 43.9% reduction in emergency visits ($p=0.0005$), and a 16.9% reduction in overall charges ($p=0.145$). Of note, the charge measure did not reach statistical significance. This is not unusual for programs with fewer than 100 enrollees. Minimally important difference studies for costs show that costs (because of their distribution and variance) may be expected to require a much greater sample size to achieve sufficient statistical power compared with outcomes, such as admissions.[4] The authors also analyzed measures of parent satisfaction and reached an exceptionally high response rate (70%); 90% of parents reported high satisfaction with the program. This study illustrates that even smaller programs can use RWD to generate RWE.

MarketScan® Data for Medicare Enrollees with Supplemental Commercial Insurance

Commercial insurance databases have an advantage when data from all three forms (the UB04, CMS 1500, and SDF) are used to construct detailed risk measures to understand their effects on outcomes. These databases often contain a very large population and can furnish a complete picture of medical conditions and resource use. One problem with using these data is that patients move in and out of the cohort as their insurance provider changes. Thus, the data may be both right and left censored. The obvious solution is to specify a specific time of coverage, but this approach may introduce its own form of selection bias, because patients with continuous coverage may be quite different from patients with interrupted coverage. However, commercial insurance data may be extremely useful for marginal comparisons or snapshots of population issues. If a study time horizon is a year or less, there may be only minor bias from censoring. Furthermore, the fact that these datasets contain data from UB04, CMS 1500, and SDF allows the researcher to measure nearly all covered care and often also care that has payment denied, because these records are retained in most datasets. The ability to have all submitted bills makes it possible to construct a very comprehensive set of baseline variables that may be used to examine how people move through a healthcare system and can be benchmarked against guidelines for continuity of care.

This approach was used in a study to examine the effect of frailty on medical care payments/costs.[5] The researchers were able to control for demographics, inpatient care during baseline, comorbidities recorded during any baseline inpatient admission (Charlson score), baseline outpatient comorbidities (Elixhauser score), polypharmacy, use of Beers Criteria drugs, rural residence, and region of residence. This is an older study, but it illustrates the power of commercial databases for research. MarketScan® Medicare data for patients with supplementary commercial health insurance from Truven Analytics was used to examine the effects of frailty on resource use and payments for patients over 12 months. A cohort of more than 3 million Medicare patients with supplementary private insurance coverage was partitioned into three groups based on the Faurot frailty score: Robust, Pre Frail, and Frail. Data from a 3-month "look-back" baseline period was used to construct all the risk variables. The remaining 9 months of data were aggregated into measures of resource use (office visits and hospital, ED, and skilled nursing facility admissions) and calculated insurance payments for each resource type as well as total payments. Patients with frailty were found to have higher costs than pre-frail and robust patients, as was expected. The researchers then estimated observed mean costs for five costing models with different numbers of baseline control variables. The mean cost difference between frail and robust individuals in Model 1 (fewest variables) was $23,117, whereas the cost difference owing to frailty in Model 5 (most comprehensive model) was $10,690. Thus, the marginal difference estimate for frail and robust patients decreased by $12,427, a 54% decrease when the risks at baseline were more stringently controlled. However, all the baseline demographic and risk measured were statistically significant in Model 5, despite some correlations between variables, and the baseline variables had different but complementary effects in the models. One major lesson from this study was that observational studies of disease risk or cost of illness for Medicare patients may be biased if a frailty measure is not included as an adjustor. However, other measures, such as polypharmacy, use of Beers Criteria drugs, inpatient admissions with Charlson score, Elixhouser score (for outpatient data), and demographic and rural residence variables may all contribute to the magnitude of the difference in observed population costs. This paper provides a nice example of the potential magnitude of omitted variable bias in cost studies using billing data.

EHR DATA STUDY EXAMPLES

Since the passing of the Health Information Technology for Economic and Clinical Health Act in 2009, the use of EHR in healthcare institutions has become institutionalized.[6] The increasing interoperability of EHR data is fueling small and large studies to assess practice patterns, facilitate practice change, and examine outcomes for patients with rare or chronic conditions. The following publications illustrate very different uses of EHR data: (1) a small study to document feeding patterns for infants who required noninvasive respiratory support (NIRS) during a hospital admission, (2) a cluster-randomized trial to implement screening for intimate partner violence (IPV), and (3) a paper comparing kidney transplant registry data to a vendor collaboration of Epic EHR system users called the Cosmos dataset.

Taken together, these studies illustrate the wide variations in how EHR data can be used to generate RWE.

In the first study, the authors were concerned about the limited safety and efficacy data available on the use of oral feeding for infants on NIRS. Barnes and colleagues[7] used a well-defined protocol approved by the institutional review board to extract data for 201 infants in one medical center. They found that a high proportion of infants (45%) received oral feeding when on NIRS, even though safety and efficacy for this approach is not clear. The study also found that swallowing and breathing issues were not recorded in the EHR, and there was a low rate (17%) of referrals of these babies to feeding specialist consults. The authors concluded that, despite limited evidence for the safety and efficacy of oral feeding for babies on NIRS, the practice is common, documentation is sparse, and experts are rarely consulted. They recommended that researchers in this area employ rigorous prospective study designs and use reliable and valid outcome measures to establish evidence-based clinical practice and reduce variability in practice. Even a small study can help to identify a high need for new evidence of efficacy and safety to improve current practice.

The second example used EHR records in a stepped-wedge randomized controlled trial to assess uptake and outcomes of a primary care program to identify and manage IPV. Lenert and colleagues[8] used a multifactorial intervention-screening function within the EHR system to identify women who were eligible for screening. They modified the system with a confidential compartment for responses to ensure patient safety and used an IPV protocol to guide clinician responses. This study used the EHR system for three tasks: (1) to identify eligible patients, (2) to field confidential questions, and (3) to collect follow-up data on outcomes. The researchers reported the rate at which eligible patients were screened and the rate at which patients at risk for IPV were detected by the screening intervention. The intervention had significant effects on the overall rate of screening for IPV, increasing the rate of screening from 45.2% to 65.3% when the noninterruptive alert was active. They concluded that a highly private approach to screening for IPV that addresses potential patient safety issues may be necessary to achieve adequate screening rates for IPV.

Real-world evidence studies are increasingly leveraging the vast, integrated clinical data within Epic's Cosmos to study various health conditions and outcomes.[9] These studies complement traditional randomized controlled trials by offering insights into real-world practice and patient populations. However, data in Cosmos have been standardized and recoded, so it is important to understand the strengths and limitations of these new "Big Data" resources. Mankowski and colleagues[10] compared the characteristics of kidney transplant recipients (KTR) identified among the 274 million patients included in Cosmos in 2022 to the 69,418 KTR recorded in the Scientific Registry of Transplant Recipients (SRTR). The authors examined demographic and clinical variables and found that Cosmos data were consistent with the data from the SRTR cohort. They also noted that survival estimates were comparable for the two data sources, with minor differences in long-term survival at 7 years. They concluded that while Cosmos captures real-world clinical variability, which can introduce errors, and the SRTR uses structured data with standardized quality controls, the Cosmos dataset appears to be highly generalizable to the KTR population and holds great promise for future research in this area.

EXAMPLES OF REGISTRY DATA RESOURCES

Early registry data analyses tended to use a cohort study design, but today these data are used for many types of quasi-experimental studies, such as propensity score weighted analysis. Indeed, registry data may be used as part of cluster-randomized trials or other designs to explore new questions for specific patients included in registries. Because the development, access, construction, and use of registry data has evolved over decades, researchers can refer to a number of important resources. The AHRQ provides a "Registry of Patient Registries," an important resource that should be the first step of inquiry for anyone needing to access registry data.[11] They have also published a user's guide[12] that shows how the data can be used (1) to describe the natural history of disease, (2) to determine clinical effectiveness or cost-effectiveness of healthcare products and services, and (3) to measure or monitor safety, harm, and quality of care. They highlight the following details regarding patient registries: (1) data collection reflects usual care not a registry protocol; (2) the purpose of the registry is clearly defined before data are collected; (3) the variables in the registry have been clearly defined in an available code book; (4) the data collection is sufficient to define important clinical issues relevant to diagnosing, staging, and measuring clinical outcomes; (5) specific (nonroutine) clinical measures may be part of standard registry data collection (date of death, cause of death); and (6) nonclinical variables, such as admissions, length of stay, and cost, may be part of registry data, or the data may be linked to Medicare or Medicaid billing records.

RWE USE CASE FOR CANCER REGISTRY DATA LINKED TO CMS MEDICARE BILLING DATA

Booth and colleagues[13] provide an example of the use of linked registry and Medicare data in a natural experiment to provide RWE for guidelines to improve cancer survival. Clinical guidelines recommend 30 days of treatment with low molecular weight heparin (LMWH) to prevent venous thromboembolism after abdominal cancer surgery. However, utilization of LMWH after surgery is low. The authors used Surveillance, Epidemiology, and End Results cancer registry data linked to Medicare billing data from 2016–2017 to identify patients (age 65+) receiving surgery for colon cancer. They excluded cases with metastases from the sample and measured cancer-specific survival. Their premise was that LMWH has an antineoplastic effect (eg, by inhibiting angiogenesis in the tumor). They used propensity score treatment-weighted multivariable regression to compare survival in patients who received 30 days of LMWH with those who did not. Eight hundred patients (3.98%) received the LMWH prophylaxis. Overall survival and cancer-specific survival were better in patients who received LMWH prophylaxis ($p = 0.0017$ overall; $p = 0.02$ cancer-specific). A Cox regression showed improved overall survival with an adjusted hazards ratio (HR) of 0.66 (0.56–0.78) and a cancer-specific HR 0.56 (0.39–0.81) with LMWH prophylaxis. This study is an excellent example of the combined use of Surveillance, Epidemiology, and End Results registry data and Medicare billing data to identify RWE for differences in outcomes associated with adherence to guidelines.

CONCLUSION

The RWD used to produce RWE all originate from a medical care contact. Archival billing data are the footprints of the care process, and their content depends on how such data are structured. Three common forms—the UB04, the CMS 1500, and SDF—provide the structure and coding conventions for diagnoses and procedures. These forms are usually embedded in the billing software used by the facility or the provider. An important point is that the software or form used determines the data content, and that some data sources contain data from only one form. This means that the researcher and the reader of a study must recognize that each database will have its specific strengths and weaknesses, which are limitations to the results. The EHR and registry data usually draw data from clinical encounters and contain actual medical test results and discussions of symptoms, diagnoses, and the recommended or provided treatments. Their limitations lie more in the variations owing to the clinician who elicited and recorded the data. They include richer clinical content but may be less complete in terms of capturing all medical services provided for an episode of care. A patient who leaves the ED against medical advice and goes to another ED the next day may not be captured in the medical record of the first hospital. Furthermore, a record of a drug prescription issued does not mean that the medication was dispensed or that it was taken. The documentation and code books for RWD are often sparse and/or difficult to access, so it is a good idea to seek advice from clinicians and researchers who are familiar with the diseases and data used in each study. Despite limitations in the data, RWE is essential for understanding issues in access to care, cost of care, and outcomes from different programs and treatments when they are provided in real-world settings.

REFERENCES

1. The 21st Century Cures Act. https://www.congress.gov/bill/114th-congress/house-bill/34. Accessed March 4, 2026.
2. Barron JJ, Willey VJ, Doherty BT, et al. The Healthcare Integrated Research Database (HIRD) as a real-world data source for pharmacoepidemiologic research. *Pharmacoepidemiol Drug Saf.* 2025;34(2):e70110. https://doi.org/10.1002/pds.70110
3. Curfman AL, Haycraft M, McSwain SD, et al. Implementation and evaluation of a wrap-around virtual care program for children with medical complexity. *Telemed J E Health.* 2023;29(6):947-953. https://doi.org/10.1089/tmj.2022.0344
4. Dooley M, Simpson AN, Nietert PJ, et al. Minimally important difference in cost savings: Is it possible to identify an MID for cost savings? *Health Serv Outcomes Res Method.* 2021;21:131-144. https://doi.org/10.1007/s10742-020-00233-5
5. Simpson KN, Seamon BA, Hand BN, et al. Effect of frailty on resource use and cost for Medicare patients. *J Comp Eff Res.* 2018. https://doi.org/10.2217/cer-2018-0029
6. National Library of Medicine. National Center for Biotechnology Information. https://www.ncbi.nlm.nih.gov/books/NBK562581. Accessed March 3, 2026.
7. Barnes CK, Simpson KN, Wilmskoetter J, et al. Feeding infants on noninvasive respiratory support: practice at one academic medical center. *Am J Speech Lang Pathol.* 2025;34(2):617-632. https://doi.org/10.1044/2024_AJSLP-24-00302
8. Lenert L, Rheingold AA, Simpson KN, et al. Electronic health record-based screening for intimate partner violence: a cluster randomized clinical trial. *JAMA Netw Open.* 2024;7(8):e2425070. https://doi.org/10.1001/jamanetworkopen.2024.25070
9. Tarabichi Y, Frees A, Honeywell S, et al. The Cosmos collaborative: a vendor-facilitated electronic health record data aggregation platform. *ACI Open.* 2021;5(1):e36-e46. https://doi.org/10.1055/s-0041-1731004
10. Mankowski MA, Bae S, Strauss AT, et al. Generalizability of kidney transplant data in electronic health records - The Epic Cosmos database vs the Scientific Registry of Transplant Recipients. *Am J Transplant.* 2025;25(4):744-755. https://doi.org/10.1016/j.ajt.2024.11.008
11. NCBI link: Rockville, MD: Agency for Healthcare Research and Quality (US). https://effectivehealthcare.ahrq.gov/products/registry-of-patient-registries/overview. Accessed April 6, 2026.
12. Gliklich RE, Leavy MB, Dreyer NA, eds. *Registries for Evaluating Patient Outcomes: A User's Guide* [Internet]. 4th ed. Rockville, MD: Agency for Healthcare Research and Quality; 2020.
13. Booth A, Brinton D, Donahue C, et al. Extended pharmacologic prophylaxis for venous thromboembolism after colon cancer surgery is associated with improved long-term survival: a natural experiment in the chemotherapeutic benefit of heparin derivatives. *Ann Surg.* 2024;280(4):595-603. https://doi.org/10.1097/SLA.0000000000006376

Considerations in Interpreting Real-World Evidence

12

Todd L. Wandstrat, RPh, PharmD, and
Annie N. Simpson, PhD

DEFINITIONS OF REAL-WORLD DATA AND REAL-WORLD EVIDENCE

Real-world data (RWD) relate to patient health status and/or the delivery of healthcare routinely collected from a variety of sources. Examples of RWD include data derived from electronic health records (EHRs), medical claims data, data from product or disease registries, and data gathered from other sources (such as digital health technologies) that can inform on health status.[1] A more inclusionary definition of RWD is data that are obtained outside the context of randomized controlled trials (RCTs).[2] Real-world data may be used in studies to produce real-world evidence (RWE), which can inform stakeholders of the real-world effectiveness of an intervention and provide data regarding specific patient types that may most benefit from an intervention.

Real-world evidence is generated from the analysis of RWD.[3] It can provide clinical evidence regarding the potential benefits and risk of an intervention.[1] Regardless of the origin of RWD and the subsequent analysis, there are strengths and weaknesses associated with its use.

RWE CHARACTERISTICS

Real-world data and RWE can inform clinical decision-making, aid in clinical trial construction, provide estimates of intervention effectiveness, add regulatory support to a proposed intervention, assess the quality of practice, detect medical errors, and provide data for comparative effectiveness studies. Real-world data itself can be utilized in a broader range of trial designs, such as observational, exploratory, case series, adaptive design, historical control, and prevention trials compared with data collected in the construct of an RCT. Using RWD to generate RWE offers several methodologic and practical advantages, including the following[3]:

- Eliminating strict eligibility criteria
- Conducting quicker and less costly analyses
- Expanding the scope of research possibilities
- Enabling exploration of patient behavior
- Facilitating subpopulation, generalizability, and modeling analyses

CHALLENGES OF USING RWD TO PRODUCE RWE

There are several challenges in utilizing RWD, and bias considerations are discussed later in the chapter.[4] Informatic challenges can arise from the nonstandardized data collection methods practiced in the real world, including incomplete data collections, missing data, and lack of harmonization across various data sources. Within a specific data source, data terminology, dataset ontology, and dataset construction can reduce the usability of data for a specific study and limit the data interpretability. Data access issues, owing to privacy or nefarious use concerns, can limit the aggregation of population data, thus reducing the significance and generalizability of the

DOI: 10.37573/9781585287666.012

subsequent RWE analyses. Data transfer strategies can sometimes be cumbersome and not accommodate large data transfers. Strategies to allay privacy fears have not come to practical fruition. The competitive nature of the US healthcare system restricts the partnering of data and sharing of insights.

RCTs VERSUS RWD/RWE STUDIES

Randomized controlled trials have traditionally been considered the "gold standard" in that they can establish causal evidence and accurately quantify treatment effects, albeit within a narrowly defined population and set of conditions. With generalizability limited by strict inclusion criteria, it is difficult to apply the findings of an RCT to diverse populations/situations.[3]

In contrast, RWE can only be utilized to support causal effect. As such, it should not be looked upon as a competitor or replacement for RCTs but as a complementary study strategy that more completely informs a stakeholder of the value and utility of an intervention in a diverse population. Real-world data can reduce evidence gaps that are common in newly devised interventions. Data generated by RCTs can address efficacy, whereas RWD has the potential to answer effectiveness and real practice settings questions. Additionally, RWD incorporates variable treatments, unplanned follow-ups, and a variety of comparators with minimal criteria for subject inclusion.[5] Please refer to Chapter 5 for a complete discussion regarding RCTs and their methodological components.

PERSPECTIVE AND USE OF RWE

When considering the perspective of RWE, the focus is the user or consumer of the research. The research question(s) depends on the type of audience or consumer. The use of perspective is different from that which is utilized for cost-effective analysis and pharmacoeconomic modeling where the object or subject of the analysis is the perspective.

If RWE is to be utilized for academic purposes and/or scholarly publication, there will necessarily be a higher level of scrutiny and review of the data. If the consumer of the data or evidence is a biotechnology or pharmaceutical company, the focus and reporting of the data will take on a unique approach. In an organized healthcare system, such as an integrated delivery network, certain data points or a singular analysis may be adequate.

RWD AND COMMON DATA MODEL FUNDAMENTALS

The origin of RWD is from a variety of sources, and the number and type of sources increase every year. The advent of artificial intelligence (AI) and large language models will undoubtably add to the data accessibility for RWD. Sources of RWD include EHRs, administrative and claims data, registries, patient-generated data from websites and wearable sensors, and health-related data from mobile devices.[4] Each source of RWD has its own challenges related to incomplete or missing data, lack of common structure, and extraction difficulties.

COMMON DATA MODELS AND RESOURCES

The need for common data models (CDMs) evolves from the disparate RWE data available. They combine data from multiple sources and locations into a common format, allowing for identical queries across multiple datasets and ensuring interoperability across all data sites.[6] Grouping them in this way increases the sample size and makes a more powerful analysis. There are many CDM methodologies, and we will review the most utilized ones.

The Observational Medical Outcomes Partnership (OMOP) is an open-source CDM that utilizes standardized structure and content in comparison to disparate observational databases to increase the strength of RWD analysis and the evidence derived from it. The OMOP and its resources provide tools to perform an observational patient-level data analysis. Different databases often have different nomenclatures and even separate data fields for variables of interest, such as drug names, procedure codes, hospitalization days, and physiologic endpoints. The OMOP allows for a common representation of different variables and groupings, enabling the analysis of the aggregated data.[7] The OMOP provides tools and tutorials to develop CDMs, analyze data, and extract, transform, and load (ETL) data. The ETL process allows for the alignment of disparate datasets and facilitates the development of a CDM.

Fast Healthcare Interoperability Resources (FHIR) is a standard for healthcare data exchange, published by Health Level Seven International.[8] Health Level Seven International is a not-for-profit organization that provides an integrated and comprehensive framework for health information exchange, integration, and sharing. Currently the US Centers for Medicare & Medicaid Services is considering a transition to a FHIR-based quality measurement system. Central to the FHIR system is an exchange framework that allows for EHR information to be shared between clinicians and organizations. Within its various systemic components there are tools to convert EHR data to a common architecture and a powerful quality measures development and reporting tool. Therefore, if the consumer of the RWE is a government organization or the purpose of the research is to share among clinicians, FHIR is a valuable resource with which to develop the CDM for analysis.[8]

The Clinical Data Interchange Standards Consortium (CDISC) was formed in 1997 to develop global standards in medical research for aligning data and research to positively influence global health. Membership includes researchers, government organizations, pharmaceutical companies, service providers, and regulatory agencies.[9] Central to CDISC's mission is standards expansion, reduced variability, and increased automation of data integration to deliver stakeholder value.[10] As with other CDM enablers, CDISC provides a wide variety of tools to allow for complete digitalization of a study and its results. Key to the development of the CDM in RWD studies is the ability for the CDISC tools to allow for mapping of terminology and meanings that do not match. The quality, integration, and traceability of RWD is increased throughout the CDISC process and allows for feedback on study design and execution. Feasibility studies and pilot studies can be reviewed, and methodologies can evolve to support RWD questions focused and aligned for specific research purposes.[11]

OpenEHR is a nomenclature for healthcare solutions that are interoperative. In response to a general lack of continuity of care, openEHR tools and solutions were developed in the late 1990s and early 2000s. Throughout the early 21st century, its stakeholder group grew, and in 2008, a prototype architecture was developed. Four programs make up the essence and focus of openEHR. Specification allows for the definition of query and model languages as well as the contents and overarching architecture of the program(s). Clinical modeling builds on the specification program and allows for international standards in model content and templates. Open-source coding and implementation allows the software program to build bespoke tools and healthcare information system components. Wrapped around the ecosystem is the education program, which provides users with an efficient way to use the openEHR outputs in a local language and cultural context.[12]

Before embarking on large examinations of variables across disparate datasets and committing economic and research resources, feasibility studies assist with understanding the bounds of what can be accomplished. When there has been little research published in a specific area, feasibility studies can inform future study designs by identifying areas to refine or improve upon methodological deficiencies. They can focus on the practicality of the analysis and adaptability of the RWD results to healthcare systems in general.[13] Practical feedback from feasibility studies can inform the efficiency of data extraction methods and provide insight into the architecture of CDM construction. Most importantly, feasibility studies help to refine the research question or hypothesis.

Because most RWD research involves multiple data sources gathered at a variety of physical and data sites, the use of a single pilot site can provide feedback regarding the probable success of data-gathering efforts and the extraction success of specific variables from datasets. Additionally, the use of a pilot site can increase the understanding of what data variables and architecture exist at other study locations. This can increase success of the research endeavor and the extraction success of relevant study variables and data. The many benefits of using a pilot site in conjunction with feasibility studies include the following[14]:

- Ensuring reliable data extraction from specific data sources, such as EHRs

- Assessing data quality in terms of completeness, accuracy, and consistency
- Refining research methodology and protocols
- Identifying key characteristics of the patient population
- Reducing overall study expenditures
- Enhancing generalizability of results through representative patient populations
- Determining technical capabilities required for data extraction and transfer
- Engaging stakeholders early in the research process
- Evaluating extraction methods and challenges in processing large datasets

EXTRACTION METHODOLOGY AND CHALLENGES OF PROCESSING LARGE DATA

Real-world data are collected during routine care. As a result, the exact data may not exist to answer any specific research question even though careful crafting of the research protocol and research question(s) is essential to success. Variables needed to answer the research question must be matched to the data source fields. One of the most time-consuming tasks of extracting RWD is the alignment of the variables required within the research protocol with the variables that live within the dataset. Equally important to research success is the methodology used to ETL the required RWD into an analyzable dataset. Key characteristics of the data, such as structured versus unstructured, common data fields, and where the data resides, inform the extraction methodology. For structured data, such as labs, data mining of the EHR will usually produce adequate results. Reasonable values (high and lows) should be established and programmed into data extraction to alert the researcher to spurious data, such as a patient age of 210 years. For unstructured data, such as healthcare provider notes, natural language processing can be utilized to analyze syntax and semantics, allowing for meaningful data contribution. Application programming interfaces can assist with automated data retrieval. This type of data extraction can save enormous amounts of time compared with manual extraction. For both structured and unstructured data, machine learning can be utilized to generate algorithms and patterns and extract relevant data. After extraction, the validity of the data must be carefully examined.

PRACTICAL CONSIDERATIONS FOR DESIGN AND CONDUCT OF RWE STUDIES

When designing a study to generate RWE, the research question should clarify the intent of the study but also ensure that the data will be able to support the question(s) being asked.[15] The research question should be asked in such a way that the direction of the effect being tested is clear and measurable, and the independent and dependent variables in the study are clearly stated. Often the data itself will drive what a researcher is able to study, particularly if the study is a retrospective design using data that already exist.

Prospective studies may have a broader ability to ask/answer research questions, because the data are collected after the study is developed and are often collected by the researchers. However, if the data being used in the prospective study are derived from sources not designed for research, such as EHRs, there may be limits on adding data elements specific to the study.

All studies intended to produce peer-reviewed evidence should consider and justify the sample size, the number of subjects being used for the study. For prospective studies, the sample size needed to find a difference in comparative groups may be calculated by using simple web-based calculators. However, it is important to ensure that the website being used is trustworthy. In retrospective studies, the sample size is often determined by the data that are readily available. In this case, a power analysis may be performed to estimate the power the study will have to find a difference if one truly exists (in a comparative study).

To run a sample size or power analysis, researchers must have a quantitative estimate of both the differences in outcomes expected between groups and the variation in the outcome measures. These are known measures that are used to calculate the unknowns (either the power or sample size). These estimates may come from prior peer-reviewed evidence, from sample data available to the researcher, or an educated guess of the minimum difference needed to be clinically or empirically significant.

BIAS IN REAL-WORLD STUDIES

Strengths and weaknesses exist in all study designs, but bias is one of the most important to understand, particularly because RWE studies do not randomize and include data that are generally collected for other purposes.[16] Bias in healthcare research refers to systematic errors that can occur during the design process, the conduct of the study, or the interpretation of results that leads to inaccurate conclusions.[17] A consumer of research evidence who is trying to judge whether the study is relevant for actionable change should be able to assess the bias and how the bias may influence the results.

Selection bias is the one most frequently encountered in RWE studies. It occurs when individuals included in a study are not representative of the broader population or the selection of individuals into study groups is not random. This can result in unrepresentative groups, which compromise the external validity or generalizability of a study. Selection bias may also impact internal validity if it systematically skews the results. As treatment groups are being developed in the real world, selection into a group is pragmatic as determined during clinical practice. For example, if health outcomes are being compared among individuals with type 2 diabetes who receive mono versus combination therapies, individuals receiving combination therapies may tend to have been in treatment longer and to have had more difficulty controlling their blood sugar. Thus, the monotherapy group may have less severe disease at baseline, making their treatment outcomes appear systematically better.

One way to examine whether comparison groups are similar is to look at the baseline descriptive statistics of the sample, often labeled "Table 1" in published studies. The comparison groups should be split up into columns where baseline characteristics are listed in the rows to facilitate comparisons. If the groups differ in any meaningful way, the researchers should detail how they addressed the imbalance. As mentioned above, even if the baseline characteristics of the groups are similar, if they are not representative of the general population of interest, then their external validity and ability to provide actionable evidence may be limited. There are study design and analysis techniques, such as propensity scoring, to deal with this type of bias, and these are discussed in Chapter 4.

Other common types of bias in RWE studies involve problems with the data. Misclassification bias occurs when data are entered incorrectly and patients are labeled in the wrong group for either exposure or outcome.[18] Nondifferential misclassification, which occurs equally across all study groups, biases results toward the null, making it harder to detect a true association. Differential misclassification can bias the result in an exaggeration or underestimate an association.

Attrition bias happens when participants are missing data or are lost to follow-up. Study results are distorted if those participants differ meaningfully from the ones who remained in the study.[19] Immortal time bias occurs when a study's period of observation is not long enough to capture the outcome of interest.[16,20] In RWE, this typically happens when the assignment of an individual's treatment status involves a delay or time period during which follow-up time is accrued—for example, waiting for a prescription to be dispensed after hospital discharge when discharge date defines the start of follow-up.[21] This wait period is immortal, because individuals in the treatment group, those getting the prescription, must be alive (or event-free) until this definition is satisfied.

Many other types of bias may occur in nonrandomized real-world studies; however, there are recommendations to mitigate threats of bias.[22] In fact, professional groups and societies have developed numerous sets of "study check lists" where the researcher or the consumer of research can systematically review details of a study to reduce or detect bias and confounding in nonrandomized studies.[23,24] An example of a high-quality checklist designed to evaluate nonrandomized comparative studies is the GRACE (Good Research for Comparative Effectiveness).[23] The principles listed in this checklist have been developed to help healthcare providers, researchers, journal readers, and editors evaluate key quality metrics in observational research studies of comparative effectiveness. Most checklists are specific to the type of study being evaluated, such as the CONSORT for RCTs, PRISMA for systematic reviews, STROBE for observational studies (not specific to comparative effectiveness), and EVEREST for economic evaluations.[24]

REGULATORY CONSIDERATIONS

As mentioned, US and international regulatory authorities have considered the use of RWE to supplement drug product approval applications. In the United States, the 21st Century Cures Act (2016) was designed to accelerate medical advances. The Food and Drug Administration (FDA) has developed a framework for evaluating RWE to support new indications of previously approved drugs and satisfy post-approval requirements.[25] Additionally the FDA has provided guidance for utilizing EHR and medical claims data in clinical studies to support regulatory decisions.[6]

Aligned with the FDA framework development, the European Medicines Agency initiated the Adaptive Pathways Pilot in 2014 that addresses the use of RWE in regulatory approval processes.[26] Subsequent to this project the Operational, Technical and Methodological (OPTIMAL) framework addressed how to integrate RWD/RWE into the approval process.[27] More recently, efforts have been made to standardize RWD within Europe with multinational initiatives. Guidelines issued by the Big Data Task Force Report (2019) discussed all forms of RWD, including social media, and provided recommendations for their regulatory acceptance, standardization, and harmonization.[28] These included proposed standards concerning dataset quality and RWD analytical methodologies.

The use of RWE for regulatory decision-making is a collaborative one. All stakeholders must have a voice within this evolving global regulatory environment to allow for aligned and positive contributions of RWD/RWE. That power of collaboration now includes the use of AI.

Throughout the last 50+ years, computing power and storage capacity have increased exponentially.[29] Moore's Law observes that the number of transistors on computer chips doubles approximately every 2 years, and by way of inference, so does computing power or ability. With increases in computational speed, the time to generate components of economic models has greatly decreased. Whereas it once took hours and days to "run" Markov models and sensitivity analyses, today these analyses can be completed within seconds or minutes after data are entered. Since the early 1990s, artificial neural networks have assisted in drug development and drug choice in disease states. Machine and deep learning have enabled prediction tools to assist healthcare professionals in the development of algorithm-only-based medicine and predictive diagnostic models.[30,31]

Although unstructured datasets of RWD have been a significant barrier to the generation of usable, generalizable, and adaptable RWE, there is light on the horizon. The use of natural language models can allow for divergent, unstructured datasets with missing data to be transformed into high-quality RWD and subsequent RWE. Data once unusable in RWD, such as clinical notes, laboratory data, and imaging, can now be utilized to construct variables.[32] Large language models, such as OpenAI's GPT-4, can assist researchers in translating text, interpreting images, writing code, classifying variables, and generating predictions.[33]

Recent guidelines have suggested appropriate uses for AI-based methods and the reporting of those evaluations.[34,35] Machine learning could be utilized to identify predictors of health outcomes, identify appropriate data given inclusion criteria, as well as increase the speed and decrease uncertainty of health economic analyses.[34] As with any technology or modeling method, reporting on the use of AI methods in an analysis has to be transparent. Understanding where and to what extent AI has been utilized is essential, because those methods may affect the outcome of any given analysis.[35]

CONCLUSION

As the healthcare landscape continues to evolve, the integration of RWD and RWE into research and regulatory frameworks offers unprecedented opportunities to enhance patient care, inform clinical decision-making, and support policy development. However, the utility of RWE is inherently tied to the quality, structure, and interpretation of the underlying data. This chapter highlighted the multifaceted considerations necessary for designing robust RWE studies, including the importance of CDMs, the mitigation of bias, and the strategic use of pilot and feasibility studies.

While RWE cannot replace the rigor of RCTs, it serves as a powerful complement, especially in diverse, real-world populations where traditional trials may fall short. The emergence of AI and machine learning further expands the potential of RWD, enabling more efficient data extraction, analysis, and insight generation. Yet, with these advancements comes the responsibility to ensure transparency, methodological rigor, and ethical stewardship of data.

Ultimately, the future of RWE lies in thoughtful collaboration among stakeholders, continuous methodological innovation, and a shared commitment to improving health outcomes. By embracing both the promise and the complexity of RWE, researchers and decision-makers can harness its full potential to drive meaningful changes in healthcare.

REFERENCES

1. U.S. Food and Drug Administration. Real-world evidence. Published 2020. https://www.fda.gov/science-research/science-and-research-special-topics/real-world-evidence. Accessed February 9, 2026.
2. Makady A, de Boer A, Hillage H, et al. What is real-world data? A review of definitions based on literature and stakeholder interviews. *Value Health.* 2017;20:858-865. https://doi.org/10.1016/j.jval.2017.03.008
3. Dang A. Real-world evidence: a primer. *Pharmaceuti Med.* 2023;37:25-36. https://doi.org/10.1007/s40290-022-00456-6
4. Rudrapatna VA, Butte AJ. Opportunities and challenges in using real-world data for health care. *J Clin Invest.* 2020;130(2):565-574. https://doi.org/10.1172/JCI129197
5. Kim HS, Lee S, Kim JH. Real-world evidence versus randomized controlled trial: clinical research based on electronic medical records. *J Korean Med Sci.* 2018;33(34):e213. https://doi.org/10.3346/jkms.2018.33.e213
6. U.S. Food and Drug Administration. Real-world data: assessing electronic health records and medical claims data to support regulatory decision-making for drug and biological products guidance for industry. Published July 2024. https://www.fda.gov/regulatory-information/search-fda-guidance-documents/real-world-data-assessing-electronic-health-records-and-medical-claims-data-support-regulatory. Accessed February 9, 2026.
7. Observational health data sciences and informatics. https://www.ohdsi.org/. Accessed February 9, 2026.
8. FHIR® - Fast Healthcare Interoperability Resources. https://ecqi.healthit.gov/fhir/about. Accessed February 9, 2026.
9. Chappell E. Demystifying CDISC, SDTM, and ADaM. May 22, 2024. https://www.certara.com/blog/demystifying-cdisc-sdtm-and-adam/. Accessed February 9, 2026.
10. CDISC Strategy and Roadmap Focus on Realizing the Long-Term Vision. https://www.cdisc.org/sites/default/files/2024-08/CDISC%20Roadmap%20-%20vJun2024.pdf. Accessed February 9, 2026.
11. Facile R, Muhlbradt EE, Gong M, et al. Use of Clinical Data Interchange Standards Consortium (CDISC) standards for real-world data: expert perspectives from a qualitative Delphi survey. *JMIR Med Inform.* 2022;10(1):e30363. https://doi.org/10.2196/30363
12. What is openEHR? https://openehr.org/about/what_is_openehr. Accessed February 9, 2026.
13. Bowen DJ, Kreuter M, Spring B, et al. How we design feasibility studies. *Am J Prev Med.* 2009;36(5):452-457. https://doi.org/10.1016/j.amepre.2009.02.002
14. Pearson N, Naylor P, Ashe MC, et al. Guidance for conducting feasibility and pilot studies for implementation trials. *Pilot and Feasibility Studies.* 2020;6:167. https://doi.org/10.1186/s40814-020-00634-w
15. Wang SV, Schneeweiss S. Assessing and interpreting RWE studies: introductory points for new reviewers. *Clin Pharmacol Ther.* 2022;111(1):145-149. https://doi.org/10.1002/cpt.2398

16. Acton EK, Willis AW, Hennessy S. Core concepts in pharmacoepidemiology: key biases arising in pharmacoepidemiologic studies. *Pharmacoepidemiol Drug Saf.* 2023;32(1):9-18. https://doi.org/10.1002/pds.5547

17. Pannucci CJ, Wilkins EG. Identifying and avoiding bias in research. *Plast Reconstr Surg.* 2010;126(2):619-625. https://doi.org/10.1097/PRS.0b013e3181de24bc

18. Pham A, Cummings M, Lindeman C, et al. Recognizing misclassification bias in research and medical practice. *Fam Pract.* 2019;36(6):804-807. https://doi.org/10.1093/fampra/cmy130

19. Lewin A, Brondeel R, Benmarhnia T, et al. Attrition bias related to missing outcome data: a longitudinal simulation study. *Epidemiology.* 2018;29(1):87-95. https://doi.org/10.1097/EDE.0000000000000755

20. Hanley JA, Foster BJ. Avoiding blunders involving "immortal time." *Int J Epidemiol.* 2014;43(3):949-961. https://doi.org/10.1093/ije/dyu105

21. Lavesque LE, Hanley JA, Kezouh A, Suissa S. Problem of immortal time bias in cohort studies: example using statins for preventing progression of diabetes. *BMJ.* 2010;340:b5087. https://doi.org/10.1136/bmj.b5087

22. Cox E, Martin BC, Van Staa T, et al. Good research practices for comparative effectiveness research: approaches to mitigate bias and confounding in the design of nonrandomized studies of treatment effects using secondary data sources: the International Society for Pharmacoeconomics and Outcomes Research Good Research Practices for Retrospective Database Analysis Task Force Report—Part II. *Value Health.* 2009;12(8):1053-1061. https://doi.org/10.1111/j.1524-4733.2009.00601.x

23. Dreyer NA, Schneeweiss S, McNeil B, et al. GRACE principles: recognizing high-quality observational studies of comparative effectiveness. *Am J Manag Care.* 2010;16(6):467-471. PMID: 20560690

24. Wiffen P. Reporting guidelines: checklists for specific study designs. *Eur J Hosp Pharm.* 2016;23(6):307. https://doi.org/10.1136/ejhpharm-2016-001115

25. U.S. Food and Drug Administration. Framework for FDA's real-world evidence program. Updated December 2018. https://www.fda.gov/media/120060/download. Accessed February 9, 2026.

26. Nicotera G, Sferrazza G, Serafino A, Pierimarchi P. The iterative development of medicines through the European medicine agency's adaptive pathway approach. *Front Med.* 2019;6:148. https://doi.org/10.3389/fmed.2019.00148

27. Cave A, Kurz X, Arlett P. Real-world data for regulatory decision making: challenges and possible solutions for Europe. *Clin Pharmacol Ther.* 2019;106(1):36-39. https://doi.org/10.1002/cpt.1426

28. European Medicines Agency. HMA-EMA Joint Big Data Taskforce—summary report. Published 2019. https://www.ema.europa.eu/en/documents/minutes/hma-ema-joint-task-force-big-data-summary-report_en.pdf. Accessed February 9, 2026.

29. Roser M, Ritchie H, Mathieu E. What is Moore's Law? Exponential growth is at the heart of the rapid increase of computing capabilities. March 28, 2023. https://ourworldindata.org/moores-law. Accessed February 9, 2026.

30. Kaul V, Enslin S, Gross GA. History of artificial intelligence in medicine. *Gastrointest Endosc.* 2020;92:807-812. https://doi.org/10.1016/j.gie.2020.06.040

31. Adamson B, Waskom M, Blarre A, et al. Approach to machine learning for extraction of real-world data variables from electronic health records. *Front Pharmacol.* 2023;14:1180962. https://doi.org/10.3389/fphar.2023.1180962

32. Coiera E. The last mile: where artificial intelligence meets reality. *J Med Internet Res.* 2019;21(11):e16232. https://doi.org/10.2196/16323

33. Rawlinson W. Generative artificial intelligence and the future of health economic modeling. *Value and Outcome Spotlight.* 2024;10(5):48-51.

34. Padula WV, Kreif N, Vanness DJ, et al. Machine learning methods in health economics and outcomes research: the PALISADE checklist: a good practices report of an ISPOR task force. *Value Health.* 2022;25(7):1063-1080. https://doi.org/10.1016/j.jval.2022.03.022

35. Elvidge J, Hawsworth C, Avsar TS, et al. Consolidated health economic evaluation reporting standards for interventions that use artificial intelligence (CHEERS-AI). *Value Health.* 2024;27(9):1196-1205. https://doi.org/10.1016/j.jval.2024.05.006

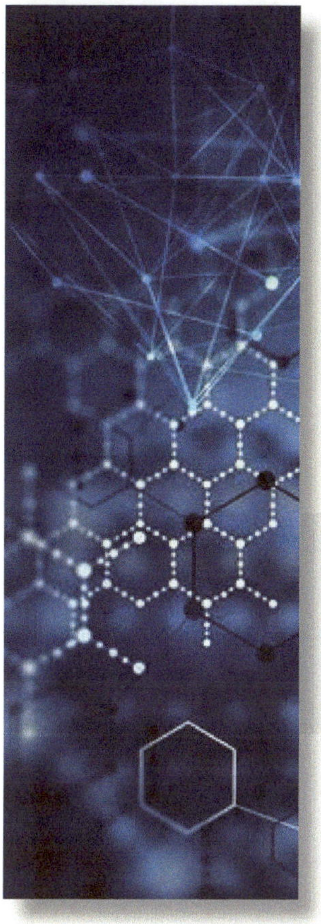

SECTION FOUR

Economic Evaluations

DOI: 10.37573/9781585287666.TITLE

Introduction to Pharmacoeconomic Evaluations

13

Elinor G. Borgert, PhD, MSc

Healthcare systems around the world face mounting financial pressures, increasing the impetus for more efficient resource allocations. Policymakers, payers, and providers need tools that can guide decisions about which interventions offer the greatest value in terms of clinical outcomes, patient preferences, and economic sustainability. Pharmacoeconomic evaluations are critical to this decision-making process, offering structured approaches to consider all of the costs and consequences of healthcare interventions.

These evaluations are grounded in the principle that healthcare resources are finite and must be used to maximum benefit. While all involve the identification and measurement of costs, the nature of the outcomes under consideration can vary significantly. Cost minimization analysis (CMA) assumes equivalent outcomes and focuses solely on identifying the least costly option and represents the most basic form of evaluation. However, because therapeutic equivalence is rare in practice, CMA is infrequently used and generally limited to narrow clinical scenarios. Much more sophisticated methods are required to capture the full range of outcomes relevant to patients, providers, and health systems.

The chapters that follow examine the principal types and components of pharmacoeconomic evaluations, beginning with integrative modeling approaches and extending through analyses of cost structures, clinical outcomes, patient preferences, and financial feasibility. Taken together, these tools offer a systematic framework for quantifying the full value of healthcare interventions and informing decisions that optimize the use of limited resources.

Routinely incorporated into pharmacoeconomic evaluations, decision analysis models play a critical role in combining and extending the utility of real-world and clinical trial data. Chapter 14 introduces some of the most common integrative modeling approaches that allow researchers to simulate long-term outcomes and cost-effectiveness when direct empirical data are limited. Markov models can be especially valuable in chronic disease contexts or when evaluating interventions with delayed or cumulative effects. By structuring clinical problems mathematically and incorporating data from multiple sources, decision models help to identify gaps in evidence, inform policy decisions, and support resource allocation strategies. When done well, their transparency and adaptability make them indispensable tools in outcomes research.

Chapter 15 introduces the foundational concepts of cost identification and classification, providing essential context for conducting meaningful economic evaluations in healthcare. Drs. Mary Dooley and Dunc Williams delve into the complexities of healthcare cost structures, offering a foundational understanding of how costs are defined, measured, and allocated. They emphasize the importance of perspective in cost analyses, as one stakeholder's cost is another stakeholder's revenue. The chapter also introduces advanced costing methodologies, such as time-driven activity-based costing, which enables precise micro-costing of healthcare services. These insights are essential for interpreting cost-effectiveness results and for designing studies that reflect the true economic impact of interventions. Understanding the nuances of cost accounting

DOI: 10.37573/9781585287666.013

and revenue recognition is critical for translating pharmacoeconomic findings into actionable healthcare decisions.

With a comprehensive understanding of cost structures and perspectives established, attention shifts to the application of these concepts in comparative analyses. In Chapter 16, Drs. Corey Morrow and Todd Wandstrat examine cost-effectiveness analyses (CEAs), which combine costs and outcomes into a single ratio. The numerator measures costs in units of currency, and the denominator measures the gain in health in natural units, such as years of life saved or cases of disease averted. Because CEAs focus on just one of a potentially wide variety of outcome measures, they are limited in both the depth of the information they provide and the generalizability of the results.

The results of a CEA are typically expressed as an incremental cost-effectiveness ratio (ICER), which represents the additional cost required to achieve one additional unit of health benefit when comparing two interventions. A lower ICER indicates a more efficient use of resources, offering greater health gains per dollar spent. Critically, the value of the ICER depends on the comparator used and can vary significantly depending on the clinical and economic context. The current standard of care or most widely accepted alternative should be used whenever possible.

While CEAs can offer insights into long-term value, healthcare stakeholders often require information on the short-term financial implications of adopting new interventions. Chapter 17 addresses this need through budget impact analysis (BIA), which complements CEAs by focusing on affordability and resource planning within specific budgetary contexts. Drs. Stephanie Earnshaw and Anita Brogan show how BIA can be used to estimate the short- to mid-term financial consequences of adopting a new intervention from the perspective of a specific budget holder, such as a payer or provider. Unlike CEAs, which focus on long-term value, BIAs help decision-makers understand how a new intervention will affect annual budgets, resource allocation, and population health outcomes. This chapter outlines the methodological framework for BIAs, offering practical guidance for their real-world application in healthcare planning and reimbursement decisions.

Economic evaluations must consider not only financial and clinical outcomes but also the preferences and lived experiences of patients. Chapter 18 introduces key methods for capturing these dimensions, including health-related quality-of-life instruments, utility estimation techniques, such as time trade-off and standard gamble, and preference-based measures, such as the EQ-5D. Drs. Caroline Vass and Sorrel Wolowacz also present advanced elicitation approaches, such as discrete choice experiments and best-worst scaling, that quantify how patients and stakeholders value different attributes of healthcare interventions. Utilities and preferences are essential for generating quality-adjusted life-years (QALYs) and for ensuring that evaluations reflect the full spectrum of value in healthcare decision-making.

Building on the measurement of patient-centered outcomes, Chapter 19 demonstrates how these metrics are incorporated into QALYs for use in cost-utility analyses (CUAs). Unlike CEAs, which rely on single, program-specific outcomes, CUAs employ a composite measure that facilitates comparisons across a wide range of interventions. Expressing value in terms of cost per QALY supports consistent evaluations across diverse health conditions and treatment strategies. In many single-payer healthcare systems, CUAs are routinely used to determine whether new treatments offer sufficient value to justify their inclusion on national formularies. Health technology assessment agencies, such as the National Institute for Health and Care Excellence (NICE) in the United Kingdom and the Pharmaceutical Benefits Advisory Committee (PBAC) in Australia, use this standardized approach to determine which treatments are most cost effective for their populations.

Although CUAs provide a robust framework for comparing health interventions, the argument can be made that certain policy and investment decisions are best addressed by valuing both costs and outcomes in monetary terms. Chapter 20 examines cost-benefit analyses (CBAs), which measure the value of all benefits from an intervention and subtracts from that the measured value of all costs (direct and indirect). Willingness to pay methods typically involve asking contingent valuation questions, thereby allowing respondents to incorporate all dimensions of value into a single currency amount. Although strongly supported by economic theory and widely used in other disciplines, CBAs have yet to reach their full potential in health economic evaluations.

Pharmacoeconomic evaluations provide a critical framework for assessing the value, affordability, and impact of healthcare interventions in an increasingly resource-constrained environment. These evaluations encompass a wide range of methodologies from CEAs to more complex models that incorporate patient preferences, quality of life, and budgetary implications. Together, these tools enable decision-makers to weigh clinical benefits against economic realities, helping to ensure that healthcare resources are allocated more efficiently. Each of the chapters that follow provide deep insights into the most current analytic techniques, modeling strategies, and stakeholder perspectives that shape outcomes research and inform evidence-based healthcare policy.

Decision Analysis Models

14

Kit N. Simpson, DrPH, MPH, and
Elinor G. Borgert, PhD, MSc

INTRODUCTION

The tremendous value of real-world evidence is most fully realized when employed in decision analysis models to inform patient care and policy predictions. These integrative or stochastic decision models enable researchers to extend their analysis beyond the data they have acquired to obtain the information they need to answer important questions facing decision-makers.[1] Data from clinical, pharmacoeconomic, or outcomes research studies are often incomplete, a result of both the enormous number of resources involved in the various study designs and the pressing need to quickly document the clinical effects of emerging interventions. Consequently, these data are limited in both the breadth of information collected and the length of time patients are followed. Patients in clinical trials are routinely observed for short-term marker or surrogate endpoints, such as blood pressure reductions, rather than long-term outcomes, such as strokes avoided, where their true value lies. Decision models use mathematical techniques to predict long-term effects and multidimensional outcomes based on available data on fewer variables and/or shorter time periods.[2] In the absence of direct primary empirical data to address key issues, the use of modeling to estimate effectiveness and cost-effectiveness is a wholly valid and value-added form of scientific inquiry.[3]

Decision models structure a clinical problem mathematically, allowing researchers to enumerate the health outcomes and costs expected from using competing treatments. Their transparency is a tremendous asset, because the process of constructing a model reveals gaps in the data that indicate areas where future research is needed. Because they integrate data and information from many sources under a clearly specified set of assumptions, decision models are useful for informing discussions for and against specific policy choices or treatment decisions. Researchers typically structure clinical problems by either summarizing the major treatment choices and their resulting outcomes in a decision tree (also called a probability tree) or describing the disease process as a series of health states that patients have a specific probability of experiencing over time (a state-transition or Markov model).

Decision trees represent a sequence of treatment decisions and probabilistic health outcomes over time in a series of chance and decision nodes. They are an extremely useful tool for representing relatively simple or acute disease/treatment processes for deciding on the best course of action. However, as we will discuss later in this chapter, one limitation of decision tree models is that they are not well suited to representing more complex events, especially those that recur and/or progress over time.

Because Markov models or state-transition models are designed to allow for event recurrence, they have eclipsed decision tree models in popularity for more complicated and chronic diseases, such as human immunodeficiency virus (HIV). Markov models depict the natural history of a disease as a sequence of mutually exclusive health states, defined to capture important clinical traits, such as acute event history. These models are based on the assumption that patients assigned to a given

DOI: 10.37573/9781585287666.014

health state incur similar economic costs and enjoy a comparable quality of life. The models then combine data about the population, the disease, and the effect of interventions to govern the transitions into and out of the various health states.[4]

USING MODELING STUDIES

Modeling studies may be useful for informing decisions at any stage of a drug's development. Simple early modeling efforts performed prior to Phase I or II clinical trials can help to identify key relationships among factors that influence the efficacy and cost of care. Modeling studies can also inform the sample size necessary to detect statistical significance regarding health-related quality-of-life or cost measures. Most importantly, such models can be used to generate the cost-effectiveness ratios for a new compound compared to drugs in current use given a range of pricing assumptions. This may be quite important if existing medications are relatively inexpensive but have low efficacy, and the new compounds are expected to be both more expensive to manufacture and more efficacious.

Modeling studies that are based on data from Phase III or IV trials may have many different purposes, and their designs must vary to reflect such differences. These studies are often used to translate efficacy results from trial data into estimates of expected effectiveness for patients under usual practice conditions. Such models may link "marker" or surrogate endpoints (eg, CD4 cell changes) to epidemiologic measures of disease, such as rates of expected opportunistic events for acquired immunodeficiency syndrome (AIDS) patients.[5] Alternatively, they may simply translate differences in resource use and outcomes reported from clinical studies into incremental cost-effectiveness ratios, given specific assumptions about practice patterns, cost of resources, or country of use. The modeling may also be used to examine expected differences for subgroups of patients, for different comparators (including other technologies, such as surgery), or for specific types of populations, such as members of a managed care group. Most importantly, modeling may be used to estimate the expected lifetime costs and effects from trial results that are limited to data collected over a fairly short time period. Because healthcare systems across the globe are challenged with allocating scarce resources to their greatest effect, modeling studies are central to support policy discussions, especially where cost-effectiveness is a key consideration.

LINKING DATA

As noted earlier, models may be used to predict long-term effects based on real-world data from a more limited time period. Dually driven by the significant resources involved and the need to document meaningful clinical effects quickly, clinical trial data often cover only a limited period of time at great expense. Patients are observed for short-term marker or surrogate endpoints, such as blood pressure reduction, rather than long-term and patient-centered outcomes, such as strokes avoided or early death. By contrast, observational data (eg, epidemiologic or billing databases) follow patients for extended periods of time and allow researchers to document the long-term health implications of the surrogate endpoints.

When short-term clinical trial data are linked with real-world data reflecting long-term outcomes and resource use, researchers must be careful to ensure that these data could have come from samples of the same population. Essentially, they must document that the incorporated datasets are similar with respect to health risks and the propensity for resource use. To do this, researchers rely on analyses of linkage variables that can be used to predict either critical outcomes or specific levels of resource use. This is often the most difficult part of modeling, and the step that is most open to challenges from critics. Thus, as always, complete transparency is essential.

Linkage variables typically include some demographic or disease-related variables that were originally used to exclude patients from enrollment in a trial. Second-level linkage variables encompass systems that classify acute episodes of care, such as International Classification of Diseases, 10th edition (ICD-10) or Current Procedural Terminology, 4th edition (CPT-4) codes. Severity of illness indices that explain either disease stage complexity or the prevalence of comorbid conditions may also be used to link datasets for modeling. One of the more commonly used indices, especially in critical care, is the Acute Physiology and Chronic Health Evaluation (APACHE). Moreover, outcome measures, such as being discharged in a dependent state either to home healthcare or to a nursing home setting, may be used to control for differences in resource use and in outcomes at the end of acute disease episodes.

Various issues should be considered when clinical and observational data are used together. First, the quality of coding in observational or billing data may be quite inferior to the coding or diagnostic descriptions found in clinical trial data. Observational data may be dirty or contaminated, with invalid observations or more than one observation for each patient. Such data also may be systematically biased in the selection of disease codes, with a high prevalence of codes for which reimbursement is favorable but few codes for patient cases associated with poor payment rules. Clinical trial data have limitations as well. Clinical episodes may be artificially mild, because adverse developments are recognized early through careful monitoring. Clinical data also may be biased if codes of particular interest to investigators appear more often than would be expected in regular practice. Finally, both the clinical and observational data may be biased against the inclusion of specific types of patients. For example, wealthier patients may be excluded from Medicaid databases, and people who do not answer their phone if the number/caller is not familiar may be excluded from surveys based on random digit telephone dialing.

DATA SOURCES

Numerous data sources have been used to supplement clinical trial data for modeling, but most of them have serious limitations that must be considered in an analysis. Hospital discharge data are commonly used to furnish data on episodes of acute illnesses. These data seem standardized, but they may exclude severe "charity" cases. The quality of coding in these types of data also may vary; some conditions may be reported in a very high proportion of cases, with others excluded.

Furthermore, hospital discharge data do not contain information on care provided by physicians, and most lack information on medications used. It is also important to note that the monetary values reported reflect billing charges, not the actual costs of care. Some observational data represent medical practice patterns that are atypical, and insurance billing data are often "right censored," because patients lose eligibility if they lose their job. Also, Medicare data must be used with caution for patients in specific age groups because of the age-dependent eligibility criteria for these programs.

When observational or epidemiologic data are used to supplement clinical trial data for modeling effectiveness and/or costs, keep in mind that, in the model, the observational or epidemiologic data are assumed to come from one population. Therefore, it often is necessary to perform direct or indirect adjustments on one or more of the datasets to ensure that important linkage variables are prevalent in the same proportion in datasets. Multivariate statistical analysis or survival analysis may also be used to adjust estimates for biasing factors. Even the best analyst, however, cannot exclude the possibility that important unmeasured or unknown factors are confounding the data.

SENSITIVITY ANALYSIS

Models are only as good as the assumptions they are based on and the data they contain. Decision-makers, therefore, need reassurance that predictions are not completely irrelevant to informing decisions. This is provided by model validation and sensitivity analysis.

Models need to have face validity, that is, they must seem reasonable to individuals who have expert knowledge in the clinical area. Models should also have predictive validity; they should be able to predict the prevalence of key conditions and costs for populations other than those they were designed to address. Unfortunately, rarely are complete data available for cost and outcomes of similar populations, or even for the therapies that are modeled. In such cases, researchers must rely on sensitivity analyses.

Sensitivity analyses evaluate a model's robustness by examining how changes in the parameters of included variables affect the model's outcomes, thereby addressing what-if scenarios. Although parameter values are usually entered into the model as discrete values, they may be drawn from a range of potential values (ie, confidence interval) based on random chance or the approach to measuring. Moreover, practitioners and researchers may want to adapt the model results to slightly different populations or scenarios, rather than those used in a model. To test the effect of these variations on the model results, the value of a single parameter may be replaced with values that are less likely but still plausible. For example, these could include values at the limits of the parameter's confidence interval or best/worst case scenario values. This is an example of one-way sensitivity analysis.

For a two-way sensitivity analysis, the values of two parameters are changed simultaneously. The stability of model predictions also may be tested by randomly varying many of the key parameter values within their confidence intervals. This type of testing may use a second-order Monte Carlo approach, which is provided in several commercially available modeling software programs.

If these extreme valuations do not affect the model's estimates enough to change the policy conclusion, then the model is characterized as stable or robust. Otherwise, the model is recognized as sensitive to changes in the given parameters, and this can be taken into consideration in policy decisions. The value of the parameter at which the model yields a different conclusion in the sensitivity is known as the threshold value.

DECISION TREES

Decision trees depict what may be expected to happen to a group of patients who receive different treatments. Each treatment choice is organized as one major branch originating from a central point, called a decision node. The population for each branch is then grouped into subgroups by (1) the process of care common to patients and (2) the intermediate and final outcomes experienced by patients over an episode of the illness.

Figure 14-1 illustrates how a decision tree may be employed with efficacy data from clinical trials to compare expected outcomes for a new drug versus usual care for a cohort of 200 patients.

Convention dictates that therapy choices are represented by square decision nodes, and probability distributions are represented by round chance nodes. The proportion of patients who fall into a group are indicated below each branch, and the type of group is written above the branch. For example, in Figure 14-1, the probability of being treated in the hospital is 20% for each type of therapy, but the probability of being discharged well is 90% for hospitalized patients who received the new drug and 80% for patients who received usual care. The average cost of care for each group is indicated at the end of each branch, as is the length of the illness episode. The total cost for each kind of therapy is then calculated by multiplying all conditional probabilities along the branches by the average cost indicated for each branch. This is called "rolling back" the decision tree.

To roll back the decision tree for Figure 14-1, we would first assume that a sample of 100 patients is taking the new drug, and another 100 are receiving usual care. We could then calculate the cost associated with the top branch (Branch 1) by multiplying the number of patients taking the new drug (n = 100) by the probability they were hospitalized (20%), then multiplying that quantity by the probability the hospitalized patients on the new drug were discharged well (0.90), and finally multiplying that quantity by the total cost associated with that experience ($10,000). The average cost per cases treated with the new drug could then be calculated and compared with the average cost of usual care as follows:

New drug: $180,000 for Branch 1 =
100 * 0.20 * 0.90 * $10,000

$30,000 for Branch 2 =
100 * 0.20 * 0.10 * $15,000

$14,400 for Branch 3 =
100 * 0.80 * 0.90 * $200 + $6,400 for Branch 4 = 100 * 0.80 * 0.10 * $800

$230,800 total (an average of $2,308 per case treated)

Usual care: $157,600 for Branch 1 =
100 * 0.20 * 0.80 * $9,850

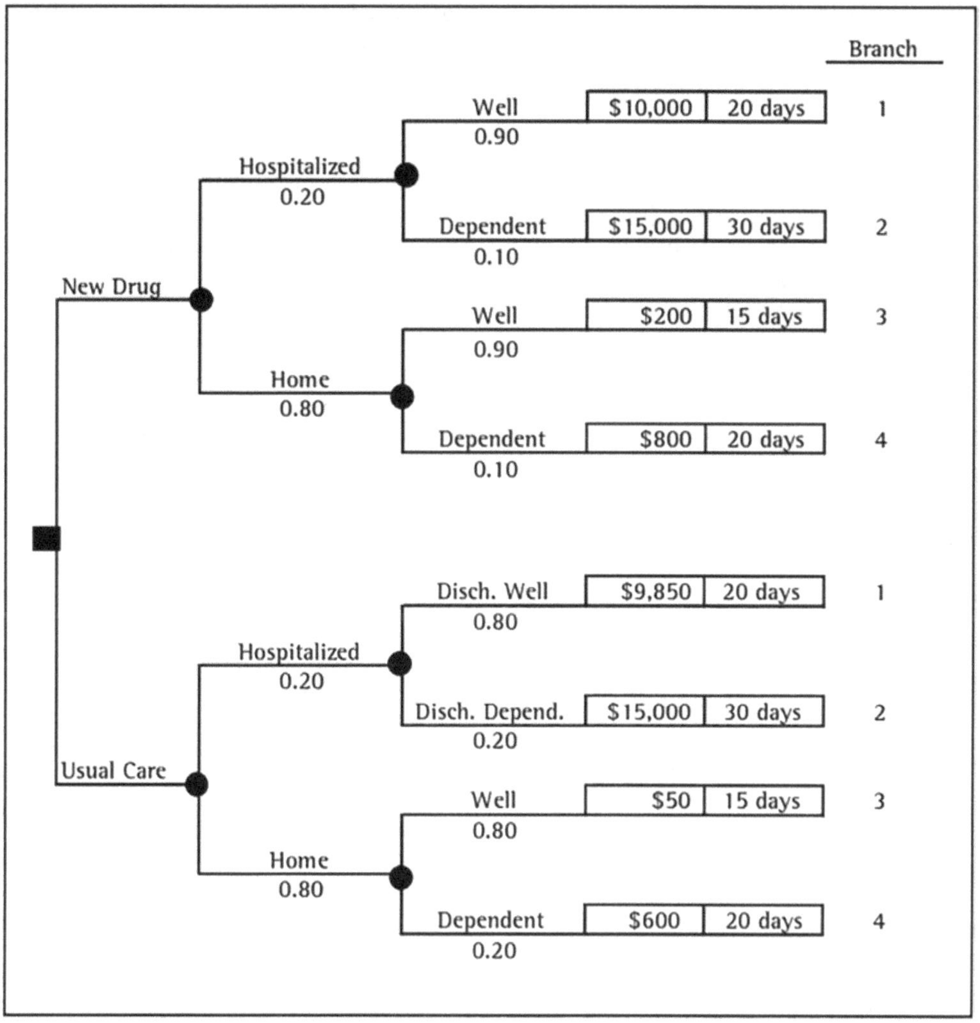

FIGURE 14-1. **Decision tree representing the choice between a new drug and usual care.**

$60,000 for Branch 2 =
100 * 0.20 * 0.20 * $15,000

$3,200 for Branch 3 = 100 * 0.80 * 0.80 * $50
+ $9,600 for Branch 4 =
100 * 0.80 * 0.20 * $600

$230,400 total (an average of $2,304 per case treated)

This cost-comparison analysis shows that, from the perspective of a healthcare system, it would cost $4 more in direct medical care costs per case for the new drug than for usual care. We can also calculate morbidity days simply by using the sick days at each terminal node instead of the costs in each calculation. Doing so reveals that 1,660 days are lost to illness for the 100 patients taking the new drug, and 1,720 days are lost to illness for those receiving usual care.

The costs necessarily vary with the perspective. For example, costs are calculated differently if the researcher is examining the issue from an employer's perspective rather than the healthcare system's perspective. If all patients are assumed to be working adults, and their employer had to hire temporary staff at a new cost of $50 per day of absence, then rolling back the tree while including the employer's cost per morbidity day (direct medical care and other direct costs) reveals that patients treated with the new drug had an average of 16.6 days absent from work, while patients treated with usual care had an average of 17.2 days absent. At a net cost for temporary help of $50 per day, the total cost per episode to an employer is $26 less for a patient treated with the new drug ($3,138 compared with $3,164 for usual treatment).

If, instead, researchers wanted to compare a new drug versus usual care from the perspective of the healthcare system (the perspective that is most often used), the investigators would want to consider the cost of medical resources used and any differences in morbidity for an average patient. One hundred patients treated with the new drug would be expected to lose a total of 1,660 days to illness, whereas 100 patients treated with usual care would be expected to lose 1,720 days being sick, or a difference of 60 days and $400, giving a cost-effectiveness ratio of $6.67 per morbidity day avoided.

If patients dislike being sick and value each day at only 50% of a day without illness, then the patients treated with the new drug gain the value of 0.5 days in full health for each of the 60 days of morbidity avoided, or 30 quality-adjusted days, at a cost to the medical care system of $400. When this is reported as cost per quality-adjusted life-year (QALY), the cost-utility ratio for new drug therapy is very reasonable at $4,867 per QALY compared with usual care.

As illustrated above, a decision tree is a useful organizing framework for calculating the different types of outcomes that would be expected for acute events under different treatment assumptions and costing perspectives. Although decision trees can be used to inform many clinical and management decisions in healthcare, published papers using decision trees often focus on comparing emerging clinical or preventive health interventions when the evidence for a new intervention is sparse. In such cases, a decision analysis can combine the limited new efficacy data available with a patient's disease history, epidemiologic data, and cost data to estimate differences in expected outcomes under a clearly articulated set of assumptions. Although the results of this type of analysis do not provide clear evidence for or against the adoption of a new therapy, the results often provide an invaluable framework for policy discussions and nearly always increase our understanding of key factors that are associated with desired outcomes from a particular therapy.[6]

An example of the use of a decision tree very early in the chain of evidence collection is illustrated in the paper by Marshall and colleagues who investigated a potential new method for screening high-risk patients for lung cancer.[7] In this policy paper, the authors used 1 year follow-up data from the first 1,000 patients to receive a helical computed tomography scan (HCT) to detect early lung cancer. Randomized clinical trials of screening for lung cancer in the United States in the 1970s using chest x-ray and sputum cytology failed to demonstrate an impact on mortality, and screening was subsequently discouraged by cancer societies and healthcare task forces. However, in 1999 Henschke and colleagues published a case series indicating a substantial "left stage shift" in lung cancer cases found through HCT.[8] This finding created new possibilities for detecting and treating lung cancer earlier and with greater success. A decision tree (**Figure 14-2**) was used to estimate the potential benefits and costs from screening for lung cancer under specific assumptions. Marshall and colleagues combined the results from the baseline screening published by the Henschke group with data from the SEER national cancer registry database to estimate the potential survival improvements, using Medicare cancer cost data to estimate the economic impacts expected if screening with HCT became current practice. The authors reported three major insights delivered by the decision model. Under the assumptions specified in the model: (1) a one-time prevalence screen for lung cancer with HCT scanning in a high-risk cohort of 60–74 years of age appears cost-effective at $5,940/LY; (2) the model estimates are sensitive to the prevalence of lung cancer in the screening population (a decrease from 2.7% to 0.7% in assumed lung cancer prevalence increased the ICER to $22,629/LY); and (3) the amount of lead-time bias assumed in the model was critical (a 1 year lead-time bias assumption increased the ICER to $58,183/LY, and the model could not identify health benefits if lead-time bias was assumed to be greater than approximately 1.5 years). This last finding made it clear that evidence on the magnitude of lead-time bias for lung cancer was needed before population-screening programs outside

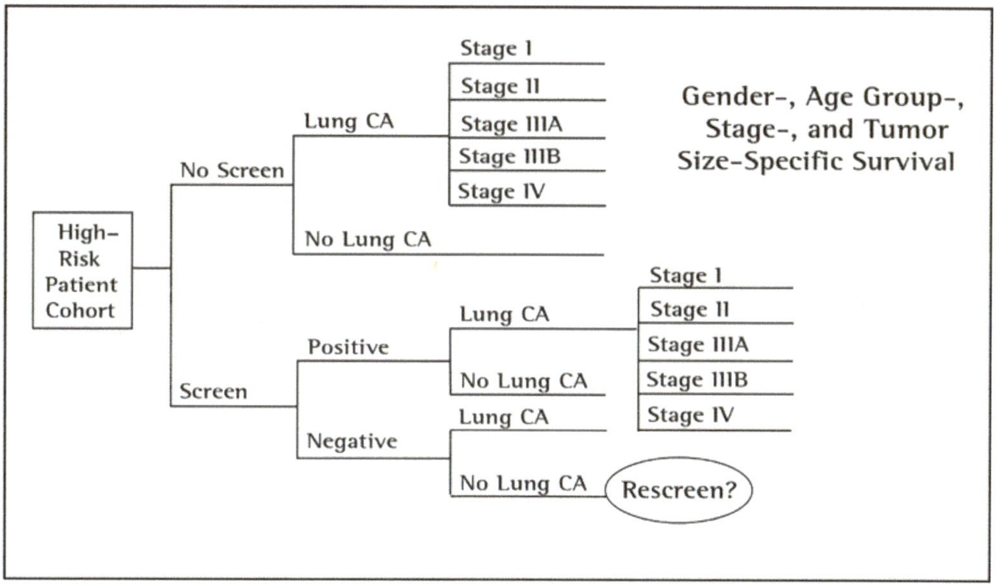

FIGURE 14-2. **Decision tree to estimate the potential benefits and costs from screening for lung cancer.**

of clinical trials should be seriously considered. When evaluating the effectiveness of the early detection and treatment of a condition, the lead time, ie, the period between early detection of disease and the time of its usual clinical presentation, must be subtracted from the overall survival time of screened patients to avoid lead-time bias. Otherwise, early detection merely increases the duration of the patients' awareness of their disease without reducing their mortality or morbidity. This modeling effort is an excellent example of how the results of a decision analysis can help to focus the attention of the scientific community on the key factors that must be better illuminated before a new intervention is implemented.

MARKOV-TYPE DECISION MODELS

A Markov or state-transition decision analysis model structure is used to organize the data for conditions where patients' health experience can be defined as a progression through different disease stages. Each stage in a Markov-type model is defined as a health state, and it may be possible to progress through stages of increasing severity, as well as from very severe stages to less severe stages, or even to be cured. Markov models are especially useful for predicting long-term outcomes, such as survival, when clinical trial results use intermediate health outcomes or surrogate markers, such as CD4 cell counts, to measure the clinical efficacy, effectiveness, and safety of treatments for complex chronic conditions. Markov-type structures are often used for modeling cases where a decision tree would have a large number of subbranches that are nearly identical except for differences in their preceding probability nodes. Thus, a Markov-type structure may be used to simplify very "bushy" decision trees.

Regardless of how many health states are included, they must be mutually exclusive and collectively exhaustive. In other words, they must be carefully defined so that a patient can only be in one health state at any given time but, taken together, capture the full disease/treatment experience. Markov models are especially useful for examining outcome differences for new treatments for conditions that already have clearly differentiated health states.[9] These states can be defined by (1) prognosis, such as in cancer stages A, B, C, and D; (2) standardized characteristics of the condition, such as CDC stages A, B, or C for patients with HIV disease; or (3) combinations of laboratory test values that have been shown to be prognostic, such as different levels of CD4 counts and RNA viral load measured in patients with HIV disease. Sometimes we can observe changes in structures used for decision models for a condition as our understanding of the condition affects the endpoints acceptable for clinical trials. The linkage between reported trial results and epidemiologic data is an important factor for selecting the structural framework for a decision model.

This relationship is readily observed in the AIDS models that have been published in the past 35 years. The efficacy measures in the early trials of antiretroviral drugs were progression from asymptomatic HIV disease to AIDS or death, and early models used simple decision trees or state-transition models with a few health states based on AIDS and death. As CD4 cell counts became a routinely reported measure of immune deficiency, and RNA viral load began to be considered a strong indicator of the risk of disease progression, the health states used in the published decision models of treatments for HIV disease became defined by these markers. Furthermore, as our understanding of HIV disease progressed and our medical armamentarium increased, published HIV disease models progressed to using Markov-type structures with many health states, even linking sequential state-transition structures to capture the complexity of a condition that was transforming from a rapidly fatal disease to a severe chronic illness requiring lifelong monitoring and therapy. The AIDS modeling papers by Schulman et al. (1991), Simpson et al. (1994), Chancellor et al. (1997), Freedberg et al. (2001), and Simpson et al. (2004) illustrate this progression.[10-14]

In a state-transition or Markov model, the disease process is carved into time periods of equal length defined by a set of health states. Each health state has a specific average quality of life, risk of progression or cure, and expected cost associated with the defining clinical markers. The progression for a specific group of patients is then defined by the length of time they spend in each health state. Some health states are final or absorbing, meaning that once a patient reaches this state no further progression or improvement will occur. Death is always an absorbing health state, but other states, such as cured or "surgical removal of . . ." may be defined as absorbing states if they are assumed to happen no more than once to any one individual. Each health state lasts for a specific time period (1 hour, day, week, month, or year); this is called the length of a cycle in the model. The choice of length for a cycle will depend on the length of the illness episode modeled, the length of time included in the efficacy and epidemiologic data available, and the average time included in cost data, which are usually reported as aggregates, such as a hospital admission. The choice of a model cycle time is an optimization process. The objective is to find the longest time period that fits the majority of the patient's natural disease episodes, the efficacy data, and the cost reporting, while making sure that the model does not inadvertently exclude differential outcomes for patients with very short episodes of care. Estimates for patient groups with very long episodes of care can be accommodated by having patients occupy a health state for more than one cycle. Thus, the selection of cycle length is often more of an art than a science.

Once a model's health states and cycle time have been defined, the available data are analyzed to populate the model. Two types of data are needed: parameters and transition probabilities. Parameters are mean values for measures of interest that are specific to each health state. For example, an AIDS Markov model would use parameters that accounted for the mean risk of experiencing an AIDS health state, the cost of treating an average patient in that health state, and mean quality-of-life weight (utility) that patients experience while in that health state.

Transition probabilities are similar to the probability nodes in the decision tree. They function like gates between connected health states. Each transition probability defines the proportion of patients in a current health state who are allowed to move to another state once the cycle time has been completed. For example, the transition probability of moving from health state A to health state B is the percentage of individuals who would progress from health state A to health state B during the time of one model cycle under the treatment conditions that are tested in the model. This seems simple, but obtaining these data can be complicated. The standard epidemiologic measures of risk, such as relative risk or odds ratios, account for the overall risk of disease progression across health states included in a model, not the contingent risk of progression from one health state to another, which is what we need to calculate transition probabilities. These transition probabilities are the critical variables that contain the differences in efficacy between the therapies compared in the model. They are the engine that drives the population through the model at different rates for different treatments. Getting the model transition probabilities right, especially the differences in transition probabilities for the treatments compared in a Markov model, are the most critical aspects of designing a Markov model. The effects of even small variations in the transition probability differences often swamp the effects of relatively large differences in parameter values for cost, events, or quality of life in most models. This characteristic of Markov models is often not recognized by reviewers of modeling papers who have not been trained in modeling.

The probabilities of moving from health state A to health state B during a model cycle, as well as the probability of moving from state B to state A, are entered into a table called a transition matrix. This table has one row and one column for each health state. Thus, a transition matrix for a model with five health states will have five rows and five columns, for a total of 25 cells. In a Markov model where patients can move from any one state to any other state at the end of each cycle, all 25 cells must contain an accurate contingent probability of a patient's movement from one health state to the next. A Markov model that has 10 health states and allows movement between all health states requires $10 \times 10 = 100$ contingent probability calculations. If we need at least 30 observations for each calculation (a good rule of thumb for such calculations), such a model would require a minimum of 3,000 patient observations to populate the transition matrix. Because the value of a decision modeling study is to inform discussions before sufficient efficacy data are available, it is essential to keep the number of model health states low and to make as many simplifying assumptions as possible to disallow movements between some model health states.

Once the health states and cycle times have been specified, and the transitions and parameters calculated, the model can be programmed. Markov models can be solved as mathematical equations using matrix algebra. They can be executed easily with spreadsheet software using one column for each health state and one row for each cycle, or they can be programmed in special software, such as TreeAge.

Our preference is to program the models in Excel, because this approach is easy and transparent, allowing the observation of patients moving through the model. Furthermore, executing a Markov model in spreadsheet software allows researchers to examine output aggregates of any parameter of interest at a specific time period. Thus, they can create graphs that illustrate the flow of funds, the cost and use of specific resources, such as drugs, or the time at which specific benchmarks are reached, such as median survival. The Markov models used by Chancellor et al. and described by Simpson et al. provide examples of a relatively simple and more complex use of the Markov modeling structure.[10,14]

USE OF MARKOV MODELS FOR CHRONIC DISEASES

Markov models have been widely used to examine the cost-effectiveness or cost consequences of antiretroviral therapy, prophylaxis treatment, or screening in HIV/AIDS.[11] Markov approaches are especially well-suited to model the progression of HIV/AIDS and typically contain health states that are defined by CD4 cell counts and viral load. These health states are associated with transition probabilities that are derived from information in the published literature based on epidemiologic studies and previous clinical trials. Markov models assume that transition probabilities are dependent only on the immediately previous health state; thus, transition probabilities can be derived from existing literature independent from the actual study time when they occurred. The proportion of patients in each health state who will have an AIDS-defining event can then be projected with its subsequent resource utilization and costs.

The model described by Chancellor et al. (1997) is a fairly simple example of a Markov structure applied to HIV disease.[10] It has three transitional health states that define an increasing deterioration in a patient's immune system: (1) A is asymptomatic, (2) B is asymptomatic but with a low CD4 cell count, and (3) C is AIDS. The model's one absorbing health state, D, is death. The cycle time in the model is 1 year. At the end of each cycle, patients can (1) stay in their current health state, (2) move to any other health state with a worse immune status, or (3) die. No improvements are allowed in the model. Thus, the transition matrix has four rows and four columns, or 16 cells. Six of these cells are empty with a value or zero. The cell indicating state D moving to state D (death) is 1.0, and the rest have actual annual transition rates derived from epidemiologic data. Costs were assigned to each health state based on the average annual costs recorded for patients in large observational databases in each health state.

If we compare the structure and parameters used in the Chancellor model that was published in 1997 to those used in the model published by Simpson and colleagues in 2004, we discover that the later model uses a far more complex Markov structure.[10,14] It has 13 health states, including death, the absorbing state. The health states are defined by combinations of values of CD4 cell counts and RNA viral load, the model includes a utility adjustment to reflect differences in health-related quality of life for each health state, and the model is not limited to capturing differences between two initial antiretroviral therapies, because it performs these differences to capture any differences that would exist for a second or third regimen.

Over the past few decades, we have seen an order of magnitude increase in the complexity and data requirements for an AIDS model. The number of cells in the transition matrix increased from 16 in the first Chancellor model (1997) to 169 in the Simpson model (2004) over just a 7-year period. We are no longer considering just the two drug treatments of interest, but also subsequent and newer therapies that have emerged in the interim. Finally, the health states in the model are now routinely defined by combinations of two laboratory measures, not by the CDC stage definition for HIV disease, and an adjustment for differences in quality of life for each health state is generally incorporated into the models.

These differences between the two models are not simply the result of differences of opinion between the two modeling groups on how best to operationalize a Markov model for HIV disease. Rather, the differences between models are dictated by the change in practice patterns and the growth in the scientific knowledge of HIV disease in the interim. The redefinition of the health states was needed, because clinical trials today report efficacy differences in terms of viral load suppression and CD4 cell gains. The large increase in the number of health states was required to enable the model to capture the fact that competing drug regimens may have the same efficacy for patients who have a relatively normal immune function, but the drugs have very different levels of efficacy for patients who are severely immune compromised. The addition of quality-of-life adjustments to the model reflects research findings in the years between the design of the two models; researchers discovered that some HIV drug regimens have significant side effects, such as nausea, diarrhea, and headache, and the survival benefit is nearly lost owing to these negative impacts on quality of life. Lastly, research has clearly shown that HIV becomes resistant to specific drug cocktails over time, and some new drug regimens are better at suppressing resistant viruses than others. Thus, it is no longer sufficient to capture the effects of the current drug treatments; a sensitive model must also be able to reflect differences in the level of resistance conferred to the virus once the current regimen has failed. This is only possible if the model extends beyond one regimen.

These two modeling papers each employed a Markov structure as an organizing framework; they were both programmed in Excel; and they based their transition probabilities and cost estimates on archival epidemiologic and cost data from large observational patient cohorts.[10,14] However, they used different definitions of health states and had vastly different levels of complexity. It would not be appropriate to use the Chancellor model to estimate differences in outcomes for the new drugs that are currently under development, because this model reflects a set of assumptions that were acceptable in 1997 but are too simple given the scientific knowledge of HIV disease that we have today. Yet, the earlier model's findings have been shown to be true, ie, that the use of a lamivudine and zidovudine cocktail gives better survival than using zidovudine by itself and that the expenditures for the additional drug give good value for the money spent. Thus, the Chancellor model provided valid information upon which to base an important clinical policy decision. Because this is the objective of any modeling study, we should consider this a valid model, even though it would not be an adequate model to use for a study of two HIV drug regimens under consideration today.

Other chronic diseases, such as diabetes, chronic obstructive pulmonary disease, and Alzheimer's disease, are also ideally suited for Markov models. With recent therapeutic advances, the existing models have been pressed into service alongside extensive critical appraisals. A perceived lack of clarity and reliability has been cited as a barrier to the use of these models by decision-makers.[15] Recurring themes are limitations in representing the natural history of the disease and a lack of empirical evidence for extrapolating trial results, such as cognition outcomes, to long-term outcomes, such as function, care needs, and mortality. In addition, real-world data on the natural progression across the disease spectrum and across various outcomes (eg, cognition, function, and behavior) are limited, as are the utility and cost data associated with these outcomes. Models also use different structures and reflect different populations/settings, and models can lack transparency around data and assumptions.[16]

Unexplained differences across models for the same disease are a threat to their credibility and could lead to inappropriate decision-making in the adoption of new interventions. Wherever possible, comparative modeling or cross-validation (ie, comparing the results of different models purporting to address the same issue) could certainly boost confidence in the modeling process if they produce similar results. Hypothetical benchmark scenarios have been successfully used to cross-validate Markov models for chronic diseases, such as diabetes, chronic obstructive pulmonary disease, and malaria.[17-19] Similar comparative modeling is urgently needed for other chronic diseases.

DISCUSSION

Modeling is a creative endeavor and at times a risky one. It should always be a multidisciplinary undertaking for several reasons. The model cannot include all clinical trial data, so the most important and valid measures must be selected. This selection process requires the involvement of those who know the clinical trials best: principal investigators, research nurses, monitors, biostatisticians, and others involved in the process. Models also use variables from real-world data. These data must be adjusted or analyzed so that the estimates that they bring to the model reflect a level of severity and risk similar to those faced by the trial population. This requires expertise in health services research and epidemiologic analysis. Thus, it is important that clinical trial team members be involved in the modeling process. They should, at a minimum, critique the model design and discuss the value of selecting specific variables and the assumptions that are valid for their data.

No ideal data sources exist to supplement clinical trial data for modeling. It is, therefore, important to cast a broad net to capture several data sources if possible. The use of more than one source of data allows for triangulation (ie, the identification of several estimates that support each other) because they identify a narrow area where the true value may be located.

The identification of a range or cluster of estimates may not seem desirable to some decision-makers. There is often a tendency among decision-makers to want the "right number"; yet finding this elusive value is never possible with a cost-effectiveness modeling study. Indeed, it is not possible for any study involving costs, because true cost is a defined concept not a measurable absolute value. Therefore, in-depth discussions of the strengths and weaknesses of a modeling estimate and of the data and assumptions embodied in this research are required for a good modeling report. In this field, pretension to excessive precision often results in a loss of face validity; it is better to be approximately right than precisely wrong, and a model that does not have face validity is useless for informing critical decisions about how scarce resources are best utilized.

REFERENCES

1. Simpson KN. Modeling with clinical trial data: getting from the data researchers have to the data decision makers need. *Drug Information J*. 1995;29(4):1431-1440. https://doi.org/10.1177/009286159502900450
2. Simpson KN. Problems and perspectives on the use of decision-analysis models for prostate cancer. *J Urol*. 1994;152:1888-1893. https://doi.org/10.1016/s0022-5347(17)32408-4
3. Gold M, Siegel J, Russell L, et al., ed. *Cost-Effectiveness in Health and Medicine*. New York: Oxford University Press; 1996.
4. Freedberg KA, Scharfstein JA, Seage GR, et al. The cost-effectiveness of preventing AIDS-related opportunistic infections. *JAMA*. 1998;279(2):130-136. https://doi.org/10.1001/jama.279.2.130
5. Simpson KN. Design and assessment of cost effectiveness studies in AIDS populations. *J Acquir Immune Defic Syndr Hum Retrovirol*. 1995;10(suppl 4):S28-S32. PMID: 7493196
6. Briggs A, Sculpher M. An introduction to Markov modelling for economic evaluation. *Pharmacoeconomics*. 1998;13:397-409. https://doi.org/10.2165/00019053-199813040-00003
7. Marshall DA, Simpson KN, Earle CC, Chu CW. Potential cost-effectiveness of one-time screening for lung cancer (LC) in a high risk cohort. *Lung Cancer*. 2001;32(3):227-236. https://doi.org/10.1016/S0169-5002(00)00239-7
8. Henschke CI, McCauley DI, Yankelevitz DF, et al. Early Lung Cancer Action Project: overall design and findings from baseline screening. *Lancet*. 1999;354(9173):99-105. https://doi.org/10.1016/S0140-6736(99)06093-6
9. Sonnenberg FA, Beck JR. Markov models in medical decision making: a practical guide. *Med Decis Making*. 1993;13:322-338. https://doi.org/10.1177/0272989X9301300409
10. Chancellor JV, Hill AM, Sabin CA, et al. Modelling the cost effectiveness of lamivudine/zidovudine combination therapy in HIV infection. *Pharmacoeconomics*. 1997;12:54-66. https://doi.org/10.2165/00019053-199712010-00006
11. Simpson K, Hatziandreu EJ, Andersson F, et al. Cost effectiveness of antiviral treatment with zalcitabine plus zidovudine for AIDS patients with CD4+ counts less than 300/microliters in 5 European countries. *Pharmacoeconomics*. 1994;6(6):553-562. https://doi.org/10.2165/00019053-199406060-00008
12. Schulman KA, Lynn LA, Glick HA, et al. Cost effectiveness of low-dose zidovudine therapy for asymptomatic patients with human immunodeficiency virus (HIV) infection. *Ann Intern Med*. 1991;114(9):798-802. https://doi.org/10.7326/0003-4819-114-9-798
13. Freedberg KA, Losina E, Weinstein MC, et al. The cost effectiveness of combination antiretroviral therapy for HIV disease. *N Engl J Med*. 2001;344(11):824-831. https://doi.org/10.1056/NEJM200103153441108
14. Simpson KN, Luo MP, Chumney E, et al. Cost-effectiveness of lopinavir/ritonavir versus nelfinavir as the first-line highly active antiretroviral therapy regimen for HIV infection. *HIV Clinical Trials*. 2004;5(5):294-304. https://doi.org/10.1310/WT81-MEM4-5C4L-CHPK
15. Handels RLH, Green C, Gustavsson A, et al. Cost-effectiveness models for Alzheimer's disease and related dementias: IPECAD modeling workshop cross-comparison challenge. *Alzheimer's Dement*. 2023;19:1800-1820. https://doi.org/10.1002/alz.12811
16. Nguyen KH, Comans TA, Green C. Where are we at with model-based economic evaluations of interventions for dementia? A systematic review and quality assessment. *Int Psychogeriatr*. 2018;30:1593-1605. https://doi.org/10.1017/S1041610218001291
17. Brown JB, Palmer AJ, Bisgaard P, et al. The Mt. Hood challenge: cross-testing two diabetes simulation models. *Diabetes Res Clin Pract*. 2000;50(3):S57-S64. https://doi.org/10.1016/s0168-8227(00)00217-5
18. Penny MA, Verity R, Bever CA, et al. Public health impact and cost-effectiveness of the RTS,S/AS01 malaria vaccine: a systematic comparison of predictions from four mathematical models. *Lancet*. 2016;387:367-375. https://doi.org/10.1016/S0140-6736(15)00725-4
19. Hoogendoorn M, Feenstra TL, Asukai Y, et al. Cost-effectiveness models for chronic obstructive pulmonary disease: cross-model comparison of hypothetical treatment scenarios. *Value Health*. 2014;17:525-536. https://doi.org/10.1016/j.jval.2014.03.1721

15 Cost Considerations

Mary Dooley, PhD, and Dunc Williams, PhD

AN OVERVIEW OF HEALTHCARE COSTS

Researchers devote great time and care to deciding outcome measures that are relevant to the intervention of interest. As discussed in Chapter 2, mortality may be the most relevant outcome for some treatments, but a measure of morbidity may be more relevant for others. The effects on quality of life or activities of daily living (ADL) may matter more than the textbook markers of disease progression. Budget constraints may limit studies to more immediately available clinical outcomes, such as lab values, rather than the longer-term disease outcomes that researchers would prefer to study. Selecting effective outcome measures is a nuanced decision-making process that directly shapes the relevance, accuracy, and impact of a study's findings.

Costs are an equally important, yet often underappreciated consideration in any cost-effectiveness analysis. In fact, "[W]hat is this going to cost?" is one of the hardest questions to answer in healthcare. This is due to several factors.

In healthcare, a charge or list price is the dollar amount a healthcare provider sets/bills for services rendered before any discounts or adjustments. Because of various discounts, this charge can be very different from the amount actually paid. In contrast, cost is defined as the dollar value assigned to resources used to create a product or provide a service. Costs are not always directly and easily associated with a product or service. As a result, cost accounting has developed as a specialized area within accounting, continually refining techniques to more accurately and practically allocate resources to the expenses associated with delivering goods or services.

Cost also depends on the perspective and period of the study.[1] Simply put, the resources that need to be included depend on the entity incurring expenses over the specified timeline. To the patient, cost is the amount paid out-of-pocket for healthcare services. This may include deductibles, copayments, coinsurance, out-of-pocket/out-of-network charges, travel costs, and wages lost in seeking care. To a healthcare provider, cost is the expense (direct and indirect) incurred delivering services to the patient. To an insurer, cost is the amount paid to the provider (or reimbursable to the patient) for services rendered. From a societal perspective, cost can be directly attributable or extend beyond to potential (although never observed) opportunity costs, such as lost quality years of life. Further complicating matters is the fact that one entity's cost can be another entity's revenue.

COST CONSIDERATIONS IN HEALTHCARE

For any business, financial viability begins with an understanding that revenue minus expenses equals profit. In healthcare, understanding revenue and expenses can be complex because of the timing of revenue and expenses. Because most healthcare reimbursement occurs through third-party payers (eg, Medicare, Medicaid, commercial insurers), most revenue is not received when services are rendered. For example, the receipt of payment for the knee replacement provided yesterday morning at your nearest hospital did not occur on the day

DOI: 10.37573/9781585287666.015

of surgery. Similarly, the money required to pay for the knee implant, surgical gloves, electricity, salaries, and other expenses incurred to provide the surgery did not leave the hospital's bank account yesterday. But the revenue and expenses associated with that surgery were recognized on the date of service.

Because it is more accurate to associate the timing of revenue and expenses with the occurrence of service provision (the revenue recognition principle and the expense matching principle, respectively), the Financial Accounting Standards Board (FASB) (for nongovernmental organizations) and the Governmental Accounting Standards Board (GASB) provide guidelines for organizational reporting under accrual accounting. Accrual accounting records revenue and expenses at the time-of-service provision and utilization. By contract, cash accounting records revenue and expenses at the time cash changes hands. For a simple lemonade stand where revenue and expenses are generally associated with the time cash is exchanged, cash accounting is simple, accurate, and may be preferred. However, for complex healthcare organizations where revenue and expenses are rarely timed alongside service provision, the more complex but also more accurate accrual accounting is generally used. Therefore, most healthcare organizations operate under accrual accounting. A specific example includes the use of Medicare Cost Reports submitted to the Centers for Medicare & Medicaid Services (CMS) Healthcare Cost Reporting Information System, where hospitals report revenues and expenses on an accrual basis to reflect the true cost and income associated with patient care during the reporting period.

Revenue is the amount of money collected for services. In hospital reporting, revenue begins with gross charges, the total amount billed for services before any contractual allowances or discounts, derived from the charge master. Gross charge amounts are rarely collected in full because of various contractual allowances and discounts. They could be compared to a car sticker price—the final payment amount is rarely, if ever, the amount listed on the sticker price. Charge master rates are set higher than an organization expects to collect for various reasons. Some organizations may (at least, historically) have used high charge master rates with commercial insurers and self-pay patients before negotiating percentage discounts. Organizations cannot collect more than a charge rate. So, setting a high rate could prevent missed revenue opportunities. Because providers may be limited to receiving payment at or below charges, many healthcare charges are set very high. Variation in charges across insurers and regions, along with variations in charges and prices actually paid, have come under increased scrutiny in recent years resulting in a number of price transparency initiatives.

Contractual allowances and discounts include amounts organizations do not reasonably expect to collect. Discounts are the difference between gross charges (the billed amount) and net patient revenue (NPR), the amount of revenue collected for services rendered. On the cost reports, CMS clarifies eight types of discounts: provision for bad debts, contractual adjustments, charity discounts, teaching allowances, policy discounts, administrative adjustments, implicit price concessions, and other deductions from revenue. Of those, three large categories are:

- Contractual adjustments
- Charity care
- Bad debt

Contractual adjustments include discounts negotiated with a payer. For example, if the knee replacement surgery was for a patient with private insurance, the difference between the gross charge and the net amount to be paid (by both the insurer and the patient) would be a contractual adjustment. Charity care represents charges that the provider (in this case, the hospital) billed for services provided to a patient whom the hospital charity care policy later determined could not pay for services. Bad debt represents charges that the provider originally expected to collect but is unable to. Bad debt may be a portion of post-contractual adjustment charges an insured individual was expected to pay but did not. The difference between charity care and bad debt is typically determined at the provider level through organization-specific policies that often consider the patient's financial situation (eg, assets, debts, income) when determining a patient's ability to pay.

Because gross charge amounts are rarely paid in full and NPR is a more accurate representation of revenue collected, a series of generally accepted accounting principles (GAAP) updates issued by the FASB and GASB over the past 50 years have transitioned away from income statements with gross charges followed by various discounts resulting in NPR. Now NPR is more explicitly reported; most discounts to gross charges are reported separately from the income statement as footnotes to the financial statements.[2,3] The amount of revenue the hospital actually collects is the NPR, where discounts are subtracted from gross charges. **Figure 15-1** visualizes those differences.

The difference between gross charges and NPR is sizeable. An evaluation of 2022 data for short-term general acute care hospitals that reported cost reports found that greater than 75% of gross charges were written off as some type of discount (**Figure 15-2**), reflecting an average charge amount of $4 for every $1 collected.[4] If a healthcare administrator reports the size of their current organization in terms of charges, divide that number by 4 to get to the national average NPR/true size of their organization in terms of collections.

Moving the discussion from revenue to expenses, expenses and costs can be defined in various ways. For purposes of this explanation, expenses represent the cost (in dollars) attributed to service provision for the reporting period, typically a year in length. Under accrual accounting, expenses generally differ from costs. Costs are the total dollar value assigned to resources used to sell a product or provide a resource. For the knee surgery example above, there was an initial cost for building the surgical suite, ie, $1,000,000. But under accrual accounting, that entire cost is not allocated as an expense on the day it is paid, rather a portion of the cost is expensed in each reporting period.

Organizations can follow a variety of allocation methods for the cost of specific items. For external financial reporting, such as annual reports and audited financial statements (AFS), items used during the reporting period are expensed during that period, such as surgical gloves. For capital items that have a useful life longer than the reporting period, such as a building, these are expensed through depreciation and amortization by a method acceptable under GAAP. External financial statements are important for stakeholders who need to access that information: banks, rating agencies, investors, and community members. Beyond external financial statements, costs are allocated internally for managerial decision-making. Internal financial documents do not need to adhere to GAAP so managers have more flexibility in how costs are allocated internally.

In our previous example, the building expense may be allocated based on an equal number of years of usage (a straight-line method); an accelerated method that expenses more of it in the earlier years; a method that expenses it based on the proportion of uses divided by the total expected uses of the asset (while less common for a building, something, such as an magnetic resonance imaging [MRI], may be expensed in this manner); or by another method.

The cost allocation method an organization uses may also vary depending on the type of cost. A building is typically a fixed cost, which means the cost occurs no matter how often it is used to generate revenue. In contrast, surgical gloves are considered a variable cost in that the number purchased varies based on the number of services provided (eg, the number of knee replacement surgeries). There may also be hybrid costs. Semivariable or mixed costs typically begin with a base fixed amount and then have a variable cost component for each use. Step costs are fixed within a range of some volume of services provided, after which they step up to a new level of fixed costs. For example, the cost of operating one surgical suite for square footage leasing would be fixed until the volume becomes too high and a second surgical suite is needed, at which point the fixed costs increase to a higher level and remain there until a third suite is needed. When possible, management generally prefer to align variable and fixed costs with the type of revenue source associated with the cost. For example, an administrator of a hospital with heavy fee-for-service reimbursement may prefer higher variable costs. They may choose to lease an MRI as a variable cost based on per-use basis rather than buying the MRI scanner, which would have been considered a fixed cost. By contrast, an administrator of a hospital that is heavily reimbursed by capitation or

Medicare Reimbursable Bad Debt Explained in the Context of Gross Charges and Net Patient Revenue	
Indicator	**Interpretation:**
Gross Charges	Billed (not collected); car sticker price - no one should pay this amount
- Contractual Allowances and Discounts	While the official CMS definition includes eight categories, we refer to them in the three largest categories: contractual allowances, charity discounts, and bad debt.
Contractual Allowances	Negotiate rate discounts with insurers.
Charity Care	Inability to pay; hospital never reasonably expected to collect
Bad Debt	Ability to pay; hospital originally reasonably expected could have collected
= Net Patient Revenues	Actual dollars collected (subtracting all contractual allowances and discounts from gross charges)

FIGURE 15-1. Gross charges, contractual allowances and discounts, and net patient revenue explained.

Gross Charges to Net Patient Revenue
Explanation with 2022 Hospital Cost Report Data
***Inclusive of all hospitals that were in US states, not VA Federal Government, and not IHS (so, a larger population that our cleaned data set).**

Financial Indicator	2022 Amount	% of Gross Charges (Billed, Not Collected)	% of Net Patient Revenue	Definition
Gross Charges (Billed, Not Collected)	$5113.0 billion dollars			Total charges billed (not collected)
- Contractual Allowances and Discounts	$3845.1 billion dollars	75.20%		Discounts between gross charges (billed) and net patient revenues (collected). CMS defines these as: provision for bad debt, contractual adjustments, charity discounts, teaching allowances, policy discounts, administrative adjustments, implicit price concessions, and other deductions from revenue.
= Net Patient Revenues	$1262.3 billion dollars	24.69%		Net patient revenue is what was collected after contractual allowances, bad debt, and charity/indigent care.

**Note: For net patient revenue, if we subtract gross charges from contractual allowances, the calculation differs slightly because it would be subtracting means, not the underlying values.*

FIGURE 15-2. Gross charges reconciled to net patient revenue: an example.

value-based reimbursement mechanisms may want higher fixed costs, allowing them to predict both revenue and expenses in a more consistent manner.

Cost allocation also depends on whether costs can be directly attributed to a service. Direct costs, such as surgical gloves, are treated differently than indirect costs, such as electricity usage. Direct and indirect costs can be a combination of fixed and variable costs.

Organizations associate costs with specific service lines. The cost of nonrevenue-generating services, such as those for hospital administrators, can be reallocated to revenue-generating service lines, such as surgery. This can be used by the organization to estimate a per-service (in the case of the knee replacement, a per-knee-replacement) cost for an organization. Ultimately, that amount can be used in conjunction with the per-knee-replacement revenue to quantify the profitability of specific services.

Regardless of the methods employed, the goal of the allocation is two-fold. It aims to associate the expenses with the period and type of usage (under accrual accounting) while using a reasonable/not overly burdensome number of resources to track allocations. It also helps the organization explain and remain consistent with its process, or if need be, reconcile any subsequent change in allocation process. The result should be consistent, documented, and adhere to GAAP.

Allocating costs in a consistent, documented manner results in more accurate profit reporting. In the knee surgery example, had the organization recorded all $1,000,000 for the building in its first year of operations when it only provided a few knee surgeries, it would have reported a very large loss in year 1 due to overreporting expenses not directly associated with the entire usage of those expenses. Then, it would have underreported expenses in subsequent years when none of the cost of the building was expensed but many surgeries were performed and generated revenue. By allocating costs through expense matching instead, organizational profits are reported more accurately. Accurate reporting is essential for all stakeholders: patients receiving care, employees, investors (eg, banks and for-profit investors), operators, and policymakers.

Example of Cost Allocation with Time-Driven Activity-Based Costing

Micro-costing is a type of cost allocation that identifies actual resource use for individual patients by directly linking their specific diagnostics, devices, and medications used in treatment; this can include identifying patient-specific treatment times to assess actual labor used. Time-driven activity-based costing (TDABC) is a method of micro-costing that looks at patient-specific resource use, factors in estimated indirect costs, and calculates true costs of production along with the patient-specific treatment times.[5,6] Time-driven activity-based costing is usually conducted by research staff in the clinic during operation hours to collect the relevant data through direct observation. These staff follow and document all activities related to a patient's treatment from the time they arrive until they leave, where time is often tracked manually with a stopwatch. Research shows that TDABC is a useful approach to calculate true costs that may uncover inefficiencies and cost drivers within processes. However, this method can be resource intensive, because staff need to be available on site and are limited to only following one patient at a time.

To address this barrier to TDABC, Dooley et. al. demonstrated a modified version of the TDABC method based on structured interviews with some of the healthcare providers at the clinic.[7] The providers described the typical process for a pediatric sick visit at their clinic and the estimated time to complete each step of the process. The study used their modified method of structured interviews to analyze the clinic's labor costs for a pediatric clinic sick visit process across three scenarios: (1) in-person visit before the COVID-19 pandemic, (2) telehealth visit during the pandemic, and (3) an in-person clinic visit during the pandemic. Through interviews with several providers (including pediatricians and nurse practitioners) from the clinic, they created workflow mapping based on providers' descriptions, having the providers review and refine the workflow until one final flowchart was approved by all providers. The estimated time spent for each step in the process provided in the interviews was then validated by using the clinic's electronic health record timestamps.

For each of the three scenarios, a flowchart was created using information from the interviews. The providers reviewed and approved the accuracy of the flowchart. In the given flowchart (**Figure 15-3**), each square represents a step in the process of the visit from the time a patient calls to schedule an appointment to the time they check out. The steps are organized in the order that they are completed with optional or alternative steps identified with decision nodes represented by diamonds. For each step of the process (square), the average time to complete the step is noted and contained within small gray circles in the bottom right corner with staff roles (eg, provider, nursing, administrative, or mix of roles) involved in completing the step identified by color-coding. Using the flowchart, they were able to estimate the total time that each role was involved in a basic clinic visit.

The authors calculated the labor cost for each minute for each of the roles involved in the clinic visit using median US salaries provided by the US Bureau of Labor Statistics salary data. An alternative approach could use the actual loaded salaries (includes their full benefits and overhead costs) of staff. The labor cost per visit was then calculated for the three scenarios based on the time in the flowchart. For example, using Figure 15-3, labor costs for an in-person clinic visit during the pandemic were calculated by using the identified staff roles and time in the flowchart with the cost per minute of labor to determine the total labor cost for each role (**Table 15-1**). The costs were then summed across all roles to get a total visit cost of $54.60. Monte Carlo simulations were used to reflect the variation of labor minutes that they expect to see by the providers and staff across various clinic visits as well as the varied median salaries for each of the roles to mimic the real world. By running 100,000 simulations across the various minutes and salaries, they created a distribution (or range) of costs for each of the scenarios. From this distribution, they derived a

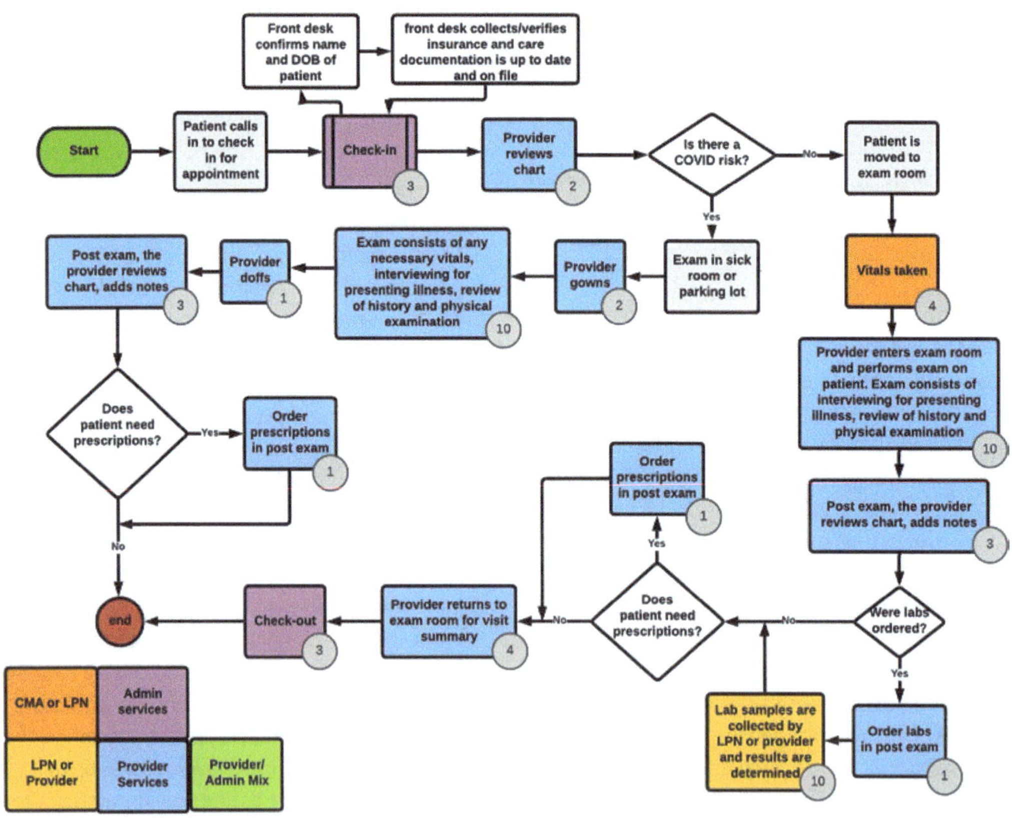

FIGURE 15-3. Pediatric clinic workflow for in-person clinic visit during COVID pandemic.[7]

*Numbers in gray circles are the average time in minutes to complete the process step.

TABLE 15-1. Labor Cost Calculation for the Workflow of an In-Person Clinic Visit During the COVID-19 Pandemic (Assuming No COVID Risk, Labs, or Prescriptions Ordered)

Staff Role	Time (min)	Cost/Min	Labor Cost (time * cost/min)
Pediatrician	19	$2.62	$49.78
Certified medical assistant	4	$0.47	$1.88
Administrative	6	$0.49	$2.94
Total labor cost			$54.60

mean labor cost with standard deviation representative of a typical clinic.

Next, to account for the differences in how care is delivered, they used a clinic-specific provider mix (physician vs. nurse practitioner) and delivery mix (percentage of clinic visits conducted by telehealth vs. in-person) based on electronic health record level data from the clinic during the respective study period. Using this information, they built decision trees (such as **Figure 15-4**) to calculate the weighted labor cost per visit. They combined decision tree weights based on the mixes with the Monte Carlo simulation results (the mean and standard deviation) to get an average weighted visit cost for labor. The weighted mean labor costs were found to be $54.47 before COVID-19 and $51.55 during.

Power Analysis for Costing Studies

As healthcare costs continue to increase, decision-makers are often tasked with controlling costs without reducing the quality of care that patients receive.[8,9] This has led to a greater focus on understanding how changes in the healthcare system may affect cost. One challenge in measuring costs is that there is no guidance in the literature for how to quantify cost savings or differences, specifically, what constitutes a "small" or "large" difference. There is no agreement of what is considered to be a small or large cost difference, even for commonly evaluated metrics, such as hospital admissions or outpatient visits. This issue is further complicated because different stakeholders look at cost differently. A finance or accounting perspective looks at fixed and variable costs and how they impact budgets, whereas the economic perspective considers opportunity costs and cost-effectiveness. Unfortunately, most studies on measuring costs do not include a formal power analysis. Another study by Dooley and colleagues evaluated three methods that potentially could be used to measure cost differences.[10]

The three approaches used to determine a minimally important difference (MID) are

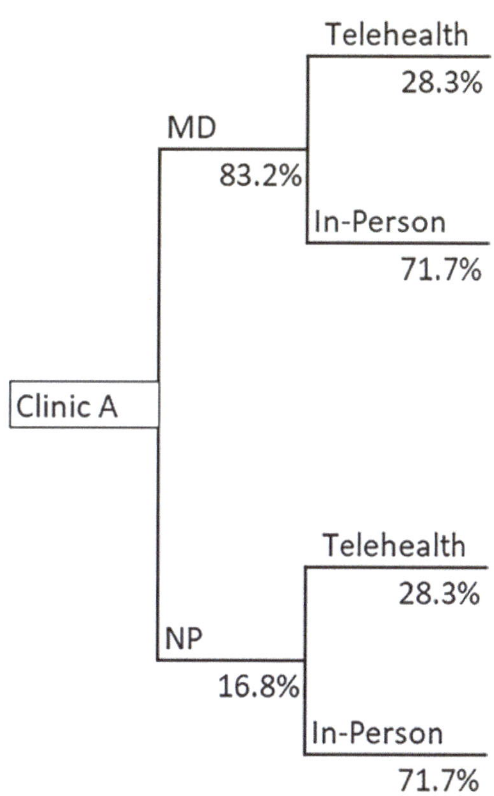

FIGURE 15-4. Decision tree weights by provider and delivery mix during COVID pandemic.

(1) anchor-based, (2) distribution-based, and (3) consensus-based. The anchor-based method maps the relationship between a change in target cost to a known, meaningful, and established difference associated with the target cost. Dooley and colleagues used an anchor-based method to estimate an effect size comparing the clinic reimbursements of adjacent Current Procedural Terminology (CPT) codes that were associated with their target labor costs. The calculated clinic reimbursement difference between a low complexity sick visit (CPT 99213—the basis of their workflow) and a moderate complexity sick visit (CPT 99214—the next level) of an established patient was $59, and this difference was used as their MID estimate. The distribution-based method estimates MID as a percentage of the standard deviation. It has become common practice to reference cut points of 20%, 50%, and 80% of the standard deviation to represent small, medium, and large effect sizes, respectively.[11] The consensus-based method uses expert opinion, typically gathered by anonymously surveying a panel of experts regarding a topic, such as what constitutes a meaningful cost difference. Returned responses are summarized and shared with the panel for reevaluation. This process is repeated until a consensus is reached. The study did not identify a superior method for estimating the MID but recommended using more than one method and assessing whether the estimates converge.

CONCLUSION

While much of the discourse in health services research emphasizes access and quality, a comprehensive understanding of cost structures is just as essential. The terminology, frameworks, and examples presented here underscore the complexity of healthcare financing and the importance of accurate cost measurement and allocation. From the nuances of accrual accounting to the application of TDABC, these tools enable more precise financial reporting and informed decision-making. As healthcare systems continue to evolve under financial pressures and policy reforms, the ability to rigorously analyze and interpret cost data remains essential for advancing value-based care and ensuring the responsible stewardship of resources.

REFERENCES

1. Gold MR, Siegel JE, Russell LB, Weinstein MC, eds. *Cost-Effectiveness in Health and Medicine*. Oxford: Oxford University Press; 1996.
2. Reiter KL, Song PH, Gapenski LC. *Gapenski's Healthcare Finance: An Introduction to Accounting and Financial Management*. 7th ed. Chicago: Health Administration Press; 2021.
3. Pink GH, Song PH. *Gapenski's Understanding Healthcare Financial Management.* Chicago: Health Administration Press; 2019.
4. Author's analysis of Medicare Cost Report data for relevant years.
5. Carroll N, Lord J. The growing importance of cost accounting for hospitals. *J Health Care Finance*. 2016;172-185. PMID: 31839701
6. Tan S, Rutten F, van Ineveld B, et al. Comparing methodologies for the costs estimation of hospital services. *Eur J Health Economics*. 2009;10:39-45. https://doi.org/10.1007/s10198-008-0101-x
7. Dooley MJ, Simpson KN, Simpson AN, et al. A modification of time-driven activity-based costing for comparing cost of telehealth and in-person visits. *Telemed J E Health.* 2022;28(10):1525-1533. https://doi.org/10.1089/tmj.2021.0338
8. Blumethal D, Abrams M. The Affordable Care Act at 10 years: payment and delivery system reforms. *N Engl J Med.* 2020;382(11):1057-1063. https://doi.org/10.1056/NEJMhpr1916092
9. Baicker K, Chandra A. Do we spend too much on health care? *N Engl J Med.* 2020;383(7):605-608. https://doi.org/10.1056/NEJMp2006099
10. Dooley M, Simpson AN, Nietert PJ, et al. Minimally important differences in cost savings: is it possible to identify an MID for cost savings? *Health Serv Outcomes Res Methodol.* 2021;21:131-144. https://doi.org/10.1007/s10742-020-00233-5
11. Cohen J. *Statistical Power Analysis for the Behavioral Sciences*. 2nd ed. Hillsdale, NJ: Lawrence Erlbaum Associates; 1988.

Cost-Effectiveness Analyses 16

Corey Morrow, PhD, MOT, OTR/L, and
Todd L. Wandstrat, RPh, PharmD

INTRODUCTION TO COST-EFFECTIVENESS ANALYSIS

In a general sense, a cost-effectiveness analysis (CEA) is used to evaluate the outcomes (consequences) and costs (resources) of interventions designed to improve health. This technique has been used to compare the economic efficiency of various medical interventions, ranging from smoking cessation and cancer screening to gene therapies.[1-3] Information from CEAs should be used as an aid to improve healthcare decision-making, rather than as the sole criterion for choice. Remember that health economics is a borrowed discipline, and the concepts of value and analysis are appropriated constructs from finance, economics, public health, applied mathematics, statistics, epidemiology, and social behavioral theory. The ultimate decision to use a particular intervention should incorporate the values of all stakeholders affected by the decision (eg, providers, payers, patients), considering a specific perspective and the goal of the analysis. The goal of improving patient outcomes while controlling costs requires data on the economic, clinical, and humanistic outcomes and costs or resources of all reasonable therapeutic alternatives available to treat the patient.[4] Cost-effectiveness analyses can also measure the efficiency of an intervention compared to a nonintervention (doing nothing). An example of this is watchful waiting for the treatment of otitis media, where many causative agents could be viruses, and the use of antimicrobial agents may not shorten the acute disease course or the intermediate-term sequelae in certain patients.[5]

A CEA is distinguished from other forms of health economic analyses by its use of nonmonetary, health-related outcome measures. Cost-effectiveness outcomes are calculated as a ratio, the difference in costs between two treatments divided by the difference in outcomes. This incremental cost-effectiveness ratio (ICER) measures the relative *efficiency* of various treatment alternatives. An efficient treatment provides the greatest quantity of the desired outcome or consequence at the lowest cost per outcome. Incremental cost-effectiveness ratios do not provide information regarding whether it is *appropriate or ethical* to spend the money (resource) to achieve the outcome, rather which treatment incurs the lowest cost to achieve the desired outcome. A CEA assumes that the funds needed to purchase the most efficient treatment are available, and it can help to identify the most *efficient* use of resources when several treatment options are available. In an era of escalating healthcare costs, it is crucial to incorporate efficiency considerations into our decision-making processes.

In a CEA, the consequences or outcomes of the treatment alternatives are measured in the same nonmonetary units, such as life-years saved, the percentage reduction in lipid levels, or cases cured. Results from different CEAs can only be compared if the alternatives are specified with the same outcome measure. For example, the effects of diet and exercise on blood pressure can be compared with those of an antihypertensive medication regimen if the outcomes of both treatments are measured on the same metric, such as systolic blood pressure or the risk of stroke. In a CEA, the outcome

DOI: 10.37573/9781585287666.016

measure used should relate to the "true" consequence of interest.[6] For example, in a CEA of patients with type 2 diabetes, HbA1c levels could be used to measure a medication's efficacy. There is little interest in the HbA1c levels per se, rather the real interest rests in how well these levels correlate with the undesired consequences of diabetes, such as diabetic neuropathy and vision loss. If controlling the HbA1c level reduces the long-term consequences of type 2 diabetes, this lab value can be used as a surrogate for treatment outcomes.

The rigorous construction of a CEA is often the first step in addressing questions centered on determining the value of a specific intervention. As crucial as perspective is to the heart of the analysis, the transparency of analytic elements and methodology is essential to determine the applicability of the analysis to a specific situation. A CEA may support or refute clinical trial results, depending on the perspective. Cost-effectiveness analysis results should always be constructed to evaluate the concept of efficiency of resource use or value from a specific perspective. As described in more detail later in the chapter, efficacy refers to the effect of an intervention under the rigorous conditions of a controlled trial. In contrast, effectiveness refers to the impact of an intervention in a real-world or real-life setting, and efficiency refers to the extent to which an output or outcome is achieved at the lowest possible cost. Notably, different perspectives may lead to very different interpretations of value.

DESIGN AND CONDUCT OF COST-EFFECTIVENESS STUDIES

As with any research approach, the thoughtful and rigorous design of a CEA influences the fidelity of the results, interpretations, and implications. The design steps are not necessarily perfectly linear and may involve an iterative improvement process before executing the analysis. Standardized approaches improve the rigor and reproducibility of scientific analyses. For example, as noted in Chapters 5 and 6, systematic reviews and randomized controlled trials (RCTs) follow the PRISMA and CONSORT guidelines, respectively. In 2022, the Consolidated Health Economic Evaluation Reporting Standards (CHEERS) were updated to provide guidance for CEAs.[7-9] The Second Panel on Cost-Effectiveness in Health in Medicine also offers specific guidelines for CEAs.[10]

To represent the vast implications of a CEA, this chapter outlines three hypothetical CEA scenarios and tracks their progression through the study design. In scenario 1, a hypothetical new rehabilitation medical device, device A, is being introduced to the fields of occupational and physical therapy to improve the chronic hand function deficits of patients who survived a stroke. Scenario 2 aims to evaluate the integration of telehealth to address rural healthcare provider shortages. Finally, scenario 3 compares various wheelchair types for people with a spinal cord injury.

Identification of the Problem

The first step in conducting a CEA should be the identification of the research problem and proposed solution(s). Analysts should aim to address issues with relevant (positive or negative) results to inform decision-makers. Appropriate literature should be reviewed to support the nature and scope of the problem, including the intervention(s) of interest.

In addition to identifying the problem and proposed solution(s), the specific objectives of the study should also be stated clearly in the problem step. For example, is the purpose of the study to compare all myocardial infarction treatment options or only those administered directly in the emergency department? Will the study include all myocardial infarction patients or specifically examine adults older than 65 living in rural counties of Montana?

Importantly, CEA study teams should engage stakeholders early in the design process to help identify clinically relevant problems and variables, refine comparator selections, and prioritize outcomes. Stakeholders may include patients, clinicians, government officials, or veteran researchers familiar with the problem. They may assist with identifying specific and impactful outcome measures, comparator groups, direct and indirect cost variables, and other considerations.

For scenario 1, hypothetical device A has been created by a rehabilitation device company to improve the upper extremity function of patients with neurological deficits.

This scope is too broad for a CEA, which requires a more focused clinical and value question.

The specific problem can be narrowed to include stroke survivors who regularly experience chronic symptoms resulting in long-term deficits in upper extremity function. The possible solution is our hypothetical device A, which was developed to improve the functional use of the hand. The study team may include stroke survivors, occupational or physical therapists, device A suppliers/manufacturers, and Medicare specialists.

Determine the Study Perspective and Audience

Now that a study problem and a possible solution of interest have been identified, determining the study perspective and intended audience further drives and informs the development of the research question, associated variables, and subsequent methodology. The study *perspective* defines which costs and outcomes are relevant. The societal perspective is the broadest and includes all costs and benefits regardless of who pays for the treatment and who benefits. A societal perspective has been recommended by the Second Panel on Cost-Effectiveness in Health and Medicine as the one that should be used in health policy decisions that would affect the public. A societal perspective may also encompass the impact of intervention on sectors beyond healthcare, such as education, transportation, and labor. The Panel also recognized a healthcare sector perspective as a CEA viewpoint that focuses on healthcare-related costs and excludes other societal costs.[10]

The audience refers to the individuals or organizations that will use the CEA study results in their decision-making process. Examples of audiences are payers (ie, Medicare, vocational rehabilitation, pharmacy benefit managers, healthcare consumers or beneficiaries—patients/groups of patients or caregivers/family members), integrated delivery networks (ie, health plan and specialty pharmacy), group purchasing organizations, health systems, pharmacies, hospitals/individual clinics, employers, and providers (**Table 16-1**).

Specifying a perspective and audience ensures that all relevant costs and outcomes are included in the analysis. **Table 16-2** provides examples of various costs included within a CEA.

TABLE 16-1. Examples of CEA Audiences for Scenario 1

Audience		Research Interest Example
Payers	Medicare	Does the use of device A reduce Medicare expenditures on falls for stroke survivors?
	Vocational rehabilitation	Does the use of device A improve work productivity for stroke survivors?
	Veterans affairs	Is the additional cost of device A justified by greater effectiveness compared to a standard resting hand splint?
Healthcare consumer	Patients	Does device A provide sufficient therapeutic value to justify its high out-of-pocket cost to the patient?
	Caregivers	Does the use of device A lead to a measurable reduction in caregiver labor hours and associated costs?
Provider	Health system	Does the purchase of device A result in improved patient outcomes that translate into shorter hospital stays and reduced inpatient costs?
	Facility	Will the patient outcomes from device A be substantial enough to lead to increased referrals, thereby justifying its purchase at the facility level?
	Clinician	Does the therapeutic benefit of increased at-home use justify a patient's out-of-pocket purchase of device A?

CEA = cost-effectiveness analysis.

TABLE 16-2. Examples of Resource Costs

Resource Cost Category	Examples
Direct medical costs	Physician office visits Hospital care Pharmaceutical products and services Outpatient medical care Laboratory tests Diagnostic tests and procedures
Direct nonmedical costs	Transportation costs to obtain care Housekeeping costs Custodial care for dependents
Indirect costs	Lost productivity due to death or illness Absenteeism
Intangible costs	Changes in productivity due to morbidity Changes in health-related quality of life Social and emotional well-being Life satisfaction

Specify Interventions, Comparators, and Outcomes of Interest

Once the research problem has been identified, the next step in designing a CEA is to specify the intervention(s), comparator(s), and outcome(s) of interest. A commonly used structure to guide this process is the PICO framework, which stands for Population/ Problem (P), Intervention (I), Comparator (C), and Outcome (O).[11] This framework helps to define the clinical and economic question in a way that aligns with the intended audience and study perspective. In a CEA, PICO ensures that the alternatives being compared are both relevant and grounded in practice and that the outcomes being measured, whether clinical or economic, are meaningful to patients, providers, and payers. **Table 16-3** outlines examples using the PICO format to compare interventions for three scenarios.

The problem statement guides the selection of relevant comparators. A robust CEA always compares two or more treatment alternatives, which may include standard care, competing interventions, or even a "do nothing" approach. The most useful analyses compare a new intervention with the current standard of care, often referred to as a head-to-head or active control comparison.

Whether a comparator is appropriate depends on both the clinical context and the study's perspective. For example, scenario 2 aims to enhance diabetes management in rural populations with limited access to in-person endocrinology services. In this scenario, the intervention might involve quarterly telehealth visits with a remote specialist. Relevant comparators could include the current standard of care, such as annual in-person endocrinology visits, or primary care-based diabetes management with limited specialty input. From a societal perspective, indirect costs, such as travel time, lost wages, and caregiver burden, may influence the selection and evaluation of these alternatives.

Outcomes in a CEA can be categorized into two main types: resource outcomes and health outcomes. Resource outcomes reflect changes in healthcare utilization, such as physician visits, emergency department use, or medication costs that result from the intervention. Health outcomes measure the intervention's effect on biomedical indicators (eg, HbA1c levels), clinical endpoints (eg, diabetes-related hospitalizations), or broader humanistic outcomes, such as health-related quality of life and patient satisfaction. In the telehealth scenario, relevant outcomes might include reduced complication rates, improved glycemic control, fewer hospitalizations, and better patient-reported access to care. **Figure 16-1** depicts the concept of a healthcare production process.

Classify the Time Horizon and Discounting

The time horizon in a CEA refers to the length of time over which costs and health outcomes are measured. This duration may be short- or long-term, depending on the research question, the intervention being evaluated, and the intended audience or perspective. Several factors influence the appropriate choice of time horizon. For instance, the type of condition and nature of the intervention often dictate

TABLE 16-3. PICO Questions with Integrated Time Horizons

Scenario	Problem/ Population	Intervention	Comparison	Outcome	Full PICO Question
Scenario 1: medical device	Adult stroke survivors with chronic functional hand deficits	Device A with standard outpatient occupational therapy	Standard outpatient occupational therapy alone	ICER expressed as improvement in functional hand use	Among adult stroke survivors with chronic functional hand deficits, does the addition of device A to 25 standard outpatient occupational therapy sessions, compared with standard therapy alone, result in a favorable ICER based on functional hand use improvement over 6 months?
Scenario 2: telehealth	Medicare beneficiaries with type 2 diabetes in rural areas with limited access to endocrinologists	Quarterly endocrinology telehealth visits covered by Medicare	Annual in-person endocrinology visit (requiring patient travel)	ICER based on reduction in diabetes-related complications and ED visits over 10 years	Over a 10-year time horizon, does Medicare coverage of quarterly endocrinology telehealth visits for rural adults with type 2 diabetes, compared with a single annual in-person visit, result in a favorable ICER based on reduced complications and ED visits?
Scenario 3: wheelchair selection	Adults with spinal cord injury at high risk of pressure injuries	Customized power wheelchair with powered tilt-in-space functionality	Noncustomized power wheelchair without tilt-in-space	ICER based on reduction in hospitalization due to pressure injuries over a 5-year period	Among adults with spinal cord injury at risk of pressure injuries, does a customized power wheelchair with powered tilt-in-space, compared to a noncustomized power wheelchair without tilt, reduce pressure injury-related hospitalizations and result in a favorable ICER over 5 years?

PICO = Population/Problem (P), Intervention (I), Comparator (C), and Outcome (O); ED = emergency department: ICER = incremental cost-effectiveness ratio.

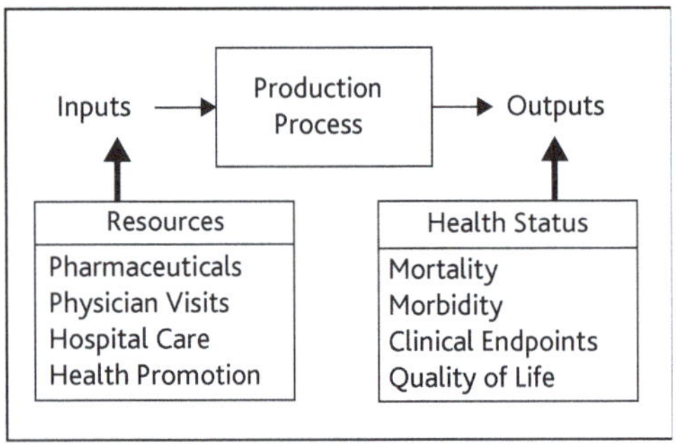

FIGURE 16-1. The healthcare production process.

whether a shorter or longer time frame is justified. A one-time preventative vaccine may require only a short-term horizon, whereas a series of vaccines administered over several months may necessitate a broader perspective.

Similarly, the expected benefit trajectory of an intervention plays a critical role. For example, a new pharmaceutical treatment for myocardial infarction may be evaluated for its immediate impact on emergency department mortality or for its long-term effect on reducing hypertension and preventing rehospitalization over a 5-year period.

The intended perspective and audience must also be taken into consideration. Different stakeholders prioritize outcomes over varying time frames. Insurance providers may place greater value on short-term cost savings, whereas physicians and patients may justify higher upfront costs based on the sustained clinical benefits they provide over time.

For example, in scenario 3, a standard wheelchair may offer immediate quality-of-life improvements for a person with a new spinal cord injury. From Medicare's perspective, the higher cost of a customized power wheelchair may be justified when considering 5-year outcomes, such as reduced falls, improved community access and return-to-work potential, and greater device durability resulting in fewer repairs. Additionally, a powered tilt-in-space feature available for customized wheelchairs may allow patients to periodically recline and redistribute their body weight, thereby reducing the risk of pressure injuries. These long-term outcomes have implications not only for healthcare costs but also for broader societal value.

Related to a study's time horizon is the change in the value of the variables over time. When costs and consequences occur over an extended period (usually more than 1 year), then these amounts need to be adjusted to reflect the "time value of money." To accurately compare the costs and benefits of a medical intervention, both must be related to the same point in time. The time value of money is influenced by inflation and interest rates on monetary value. In simple terms, a dollar today is worth more than a dollar received in the future. For example, suppose someone has a choice between receiving a payment of $10,000 today or the same $10,000 payment a year from now. In that case, it is financially preferable to take the money now, given interest rates and inflation.

The technique used to account for the time value of money is called discounting. In discounting, the net present value of future cash (inflows or outflows) is calculated. Adjusting the value of future costs and consequences to account for inflation and interest portrays these amounts in today's dollars. For instance, with a 4% annual interest rate, accepting $9,615 today would be financially equivalent to receiving $10,000 at 1 year from now. Why? Because $9,615 invested at 4% interest over 1 year would grow to $10,000 ($9,615 × 1.04 = $10,000). Discounting ensures that future costs and benefits are accurately compared by adjusting for the time value of money.

For example, two vaccines, X and Y, may be used for the prevention of "epizuditis." Both are expected to save a total of $30,000 in medical costs over the next 3 years; however, the timing of these savings differs. Vaccine X yields consistent annual savings of $10,000 per year, whereas vaccine Y produces $20,000 in savings during the first year, followed by $5,000 in each of the second and third years. Although the total savings are identical, vaccine Y may be preferred, because a larger portion of the savings occurs earlier, increasing its discounted present value. When future costs or savings are brought into today's dollars using discounting, earlier benefits are worth more than later ones. Discounting is very important when costs and benefits of treatments accrue unevenly over time (as in the vaccine example), inflation and interest rates are high, or the time horizon for the comparison exceeds 1 year.

Determine the Model Design

Once the problem has been stated clearly and relevant alternatives are specified, the next step is to describe the relationship between resource inputs and outcomes. Health economists refer to this relationship as the "production process" for treatment; clinicians might explain the production process in terms of a clinical pathway or treatment algorithm. In a production process, resource inputs refer to the products and services required to produce a specific outcome or output. Examples of inputs to medical care production include medications, physician visits, hospitalizations, laboratory tests, and nursing care. These inputs are combined in the production process, where outcomes are generated. The "production" takes place in a variety of settings, such as the physician's office, ambulatory clinic, hospital, emergency department, pharmacy, or the patient's home. Figure 16-1 depicts the concept of a healthcare production process.

A decision tree is a useful technique for depicting the clinical relationship between resource inputs and outcomes. The decision tree in **Figure 16-2** models the clinical decision-making process and related outcomes. Inputs are ordered chronologically from left to right and lead to the possible outcomes (outputs) of treatment. These outcomes may be desired outcomes (increased survival) or unintended outcomes (adverse medication events). The decision tree in Figure 16-2 compares the cost and outcomes of two antibiotics (A and B) for treating community-acquired pneumonia. Each treatment branch includes probability of cure or no cure, followed by downstream outcomes, such as gastrointestinal upset, the need for hospitalization, or home infusion, each with associated costs. More complex models, such as those with recurring events or ongoing disease progression, may be better represented by using a Markov model. For more information on decision trees and Markov modeling, see Chapter 14.

Establish Model Parameters

Once the clinical treatment pathway (decision tree/Markov model) is specified, resource costs and outcomes for each alternative can be incorporated. Identifying relevant costs and consequences associated with the use of the intervention of interest is an essential task in any CEA and is influenced by the study

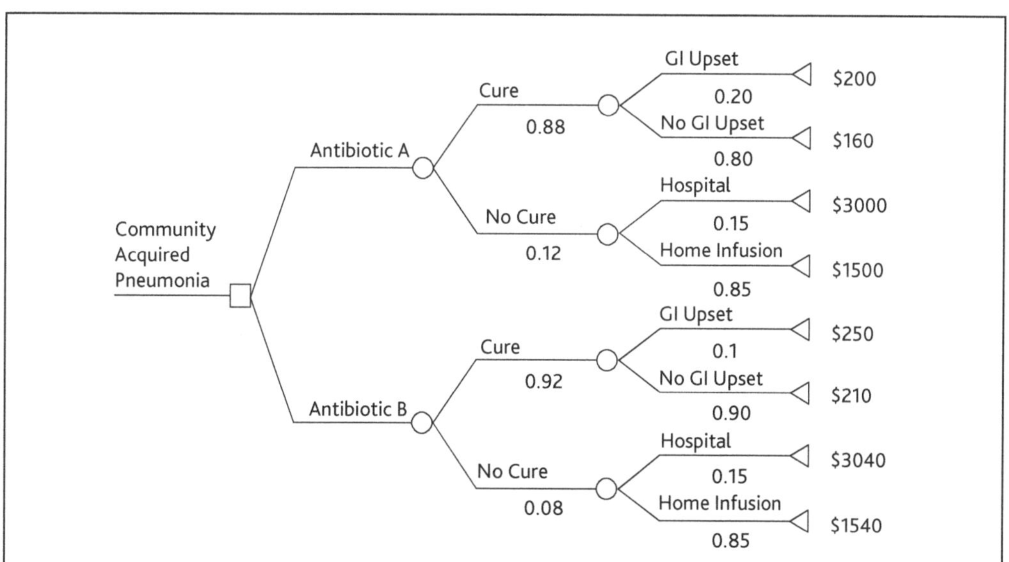

FIGURE 16-2. **Decision tree diagram comparing antibiotic outcomes.**

audience/perspective, time horizon, and comparators. As previously discussed, the broadest perspective is societal and encompasses the full range of costs and potential consequences listed in Table 16-2. If the study is conducted from a narrower perspective, such as that of a healthcare payer or provider, cost and consequences in the indirect and intangible categories may not be included in the analysis. In contrast, a study conducted for an employer or patient audience might consist of the effects of treatment on productivity and quality of life.

Costs and consequences (outcomes) may be classified into three major groups: direct, indirect, and intangible.[12] Table 16-2 provides some frequently encountered examples of these types of costs and outcomes, while **Table 16-4** applies these costs to scenarios 1, 2, and 3.

Direct costs include both medical and nonmedical expenditures for the detection, treatment, and prevention of disease. Direct medical costs reflect resources consumed in the "production" of medical care, such as pharmaceutical products and services, physician visits, laboratory monitoring, and hospital care.

Direct nonmedical costs refer to expenditures for products and services that are not directly related to disease treatment but are still closely related to patient care. Examples of direct nonmedical costs include transportation costs to a pharmacy or physician's office and caregiver costs during the illness period. Frequently, direct nonmedical costs are paid out-of-pocket by the patient or assumed as an unreimbursed cost of care.

Indirect costs account for changes in an individual's productivity, as illness leads to both absenteeism and presenteeism. Absenteeism refers to the time a person is away from their job, whereas presenteeism represents the decrease in productivity that occurs when an individual works while ill. The monetary value of lost or altered productivity is typically used as a measure of indirect costs.

Intangible costs and consequences are nonmonetary, and they reflect the impact of a disease and its treatment on the social and emotional functioning of individuals as well as their quality of life. These humanistic consequences are measured by using health-related quality-of-life instruments and patient satisfaction questionnaires.

TABLE 16-4. Scenario Resource Cost Examples

Cost Category	Scenario 1: Device A	Scenario 2: Telehealth	Scenario 3: Wheelchair Selection
Direct medical	Outpatient therapy visits	Physician office visits	Wheelchair base cost
	Device A and training	Telehealth equipment and maintenance	Wheelchair pressure relief cushion
Direct nonmedical	Electricity usage for charging	Transportation/hotel costs to obtain distant care	Transportation to seating clinic
	Device storage modifications (ie, locked cabinet)	Reduced physical building costs	Home modifications: wheelchair ramp
Indirect	Increased work productivity due to improved hand function	Patient absences from work due to long travel distances	Increased productivity at work due to increased wheelchair function
	Decreased caregiver burden for functional activities	Missed opportunities for chronic disease management	Reduced caregiver burden for transfers and mobility
Intangible	Improved sense of independence	Reduced stress from long travel distances	Improved life satisfaction
	Increased confidence	Increased perception of control in managing condition	Increased social participation

Valuing Resource Costs and Outcomes

Once all relevant costs and consequences for a treatment pathway have been identified, the value (cost) of each item must be determined. Resource and outcome costing has two components: the quantity of resources consumed and the price of each unit of resource.[12,13] The quantity of resources is measured as the number of resources used in the care (production) process. The price of the resource should reflect the amount paid (ie, the cost) to purchase the resource or input.

There are several methods for measuring and determining resource use and costs in an economic study. First, resource use and costs can be collected concurrently as part of a clinical trial protocol. With this approach, the quantities of resources used in treatment are collected alongside the clinical data. When economic data are collected as part of a clinical trial, there may be resources consumed that would not be used in routine daily practice. These are known as protocol-induced costs. When economic data are not collected as part of a clinical trial, resource use may be determined by examining patient charts or databases. Second, resource use may be determined by patient or provider interviews. Patient diaries are frequently used to track the types and quantities of resources consumed by patients throughout their treatment. Healthcare providers, such as physicians, pharmacists, and nurses, can also provide information on the resources used and the outcomes of treatment. Third, administrative databases can be used to extract utilization and cost data. Health plans maintain claims files for all services paid for by the plan. To the extent that these files contain diagnosis and procedure codes, they can be used to determine resource use patterns for the treatment of specific diseases.

Once the quantity of resources is determined, a relevant price must be attached to each unit of the resource that is consumed. For example, if a hospitalized patient receives two vials of an intravenous antibiotic per day for 5 days, the total consumption is 10 vials. Next, a price must be determined for each vial. The relevant price that is used is a function of the study perspective. If the study were being conducted for a provider's (hospital's) audience, the price would be what the hospital paid for the medication. If this were $120 per vial, the resource cost for this medication would be $1,200. If the study occurred for a payer audience, such as the health plan or patient, the relevant price would be the amount paid by the plan or patient. So, if the hospital charged the patient $200 per vial, the relevant price of the medication to the patient would be $2,000. As illustrated by this example, the decision to use costs or charges in an economic evaluation should be determined by the study's audience.

There are two approaches to assigning a price to resource use: market price and reference price. The market price reflects the amount paid by the producer to acquire the resource. In the example above, this would be $120 per vial of antibiotic. The second approach, a reference price, is used when actual market prices are unknown and must be estimated. Reference prices are obtained from external sources and reflect prices that are available in the general marketplace. A commonly used reference price for pharmaceuticals is the average wholesale price, which is a readily available, standard price in the public domain. When studies include data from administrative claims, it is often difficult to determine the actual cost of resources, because these databases typically contain charge data that may not accurately reflect the actual amounts paid. In these cases, reference prices can be used to provide a more realistic estimate of the actual price.

For example, a study to evaluate which of several lipid-lowering agents is most cost-effective for a state Medicaid program formulary should include all costs that the Medicaid program would incur for lipid reduction treatment as well as all the benefits (in terms of future cost savings from a reduced rate of cardiovascular disease) expected to accrue to Medicaid as a result of coverage. Because Medicaid is a public program that covers most of the medical care for program participants, a broader societal perspective may be appropriate. In contrast, a private health plan (insurer) might only be interested in the direct costs and benefits from paying for any given treatment. Refer to Chapter 15 for more on cost considerations.

Data Sources

To build a CEA, data are extracted from other studies and plugged into a model. The results of a CEA model are only as strong as the quality of data inputs. Establishing evidence of efficacy and effectiveness is critical to conducting a valid CEA. Evidence of efficacy and effectiveness can be gathered from a variety of sources, which can differ in the strength and quality of the evidence they provide. The most common sources of efficacy and effectiveness data for CEAs are RCTs, effectiveness trials, meta-analyses, observational studies, and database studies. Results from clinical trials, effectiveness studies, and meta-analyses are used to determine the probabilities of events and outcomes in economic studies. These data are used to populate decision tree models, which are then used to estimate the average treatment cost.

The distinction between efficacy, effectiveness, and efficiency is crucial in understanding how broadly the results of a CEA can be generalized. Efficacy measures the direct effect of a medical treatment (ie, pharmaceutical, surgical, or device interventions) under well-controlled scientific conditions, such as those found in RCTs. The adoption of new medication therapy has historically been based on the results of RCTs, which show that the medication is safe and efficacious compared with either a placebo or current practice. Little to no consideration was given to the cost of the medication. As the cost of healthcare and pharmaceuticals increased, the emphasis shifted from solely efficacy to the inclusion of effectiveness and efficiency.

Effectiveness measures the outcomes of medical interventions under real-world practice conditions. Real-world effectiveness differs from efficacy, because the daily use of prescribed treatments can differ considerably from how they were used in clinical trial protocols. Factors, such as compliance, age, ethnicity, genetics, and comorbidity, influence patient response to treatment. Consequently, the effectiveness of a new medicine is typically less than its efficacy.

When costs are considered along with efficacy and effectiveness, the question of efficiency arises. Efficiency refers to the effective use of resources in producing healthcare outcomes. In CEAs, the most efficient treatment delivers the desired outcome for the lowest possible cost. Cost-effectiveness analyses use data from both efficacy and effectiveness trials to estimate efficiency.

Meta-analyses have become a popular source of efficacy and effectiveness data for CEAs. As explained further in Chapter 6, a meta-analysis is a systematic approach to identifying and synthesizing the results of multiple clinical trials into a comprehensive summary. By pooling efficacy data from similar clinical trials, meta-analyses can provide more precise estimates of intervention efficacy than those reported in individual trials. Because meta-analyses incorporate the results from multiple studies, the efficacy and effectiveness results are considered more reliable than those from a single clinical trial.

Healthcare databases are another valuable source of data, as detailed in Chapter 11. Paid claims databases from private insurers, healthcare plans, and employers provide a rich source of information on utilization and cost of treatment in the daily practice of medicine (ie, effectiveness). While not as scientifically rigorous as RCTs, database analyses employ epidemiological and statistical methods, along with large numbers of patient records, to provide reasonably valid and reliable estimates of effectiveness and treatment outcomes.

Referring to the hypothetical device A in scenario 1, data inputs for a CEA could be extracted from various sources, depending on the availability and quality of existing evidence. Cost-of-care estimates can be obtained from large administrative datasets, such as Medicare claims, which reflect real-world spending patterns on hospitalizations, outpatient visits, and durable medical equipment. Clinical trial data could provide measures of efficacy under controlled conditions, whereas meta-analyses might offer more robust pooled estimates of both efficacy and effectiveness across multiple studies. For real-world effectiveness data, observational studies or claims-based analyses could be used to estimate actual outcomes associated with device A, such as improvements in hand function. Importantly, analysts must critically assess the strengths and limitations of each data source, recognizing that no single source is likely to provide all the necessary inputs. The validity and transparency of a CEA ultimately depend on how well these inputs are selected, justified, and interpreted within the context of the clinical and policy question at hand.

INTEPRETATION AND PRESENTATION OF RESULTS

Once all costs and consequences have been measured and the effectiveness of the treatment alternatives is determined, the relative cost-effectiveness of the treatments can be estimated. This is done by ranking the treatments in order of their cost and effectiveness and eliminating those options that are most costly and least effective (ie, dominated). Next, the ratios can be calculated and ranked to determine which alternative is most efficient.

The idea of relative cost-effectiveness and dominance is illustrated in **Table 16-5**. Treatment may be considered cost-effective in three cases: (1) when it is more effective and less costly than the others; (2) when it is more effective and higher cost but adds additional value, such as improved access; and (3) when it is less effective and less expensive. Dominant alternatives are those that are more effective and less costly than other treatments (case 1). In cases 2 and 3, trade-offs are made regarding whether the increase (or decrease) in cost is worth the increase (or decrease) in effectiveness.

Before drawing conclusions from a CEA, however, it is essential to understand the study's limitations and how the results apply to a specific practice setting. In a simple CEA, the results may be presented as a single *average* cost-effectiveness ratio (CER), such as $28,000 per year of life saved. When used as the sole measure of efficiency, average CERs can be highly misleading.

TABLE 16-5. Average Treatment Costs and Outcomes

Medication	Average Treatment Cost Per Month	Symptom-Free Days Per Month
LowTack	$43.20	24
EZBreathe	$32.00	20

INCREMENTAL COST-EFFECTIVENESS RATIO

To be truly meaningful, the ICER should be presented instead and compared with other treatment alternatives, preferably the current standard of practice or treatment. Because ICERs are ratios, it is important to interpret both the numerator (cost) and the denominator (effectiveness) rather than just the final value. The numerator and denominator should be evaluated to ensure that the costs and effects of the treatment are meaningful to the treatment decision.

For example, if asked to name the most cost-effective medication to lower lipid levels, a logical choice, based on CERs, would be generic niacin tablets. Why? Because it works (lowers lipid levels by 5% to 10%), and it is low cost (pennies per tablet). Niacin would have a very favorable *average* CER; however, few would argue that it is the medication of choice for patients who require a substantial reduction in lipid levels. A classic example of how average CERs can be misleading is illustrated in a 1975 article in the *New England Journal of Medicine*.[14] The article compared the average CERs with the ICERs for conducting consecutive screening tests for blood in the stool (a marker for colon cancer). The average CER for conducting six consecutive tests was $2,451 per case detected, whereas the ICER for the sixth test was $47,107,214 per additional case detected. While the average CER per case detected seems reasonable, the ICER for the sixth test was astronomical. This disparity in the average and ICERs existed, because most of the benefits of screening resulted from the first of the six tests; the additional benefit of the other tests was very small, but the costs were substantial. Because the ICER compares the relative change in effectiveness of two treatments to the relative change in cost, it is a much more informative measure in assessing the relative value of alternative treatments. It is calculated by dividing the difference in costs of two treatments by the difference in effectiveness of the two treatments.

The presentation of the ICER is particularly important when one treatment is both more effective and more costly than the alternative treatment. For example, two treatments (A and B) both improve survival. Treatment A increases survival by 22 years and treatment B by 22.5 years. The average CERs are $15,000 per year of life saved for A and $16,000 per year of life saved for B. Based on these ratios, it might be tempting to pay an additional $1,000 on average more for treatment B. However, the ICER shows that an extra year of life saved would cost $60,000, not the $1,000 difference in the average cost of the two medications.

Another method for illustrating the incremental cost-effectiveness of one treatment versus another is the cost-effectiveness grid (**Figure 16-3**). The cost-effectiveness grid illustrates the incremental cost of the two treatments on the y-axis and the incremental effectiveness on the x-axis.[4,15] **Figure 16-4** illustrates the four cost-effectiveness quadrants comparing a new intervention to the current standard. In Quadrant I, the new intervention is more effective but also more costly, requiring a determination of whether the added benefit justifies the added cost. In Quadrant II, the new intervention is dominant: it is both more effective and less costly than the comparator. In Quadrant III, the new intervention is less effective but also less costly, representing a trade-off in which decision-makers must assess whether cost savings justify reduced effectiveness. Finally, in Quadrant IV, the new intervention is both more costly and less effective than the comparator, meaning it is dominated.

SENSITIVITY ANALYSES

When interpreting the results of a study, it is essential to carefully examine the estimates used for resource utilization and costs. Assumptions are made in all health economic analyses regarding the likelihood (probability) of the occurrence of desired or undesired effects, the cost or value of inputs and outcomes, and the audience of the analysis. However, these assumptions inevitably introduce uncertainties into the results.

The purpose of a sensitivity analysis is to assess how much the study's results might change if certain assumptions about utilization and cost were varied. As the costs of medical care (including medications, physician visits, and emergency department visits) increase each year and vary among suppliers and regions of the country, it is essential to account for these potential differences when estimating cost-effectiveness. In addition to variations in costs, assumptions about effectiveness should also be varied, as they can influence the results.

Sensitivity analyses can also be used to illustrate how cost-effectiveness results may change in response to variations in variables (parameters) or factors in the real-world environment, such as the cost of medications, the incidence of adverse effects, and disease progression. Specific geographical differences in variables and outcomes, when adjusted for through sensitivity

Cost of A versus B

Effectiveness of A versus B		Lower	Equal	Higher
	Higher	Choose A (*Dominant*)	Choose A	Trade-off
	Equal	Choose A	Equality	Choose B
	Lower	Trade-off	Choose B	Choose B (*Dominant*)

FIGURE 16-3. **Cost-effectiveness grid and the concept of dominance.**

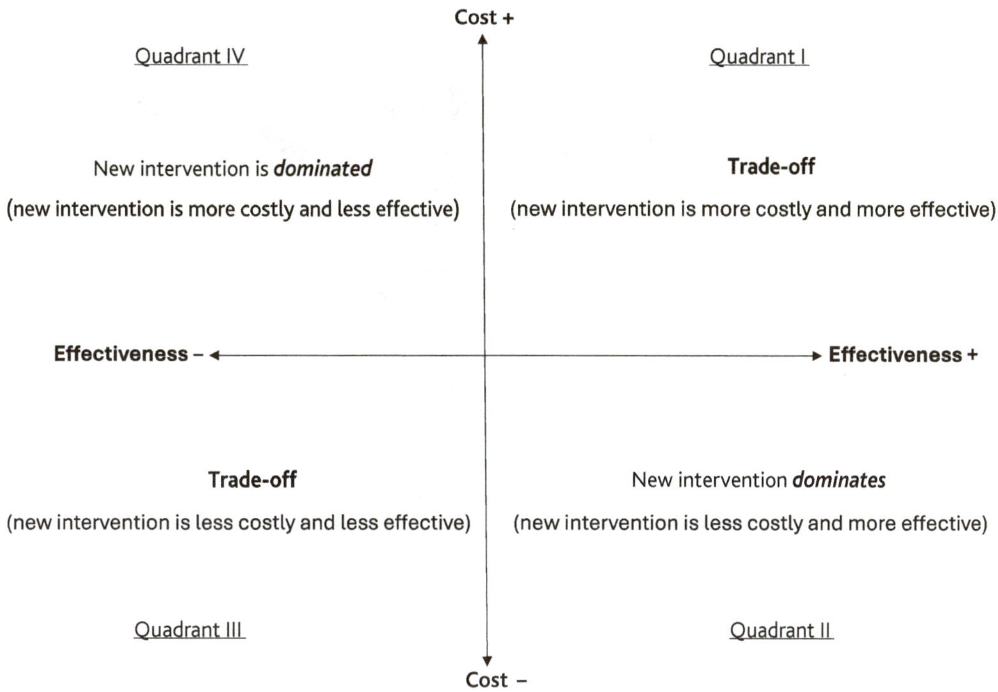

FIGURE 16-4. **Cost-effectiveness quadrants comparing a new intervention to a standard comparator.**

analysis, can enhance the applicability or generalizability of a study.[16,17] The results of sensitivity analyses can be presented in various ways, including cost-effectiveness acceptability curves, tornado diagrams (**Figure 16-5**), scatter plots, and tabular form.

What constitutes a relevant range of values over which robustness should be tested? Put another way, what change in outcomes would be deemed meaningful by a clinician? The answer to these questions helps to determine the ranges included in a sensitivity analysis. Consider a case in which compliance with a new asthma medication was reported in clinical trials to be 95%. It is unlikely that a higher compliance rate would ever be realized in actual practice. The effects of lower compliance rates, perhaps around 70%, on patient outcomes would be of more interest. If the medication remains effective when compliance decreases from 95% to 70%, clinicians can reasonably be confident that the new medication will perform well in actual practice.

Examples

Suppose a new inhaled therapy for managing acute asthma attacks has been tested in an RCT. In the trial, the new therapy (LowTack) was compared to the current standard of treatment (EZBreathe). The primary outcome of interest in the trial was the number of symptom-free days, a nonmonetary measure. Economic data were captured as part of the clinical trial, because the company thought their product might offer not only a clinical advantage but also an economic advantage. Given the nonmonetary outcome of symptom-free days, a CEA was conducted. The study was conducted for a third-party payer audience, and only direct medical costs (including medication costs, physician office visits, and emergency department visits) were included in the analysis. Market prices were used to determine resource unit costs. The patient recorded the number of symptom-free days (days without any breathing problems) over 3 months in a diary. Medical resource utilization was abstracted from patient charts and study records. The average total cost of treatment per patient and the average number of symptom-free days per patient for each medication are summarized in Table 16-5.

Average Cost-Effectiveness Ratios

The average CER is calculated for each treatment by dividing the treatment cost by

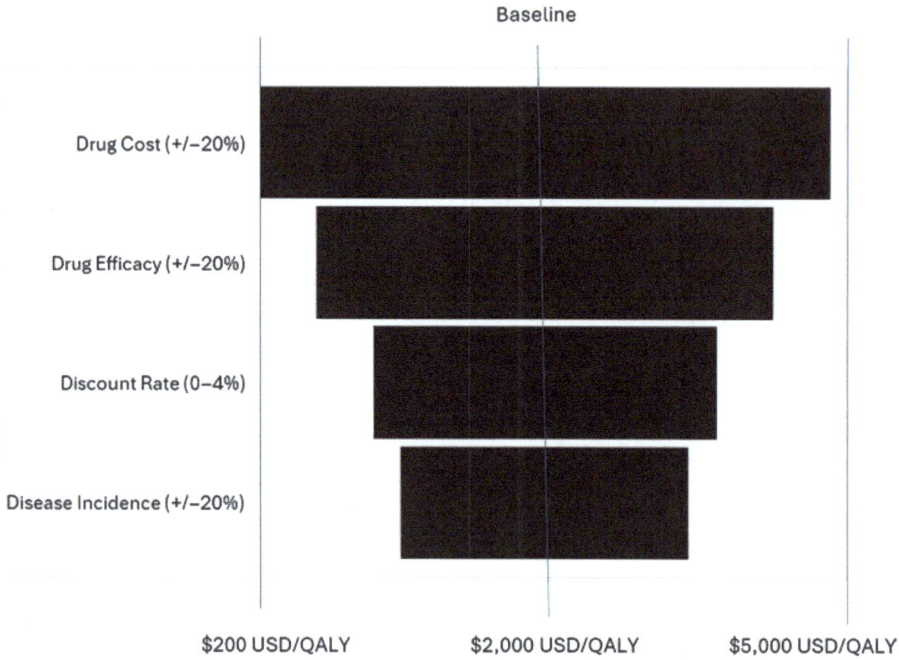

FIGURE 16-5. **Tornado diagram.**

the number of symptom-free days for each medication.

For LowTack:

$$C/E_{LowTack} = \frac{(Cost_{LowTack})}{(\text{Symptom-free days}_{LowTack})}$$

$$C/E_{LowTack} = \frac{\$43.20}{24 \text{ days}}$$

$$C/E_{LowTack} = \$1.80 \text{ per symptom-free day}$$

For EZBreathe:

$$C/E_{EZBreathe} = \frac{(Cost_{EZBreathe})}{(\text{Symptom-free days}_{EZBreathe})}$$

$$C/E_{EZBreathe} = \frac{\$32.00}{20 \text{ days}}$$

$$C/E_{EZBreathe} = \$1.60 \text{ per symptom-free day}$$

Based on these average cost-effectiveness ratios, one might assume that EZBreathe, the current standard of treatment, is the most cost-effective agent (lowest cost per outcome). The average CER reflects the cost to achieve an outcome (symptom-free day) independent of other treatments. If this was all the information available, EZBreathe would be the choice. But it is important to note that while LowTack costs more than EZBreathe, it is also more efficacious (more symptom-free days). LowTack would be in quadrant I of Figure 16-4; it is more effective than EZBreathe and more costly. The average CER is simply a measure of efficiency and does not tell us whether it is appropriate to spend more money for greater efficacy. A more informed choice can be made by examining the ICER, which indicates the amount needed to pay to achieve the additional efficacy of LowTack over EZBreathe.[10] When one treatment is both more effective and higher cost than another, the real question is how much it costs to receive the additional or incremental benefit. The ICER is calculated by dividing the incremental change in the cost of two therapies by the incremental change in effectiveness.[10]

$$ICER_{LowTack\ vs.\ EZBreathe} = \frac{(Cost_{LowTack} - Cost_{EZBreathe})}{(\text{Symptom-free days}_{LowTack} - \text{Symptom-free days}_{EZBreathe})}$$

$$\text{ICER} = \frac{(\$43.20 - \$32.00)}{(24\text{ days} - 20\text{ days})}$$

$$\text{ICER} = (\$11.20 / 4\text{ days})$$

ICER = $2.80 for each additional symptom-free day

Incremental cost-effectiveness ratios are the preferred measure of relative value, because they enable decision-makers to compare the cost of the additional benefit of one treatment with that of another. The decision now rests on clinical and economic judgment, rather than mathematics: "Is it worth $2.80 to achieve an additional day free of asthma symptoms?" In this case, it might be easy to agree. In other cases, it may be much more challenging to make a decision. Whether the extra expenditure is appropriate is a matter of choice and should be considered in terms of clinical, economic, and humanistic factors.[17]

For another example of CEAs in practice, consider a recent review of health economic evaluations of COVID-19 vaccination that combined various health economic methodologies and outcomes, providing an excellent overview of the public health implications of an invention.[18] One of the studies in this review is a CEA that utilized years of life saved (YLS) as an outcome measure, and vaccination results in an ICER that represents a cost savings compared with no vaccination. In this analysis, the COVID-19 vaccine was considered cost-effective unless there was an incidence of prior immunity to COVID-19 greater than 50% in the population.[19] This study employed a health sector perspective (public/population health sector) to inform public health policy decisions. To assess the effect of real-world influences on a vaccine program, the model in the study varied both the supply and the speed of vaccination in a population. Incremental cost-effectiveness ratios were calculated by

$$\text{ICER (specific strategy and scenario)} = \frac{\text{costs of program vaccine} - \text{costs of program no vaccine}}{\text{years of life saved (YLS)}}$$

The different parameters defining vaccines (vaccine effectiveness, vaccine acceptance, cost per person vaccinated, percentage of population vaccinated, and virus epidemic scenarios) were varied in a number of sensitivity analyses. The lowest ICER and cost savings were realized when the cost per person vaccinated was < $25 (2020 USD). This study is an excellent example of utilizing a CEA and ICER to inform public health decisions and policymaking.

CONCLUSION

A CEA is used to compare the costs and outcomes of two or more treatments when the outcomes are measured in the same nonmonetary unit. An average CER measures the cost per unit of health outcome for a single intervention, without considering any alternatives. In contrast, an ICER compares two interventions and shows the additional cost required to gain one additional unit of health benefit, providing a measure of relative efficiency more useful for decision-making.

When presenting the results of a CEA, researchers should make every effort to transparently include study limitations and assumptions. Sensitivity analyses should be conducted for all key assumptions in the analysis, allowing the reader to understand how robust the results are to variations that are likely to occur in real-world practice.

Cost-effectiveness analyses provide us with one tool to improve our treatment decisions and should not be used in isolation from other factors in the treatment process. Rather than dictating which medication or treatment to use, CEAs inform about the circumstances under which a particular treatment is likely to be most efficient. Incorporating efficiency criteria in our decision-making is necessary and desirable, given the escalating demand for newer, higher-cost treatments and the constant pressure to control healthcare costs.

REFERENCES

1. Levy DE, Klinger EV, Linder JA, et al. Cost-effectiveness of a health system-based smoking cessation program. *Nicotine Tob Res*. 2017;19(12):1508-1515. https://doi.org/10.1093/ntr/ntw243
2. Ratushnyak S, Hoogendoorn M, van Baal PH. Cost-effectiveness of cancer screening: health and costs in life years gained. *Am J Prev Med*. 2019;57(6):792-799. https://doi.org/10.1016/j.amepre.2019.07.027

3. Garrison Jr LP, Jiao B, Dabbous O. Gene therapy may not be as expensive as people think: challenges in assessing the value of single and short-term therapies. *J Manag Care Spec Pharm*. 2021;27(5):674-681. https://doi.org/10.18553/jmcp.2021.27.5.674
4. Deng Z-J, Gui L, Chen J, et al. Clinical, economic and humanistic outcomes of medication therapy management services: a systematic review and meta-analysis. *Front Pharmacol*. 2023;14:1143444. https://doi.org/10.3389/fphar.2023.1143444
5. Sun D, McCarthy T, Liberman DB. Cost-effectiveness of watchful waiting in acute otitis media. *Pediatrics*. 2017;139(4):e20163086. https://doi.org/10.1542/peds.2016-3086
6. Berger ML, Bingefors K, Hedblom EC, et al. *Health Care Cost, Quality, and Outcomes: ISPOR Book of Terms*. Baltimore, MD: ISPOR; 2003.
7. Page MJ, McKenzie JE, Bossuyt PM, et al. The PRISMA 2020 statement: an updated guideline for reporting systematic reviews. *BMJ*. 2021;372. https://doi.org/10.1136/bmj.n71
8. Moher D, Schulz KF, Altman DG. The CONSORT statement: revised recommendations for improving the quality of reports of parallel-group randomised trials. *Lancet*. 2001;357(9263):1191-1194. PMID: 11323066
9. Husereau D, Drummond M, Augustovski F, et al. Consolidated Health Economic Evaluation Reporting Standards 2022 (CHEERS 2022) statement: updated reporting guidance for health economic evaluations. *MDM Policy & Pract*. 2022;7(1). https://doi.org/10.1177/23814683211061097
10. Sanders GD, Neumann PJ, Basu A, et al. Recommendations for conduct, methodological practices, and reporting of cost-effectiveness analyses: Second Panel on Cost-Effectiveness in Health and Medicine. *JAMA*. 2016;316(10):1093-1103. https://doi.org/10.1001/jama.2016.12195
11. Miller SA, Forrest JL. Enhancing your practice through evidence-based decision making: PICO, learning how to ask good questions. *J Evid Base Dent*. 2001;1(2):136-141. https://doi.org/10.1016/S1532-3382(01)70024-3
12. Neumann PJ, Ganiats TG, Russell LB, et al. *Cost-Effectiveness in Health and Medicine*. 2nd ed. Oxford: Oxford University Press; 2016.
13. Neumann PJ, Sanders GD. Cost-effectiveness analysis 2.0. *N Engl J Med*. 2017;376(3):203-205. https://doi.org/10.1056/NEJMp1612619
14. Neuhauser D, Lewicki AM. What do we gain from the sixth stool guaiac? *N Engl J Med*. 1975;293(5):226-228. https://doi.org/10.1056/NEJM197507312930504
15. Black WC. The CE plane: a graphic representation of cost-effectiveness. *Med Decis Making*. 1990;10(3):212-214. https://doi.org/10.1177/0272989X9001000308
16. Simpson KN, Fossler MJ, Wase L, et al. Budget impact and pharmacy costs with targeted use of oliceridine for postsurgical pain in patients at high risk of opioid-related adverse events. *Expert Rev Pharmacoecon Outcomes Res*. 2022;22(4):671-681. https://doi.org/10.1080/14737167.2022.2038137
17. Simpson KN, Fossler MJ, Wase L, Demitrack MA. Cost–effectiveness and cost-benefit analysis of oliceridine in the treatment of acute pain. *J Comp Eff Res*. 2021;10(15):1107-1119. https://doi.org/10.2217/cer-2021-0107
18. Utami AM, Rendrayani F, Khoiry QA, et al. Economic evaluation of COVID-19 vaccination: a systematic review. *J Glob Health*. 2023;13:06001. https://doi.org/10.7189/jogh.13.06001
19. Reddy KP, Fitzmaurice KP, Scott JA, et al. Clinical outcomes and cost-effectiveness of COVID-19 vaccination in South Africa. *Nat Commun*. 2021;12(1):6238. https://doi.org/10.1038/s41467-021-26557-5

Budget-Impact Analysis 17

Stephanie R. Earnshaw, PhD, MS, and
Anita J. Brogan, PhD, MS

Budget-impact analysis (BIA) is an economic assessment that estimates the financial (and possibly health) consequences of adopting an intervention. Based on forecasted rates of use of the intervention along with the rates of use of competing interventions, short- and medium-term effects on financial statements and other resources are calculated. In healthcare, BIA is used by budget holders to understand the affordability of interventions, inform reimbursement recommendations, and support requests for additional healthcare funds, all along with estimating the impact on the health of their population (if considered). These results help budget holders with budget planning, reaching target population health outcomes, and planning health resource needs.

For the purposes of this chapter, we define a few key terms below:

- An **intervention** may be a new or existing pharmaceutical, vaccine, medical device, diagnostic, surgical approach, digital application, or anything else that may be used to support the medical treatment of a patient. For brevity, we will refer to the intervention of interest for the BIA as the "new intervention," remembering that the actual intervention of interest may be a new intervention or an intervention that has been on the market for some time. In either case, we are interested in understanding the impact to the budget holder's budget of adding, increasing, or changing the intervention's projected use.
- A **budget** is an estimate of income and expenditures for a fixed period of time. It is used to plan and manage finances. In a broader sense, it also refers to the amount of money needed/available for a specific purpose.
- A **budget holder** is the audience for or the perspective of the budget. In the world of economic analysis of healthcare interventions, the budget holder is typically a payer such as a health plan or government body that is responsible for paying for the intervention. The budget holder could also be a provider, such as a clinic or hospital, that may observe financial or clinical changes to their system due to the introduction of the intervention.

Budget-impact analyses are set up as a comparison of financial statements or budgets. **Table 17-1** shows the comparison of a budget with and without a new intervention and provides a listing of the typical components of a BIA.

Many reimbursement/health technology assessment agencies require BIAs along with a cost-effectiveness analysis as part of the comprehensive economic evaluation. As such, the International Society for Pharmacoeconomics and Outcomes Research (ISPOR) issued guidelines in 2007 with an update in 2014 specifically for building BIAs.[1,2] Additionally, some reimbursement agencies have their own BIA guidelines, such as Canada's Patented Medicine Prices Review Board (PMPRB), Australia's Department of Health, Belgium's Health Care Knowledge Centre, and Portugal's National Authority of Medicines and Health Products.[3-6] These guidelines are helpful in that they provide jurisdiction-specific guidance as well as general guidance on the estimation framework and types of input data to be considered. Most other organizations provide less detailed guidance, often focusing on how they prefer

DOI: 10.37573/9781585287666.017

TABLE 17-1. Budget-Impact Analysis Construct

Budget Component	Budget Without New Intervention	Budget with New Intervention
Perspective	All costs/outcomes of interest to the budget holder Consider costs or revenue	
Population	All new and existing individuals who are eligible for the new intervention	
Time horizon	Annual budgets projected out for several years	
Interventions	Current: Mix of currently used interventions	Current: Mix of currently used interventions plus the new intervention
	Projected future: Projected mix of interventions for each budget year without the new intervention	Projected future: Projected mix of interventions for each budget year with the new intervention
Health outcomes	Identify health benefits and risks that the new intervention may impact	
	Health benefits and risks of currently used interventions	Health benefits and risks of currently used interventions and the new intervention
Costs	Intervention-related costs: Cost of the currently used interventions and associated resources	Intervention-related costs: Cost of the currently used interventions, the new intervention, and associated resources
	Nonintervention-related costs: Cost of the nonintervention-related outcomes for the currently used interventions and associated resources	Nonintervention-related costs: Cost of the nonintervention-related outcomes for the currently used interventions, the new intervention, and associated resources
Results	Aggregated and disaggregated costs (total annual, per member per month) Health outcomes	

analyses and results to be reported. A comprehensive review of BIA methods, reporting, and applications can be found in the book *Budget-Impact Analysis of Health Care Interventions: A Practical Guide.*[7]

PERSPECTIVE

The perspective of a BIA is typically that of the budget holder, focusing on the actual costs and outcomes that will impact their financial obligations within their jurisdiction. This approach ensures that budget holders can assess affordability and make informed decisions that balance financial considerations with the health impact on their population.

Specifically, a budget holder could be a payer, in which case the values of interest are the costs and outcomes for which the payer is responsible. Indirect costs, such as caregiver burden or lost time from work, do not impact the payer's financial obligations and so may not be included. In contrast, a self-insured employer may have interest in including these indirect costs in their BIA, because they impact the employer's obligations (although these costs may be included in different budgets within the organization).

Up to this point, we have been discussing budget impact in terms of costs. Another perspective is that of revenue. When adding a new intervention or increasing its uptake, the budget holder's costs and revenue are both likely to change, and although a budget holder is still interested in the impact on their costs, they may also be interested in understanding the financial impact from a revenue perspective. For example, a hospital budget holder could be interested in the impact of a new intervention on costs within their organization to ensure that they can afford materials and services, but they may also be interested in the impact of the new intervention on their revenue stream, which influences their profits and ability to cover operating expenses. Will the introduction of the new intervention reduce the hospital's revenue, creating a concern about profitability, or will revenue increase, thereby allowing the hospital to increase profits? In general, the cost and revenue perspectives are very different, and we highly recommend separating them into distinct analyses so that one does not confuse costs with revenue.

POPULATION STUDIED

The budgets for a BIA are built on a population of individuals who are eligible for the intervention within the jurisdiction of the healthcare budget holder. Identifying this population is crucial for the BIA, because it is the population of individuals upon which changes in costs and outcomes will occur due to the changes in the uptake of this intervention.

The BIA population is made up of two types of individuals: the **prevalent population**, individuals who meet the eligibility criteria for the intervention before the intervention is available, and the **incident population**, individuals who are newly eligible for the intervention. Individuals in the prevalent population may have received a competing intervention or no intervention prior to switching to this new intervention, whereas individuals in the incident population are receiving an intervention for the condition for the first time. As a result, the prevalent population has likely been diagnosed with the condition for a longer period of time and thus could have important differences from the incident population, such as older age or more severe disease.

To identify the BIA population, it is common to use what is often referred to as a "funnel-down approach." In this approach, the funnel starts with the broadest population, such as all patients within the jurisdiction or health plan. The population is then progressively narrowed using epidemiologic information (data such as age and sex distribution, prevalence and incidence rates, and the percentage of individuals with a diagnosis who are under a physician's care) to the point that only patients who are eligible for the intervention are identified. See **Table 17-2** for an example of this approach for a prevalent adult population with human immunodeficiency virus (HIV).

While identifying the BIA population, it may be important to consider issues, such as:

- Acute versus chronic: For acute conditions, typically only the incident population is considered (because there may be no prevalent population or the duration of the condition is shorter than the annual budget period), whereas for chronic conditions, both prevalent and incident populations are typically included, either separately or combined.
- Disease severity: Populations with more severe disease may receive the intervention for shorter or longer periods of time and may have different outcomes than those with mild disease.
- Changes in population size: The size of the eligible population can change over time due to factors such as demographic shifts, changes in disease incidence, and the introduction of new interventions.

TABLE 17-2. Prevalent Population Eligible for Add-on Antiretroviral Treatment: Funnel-down for Adults with HIV Who Are Highly Treatment Experienced and Failing Current Treatment

Population	Percentage	Persons	Source Information
Health plan members		1,000,000	Assumption
Adult population (18+ years)	78.5%	785,000	US Census Bureau, 2024 estimate[8]
Adults living with diagnosed HIV-1 infection	0.4%	3,140	CDC, derived from 2022 estimates (Table 15a)[9]
Diagnosed individuals who are HTE	6.0%	188	Composite definition of HTE[10]
HTE individuals who are failing their current antiretroviral regimen	15.6%	29	Among HTE individuals, percentage with viral load ≥ 200 copies/mL at 12 months[11]

CDC = Centers for Disease Control and Prevention; human immunodeficiency virus = HIV; HTE = highly treatment experienced.

TIME HORIZON

The time horizon of a BIA should be relevant to the budget holder's situation. Typically, annual budgets are compared and projected for 3 to 5 years due to uncertainty associated with budgets beyond that point. Budget holders are interested in actual costs and outcomes that may occur during the time period of interest, which means discounting (ie, reduction of future costs to account for the time value of money) is not applied. In fact, theoretically, budget holders might consider applying inflation rates. However, in practice, inflation is not often incorporated in BIA, because inflation rates can be difficult to predict and can vary based on the type of cost.

While most BIA time horizons are relatively short, there are cases when longer time horizons or alternate analyses may be considered. For example, for preventive interventions and for chronic diseases, it is not uncommon to see increased short-term budgets with no or limited cost offsets, which result in immediate budgets that are unfavorable to the new intervention. For these situations, if substantial cost offsets occur beyond the primary time horizon, longer time horizons may be considered. However, BIA is intended to support decisions in the short-term, and longer time horizons may not be of interest to the budget holder. As a result, it may be helpful to conduct a cost-effectiveness analysis to complement the BIA.

INTERVENTION MIX

Creating and comparing budget scenarios is the central focus of BIA and is essential for understanding the financial implications of introducing a new intervention. The budget scenarios consider all patients eligible for the new intervention within the jurisdiction of the healthcare budget holder and capture use of the new intervention and of competing interventions among these patients over the analysis time frame. The budget scenarios are typically constructed as a budget in which patients receive a mix of competing interventions in a world without the new intervention (ie, the current intervention mix) and a budget in which patients receive a mix of competing interventions in a world with the new intervention.*

The competing interventions and the new intervention do not have to be of the same type. For example, the introduction of a new drug could replace treatment with other drugs, a surgical intervention, best supportive care, or no intervention at all. When constructing the full analysis over a designated time horizon, it is important to consider multiple issues around the intervention mix. These issues include the following:

- The current intervention mix should include all relevant interventions currently used in the population and that might be affected by the new intervention. This involves careful selection of competing interventions and understanding the current mix of these interventions.
- Over time, the current intervention mix (without the introduction of the new intervention) may change because of factors such as new clinical information, marketing, patent expirations, and the entry of generics (**Figure 17-1A**). The analysis will need to project changes to this intervention mix over time.
- The introduction of the new intervention will impact the current intervention mix. Several questions may help to identify appropriate projections, such as: What will the initial uptake of the new intervention be? What will the trajectory of that uptake look like over time? How will the mix of the competing interventions in the presence of the new intervention change over time (**Figure 17-1B**)? For example, will the new intervention draw market share primarily from one competing intervention, equally from all competing interventions, or something in between?

* Although we denote the scenarios as a "world without" and a "world with" the new intervention, it is important to recognize that scenarios may represent other situations as well. For example, a budget holder may wish to understand the impact of encouraging use of interventions that have been in the marketplace for some time. In this case, the scenarios could be thought of as "world with current use" and "world with expanded use." Although not a requirement, it is typical for the first scenario to represent the status quo and the second scenario to represent a potential change.

Budget Scenario Year 1 World Without New Intervention	Budget Scenario Year 2 World Without New Intervention	Budget Scenario Year 3 World Without New Intervention
• 20% receiving intervention 1 • 30% receiving intervention 2 • 50% receiving intervention 3	• 25% receiving intervention 1 • 30% receiving intervention 2 • 45% receiving intervention 3	• 27.5% receiving intervention 1 • 32.5% receiving intervention 2 • 40% receiving intervention 3

A. Projection of the mix of competing interventions over a 3-year BIA time horizon in a world without the new intervention.

Budget Scenario Year 1 World With New Intervention	Budget Scenario Year 2 World With New Intervention	Budget Scenario Year 3 World With New Intervention
• 5% receiving new intervention • 20% receiving intervention 1 • 30% receiving intervention 2 • 45% receiving intervention 3	• 10% receiving new intervention • 23% receiving intervention 1 • 28% receiving intervention 2 • 39% receiving intervention 3	• 15% receiving new intervention • 22.5% receiving intervention 1 • 27.5% receiving intervention 2 • 35% receiving intervention 3

B. Projection of the uptake of the new intervention and the mix of competing interventions over a 3-year BIA time horizon in a world with the new intervention.

FIGURE 17-1. **Construct of budget scenarios.**

Note that projections of future intervention mixes are needed for both the world without the new intervention and the world with the new intervention. As usual, predicting the future is challenging! Furthermore, sources for these data differ from published sources typically used for other BIA parameters. Options include data from past product launches, sales projections developed by manufacturers, or input from clinicians or payers about what they expect to see.

HEALTH OUTCOMES

The introduction of a new intervention will often increase the budgets of a budget holder, because the new intervention may be more expensive than existing, competing interventions. However, when introducing or encouraging the use of an intervention, outcomes within the population will also change due to the benefits and risks associated with the interventions. As a result, it is important for the BIA to capture the impact of efficacy and safety to estimate changes in health outcomes (ie, What impact can we expect on the budget holder's population given the financial change?). Furthermore, these changes in health outcomes may lead to offsetting costs to the budget holder that are also important to capture. Budget-impact guidelines recommend that if changes in health outcomes or condition-related costs are likely to occur within the analysis time horizon and are supported by credible clinical data, then they should be incorporated into the analysis.[2]

Health outcomes that might be impacted include the number of hospitalizations in the population, hospital length of stay, the number of episodes or exacerbations that require intensive healthcare resource use, the number of patients who acquire a condition (for preventives), reduced progression of a disease, or the number of patients cured. Accounting for these changes in health outcomes will not only inform a budget holder about the population health benefits they can expect for the added cost (assuming an increase in budget) but may also reveal cost offsets (areas in which money is saved), as the need for healthcare resources may be reduced.

Health outcomes might occur at various points within the time horizon of the analyses. For example, for interventions to treat acute diseases, it is likely that the health events will occur within the time horizon of the analyses; thus, they are easy to capture. However, some preventive interventions or interventions to treat chronic diseases may have clinical benefits or risks that occur well after the time horizon of the analysis. For example, preexposure prophylaxis for HIV may prevent HIV acquisitions in the short term, yielding health benefits within the analysis time horizon as well as health benefits for many years into the future. Interventions that reduce disease progression may not change the severity of a patient's disease, but preventing progression to a more severe disease state could lead to less resource use or reduced mortality years after initiation of treatment. All in all, it can be beneficial to capture these elements especially if there is credible supporting evidence. As discussed in the section on time horizon above, potential options to incorporate these benefits include use of a longer BIA time horizon or development of a complementary cost-effectiveness analysis.

To capture the impact of interventions on health outcomes, the approach and data needs may vary. For conditions where changes occur almost immediately, clinical trials can provide data to estimate changes in condition outcomes and associated costs directly. Population health outcomes are then estimated by applying these clinical trial data to the intervention mix for incident populations starting the intervention each year of the BIA time horizon. On the other hand, for chronic conditions where changes occur gradually within the BIA time horizon, a decision-analytic model, such as a Markov model or simulation model, might be needed to capture the effects on condition outcomes over time. For example, natural history data might be used to model disease progression among patients not receiving any intervention, and clinical trial data could be applied to examine the impact of the new and competing interventions on disease progression. Reduced disease progression would then yield reduced disease severity in the modeled population and ultimately impact healthcare resource use, as more advanced disease typically requires more intensive resource use. When incorporating these more advanced analysis structures, it is important to remember that the approach to BIA (eg, identifying the eligible population and comparing budget scenarios) remains the same.

COSTS

Naturally, the budget scenarios are made up of costs. There are two primary types of costs to consider in a BIA: intervention-related costs and nonintervention-related costs.

Intervention-Related Costs

Intervention-related costs include costs for acquisition, administration, and adverse event management. Acquisition costs include the price of the intervention itself, whether it is a drug, vaccine, diagnostic, surgery, or other intervention. Acquisition costs can vary based on national or regional price lists and negotiated discounts and rebates. Administration costs depend on the method of delivery. For example, oral medications have minimal administration costs, while injectable or intravenous drugs may require involvement of healthcare professionals. A self-administered diagnostic, such as a COVID or pregnancy test, may have no administration cost, whereas other diagnostics, such as magnetic resonance imaging, require administration by a healthcare provider at significant cost. Adverse events may also be factored in, as they can lead to additional costs for monitoring and/or treatment.

Nonintervention-Related Costs

Nonintervention-related costs refer to all other costs related to managing the condition, including any impact of interventions. These include costs associated with managing symptoms and consequences of the condition. Symptoms and consequences may include events, such as infections, exacerbations, episodes, or crises, and the resource use, such as physician visits and hospitalization, that may be associated with the events. If available, the cost of these events may be derived in aggregate through an analysis of healthcare claims. Otherwise, the components to derive the costs of events may need to be defined, with each component of the event costed individually

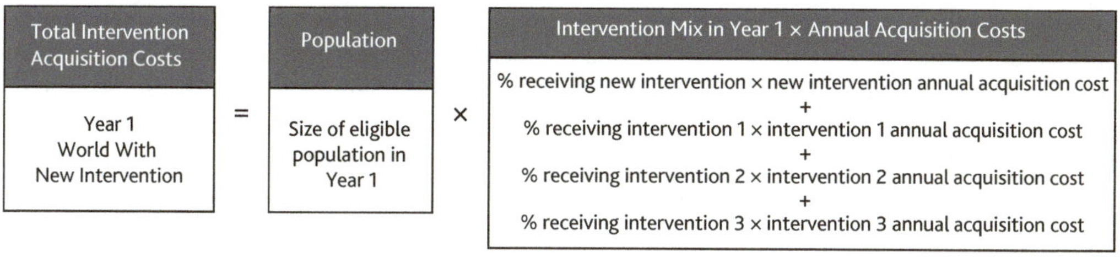

FIGURE 17-2. **Example calculation: total intervention acquisition costs in year 1 for the scenario with the new intervention.**

to derive the overall cost. In this case, unit costs for resources (eg, the cost of one physician visit) may be obtained from jurisdiction-specific costing sources.

When considering costs, it is important to consider the perspective of the budget holder and to include costs that impact them. For example, a payer, such as a managed care plan, may be interested in costs associated with hospitalizations, physician visits, and lab tests but may not be interested in patient out-of-pocket expenses, such as those for over-the-counter medications or transportation costs incurred by a patient's family to bring them to a treatment center.

It may be important to consider other factors that may impact costs, such as medication adherence and persistence. High adherence and persistence rates can improve health outcomes but may also be associated with higher costs due to more intensive and prolonged intervention use. Additionally, copayments, coinsurance, discounts, and rebates can significantly impact the net cost to the budget holder. Copayments and coinsurance paid by patients can reduce the budget holder's expenses, while manufacturer discounts and rebates can lower the acquisition costs. It is essential to account for these factors to provide an accurate estimate of the total cost over the budget horizon.

BIA CALCULATIONS

Once the analysis is planned and credible data are collected for each of the BIA elements above, the budgets and health outcomes can be calculated for each budget scenario (eg, the world without and the world with the new intervention). In essence, this calculation involves multiplying the eligible population by the intervention mix and the costs or health outcomes associated with each intervention. **Figure 17-2** provides an example of the calculation for intervention acquisition costs.

RESULTS

When presenting BIA results, it is customary to show outcomes for each budget scenario separately (ie, the scenario without the new intervention and the scenario with the new intervention) and then to show the budget impact, calculated as the difference between these two scenarios. Within this framework, it is important to consider costs that are applicable to the budget holder. For example, to understand short- to mid-term affordability, it is often helpful to consider total annual costs over 3 years or 5 years. Or per-member-per-month costs may be preferred because they inform the increase in member premiums needed to cover the introduction of the new intervention. In either case, costs may be categorized into pharmacy versus other medical costs.

Health and population outcomes are also important to present, because they demonstrate to the budget holder what they are getting in exchange for the change in budget. The BIA should highlight relevant outcomes, such as fewer symptom days or more people alive, and distinguish between short-term and longer-term outcomes. This comprehensive approach ensures that budget holders can estimate the likely budget impact for their jurisdiction, understand the health impact, and make informed decisions. **Table 17-3** provides an example of BIA results for a new asthma treatment (Drug D) presented in a tabular format.

Along with base-case results, it can be beneficial to provide one-way sensitivity analyses and results for alternative scenarios. These analyses help to demonstrate the impact on the BIA results of uncertainty in the input parameters and different clinical or modeling assumptions.

TABLE 17-3. Example Tabular BIA Results: Drug D for Asthma Joins the Market

Outcome	Year 1	Year 2	Year 3
Annual Costs			
Scenario 1: Drug A, B, and C only			
Drug costs	$9,511,735	$9,504,463	$9,497,190
Asthma care costs	$8,899,958	$8,900,111	$8,900,263
Total costs	$18,411,694	$18,404,573	$18,397,453
Scenario 2: Drug D joins the market			
Drug costs	$9,604,272	$9,689,537	$9,774,801
Asthma care costs	$8,898,792	$8,897,778	$8,896,764
Total costs	$18,503,065	$18,587,315	$18,671,565
Budget impact			
Pharmacy budget impact	$92,537	$185,074	$277,611
Asthma care budget impact	–$1,166	–$2,332	–$3,498
Budget impact (annual)	$91,371	$182,742	$274,112
Per-Member-Per-Month Costs[a]			
Scenario 1: Drug A, B, and C only	$1.53	$1.53	$1.53
Scenario 2: Drug D joins the market	$1.54	$1.55	$1.56
Budget impact (per member per month)	$0.01	$0.02	$0.03
Health Outcomes			
Scenario 1: Drug A, B, and C only			
Rescue medications (30-day supply)	38,896	38,999	39,103
Unscheduled physician visits	34,271	34,340	34,408
Scenario 2: Drug D joins the market			
Rescue medication use (30-day supply)	38,103	37,414	36,725
Unscheduled physician visits	29,930	29,623	29,316
Health impact			
Rescue medication use (30-day supply)	–793	–1,585	–2,378
Unscheduled physician visits	–4,341	–4,716	–5,092

[a] Per-member-per-month cost outcomes are calculated by dividing annual cost by 12 (to convert from annual to monthly costs) and by the number of members in the health plan.

THE PHYSICAL BIA MODEL

A BIA is typically created using decision-analytic modeling techniques. As such, a BIA may be referred to as a "budget-impact model." Model users and model developers alike can benefit from understanding best practices for building a physical BIA model. This section describes the model-building process, with emphasis on the importance of customizability, programming platform, model design, and quality checking.

BIA Customization

Programming a BIA is similar in many ways to building other types of health economic models. Choice of software, transparency, user-friendliness, and presentation of results are all common considerations. However, while analyses such as cost-effectiveness analysis might demonstrate the value of a new intervention in a jurisdiction generally (eg, in the United States), BIA is unique in that it is meant to represent the financial perspective of a specific budget holder, and as such, the BIA inputs and results will be specific to that budget holder. Thus, the programmed BIA must be flexible to allow users to easily change input parameter values to align with their specific population size and characteristics, treatment patterns and market projections, and costs. While health economic models in general often allow users to change input values, it is especially important in BIAs to ensure that these changes are easy to make and that the impact on the results is clear.

Programming Platform

As with other health economic analyses, BIAs can be programmed within any software that can handle mathematical calculations. However, with the budget holder in mind, basic spreadsheet software, such as Microsoft Excel, is a good choice most of the time. Spreadsheets are flexible, transparent, and accessible. (Most users have at least basic proficiency with spreadsheets, and budget holders in particular often manage budgets by using spreadsheets.) Furthermore, in a spreadsheet platform, programmers can develop BIAs with an aesthetic design and intuitive user interface. These considerations are particularly important for BIA, because customization will be needed for each individual budget holder; thus, users will often need to interact with the physical model itself.

In rare instances, BIAs may be very complex and require efficient computations to reduce run time. In these cases, software platforms such as R, Matlab, TreeAge, or specialized simulation software (eg, Simio, Simulink) might be considered. Trade-offs in user-friendliness can sometimes be mitigated with these applications by creating a spreadsheet interface that interacts with the underlying software platform. Reduced transparency of calculations is more challenging to overcome, however.

Model Design

Planning the model design includes consideration of several elements, including general layout, introductory information, input parameters, model calculations, and presentation of results. **Table 17-4** provides recommendations for each of these elements. Overall, the model should be organized with the user experience in mind.

Quality Checking and Pressure Testing

Quality checking is important for all health economic analyses, and BIA is no exception. Even one error in the inputs or calculations can affect the analysis results and undermine the credibility of the analysis. While quality-checking may be covered in other chapters of this book, it cannot be overemphasized, so we provide our preferred process as follows:

- Both the programmer and ideally one or more additional reviewers should check all links and calculations for logic and accuracy.
- All default input values should be checked against source information, and all text in the model should be reviewed for clarity, accuracy, and correctness (eg, spelling and grammar).
- Various analyses should be run to ensure that the model results change as expected, including analyses testing both plausible and extreme values of input parameters.
- Following a predetermined quality review protocol is good practice.

TABLE 17-4. Guidance for BIA Physical Model Design

Model Element	Recommendation
Model layout	The model layout should balance a clean interface with an appropriate level of written information and detail. Positioning some of the detail on background worksheets or in pop-up boxes can help achieve both objectives. The user experience can also be enhanced with clear navigation through the model and features such as buttons to restore default values after changes have been made.
Introductory information	Introductory information may include background about the disease area and available interventions; description of the model objective, structure, and assumptions; and clear instructions for using the model.
Input parameters	For BIA, input parameters are often organized onto several worksheets, such as Population, Intervention Mix, Health Effects, Intervention-related Costs, and Other Costs. On each worksheet, input parameters should have well-labeled entry points so that users can tailor the inputs to their specific population and data. All input parameters should also have a default value and a clear reference. Users will likely appreciate suggested default values from appropriate sources in case they do not have their own data on hand. Relevant, credible data that can be easily verified from the source information also enhances the reliability of the analysis.
Model calculations	Model calculations are often included on background worksheets, because they may not be of interest to all users. Organized tables of equations and clear labeling are critical to the transparency and credibility of the analysis, as some users will want to understand and verify the calculations.
BIA results	Results should be presented to allow for ease of use and interpretation. For example, results presented in graphs allow users to quickly interpret and visualize trends, and results presented in tables allow users to dig into the details of disaggregated costs and small differences. While it may be tempting to present as many outcomes as possible to provide the full picture of the analysis, careful consideration of the user and audience is important. There may be trade-offs between overwhelming users with information and providing sufficient detail. Including a summary of key results at the top of the screen can help users focus on top-level outcomes. Additionally, drop-down boxes can be included to allow users to select information they would like to view (eg, annual results or per-member-per-month results).

Once the quality check is complete, pressure testing should continue while running analyses and developing reports. Keeping watch for unexpected results or inconsistencies is a good way to identify errors or unexpected assumptions in the inputs or calculations. Once identified, they can be remedied during this pressure-testing phase.

VALIDATION WITH STAKEHOLDERS

Depending on the jurisdiction, it is often helpful to discuss the BIA with key stakeholders, such as clinicians familiar with the condition, and potential users, such as payers. These discussions can be used to identify important concepts to include in the analysis, obtain feedback on the modeling approach and input data, and identify objections. This process can occur at any stage of BIA development. Early input can help identify and shape key elements to be included in the analysis. Feedback provided after the analysis approach is planned but before it is built can be incorporated into initial versions of the physical model. Sharing the analytical approach, inputs, and results after the BIA is constructed allows stakeholders to understand, evaluate, and validate the full model. Regardless of the timing of feedback, obtaining input and buy-in from a sample of stakeholders or decision-makers can be very helpful for BIA because budget holders can be particularly skeptical, especially if the BIA was developed by the intervention's manufacturer. Review and endorsement by clinicians and peers can help to ensure the credibility of the analysis.

INTERPRETATION OF RESULTS AND REPORTING

Interpretation of results and reporting recommendations differ for BIAs compared with other types of economic analysis in important ways. The following sections cover these topics.

Interpretation of Results

Interpretation of BIA results involves first remembering that this type of analysis helps to estimate the impact of a new intervention on a payer's budget and population and to assess the affordability of the new intervention. Budget-impact analysis is not intended to provide a head-to-head comparison, like in cost-effectiveness analysis, between new and existing interventions. Keeping this in mind, the next step is to examine the budget and health outcomes that have been calculated, identify a few key messages associated with these outcomes, and then communicate these messages in a simple way for the intended audience. The ability to effectively summarize comprehensive BIA results into key value messages for the new intervention is crucial to communicate the value story and hence to ensure that the analysis attains the goal of appropriately informing decision-making.

Typically, budget-impact results fall into one of three primary interpretation categories when the new intervention is expected to be more costly than the existing, competing interventions. Specifically, a new intervention could yield results as follows:

- *The cost budget is predicted to increase while health outcomes improve.* This situation often arises when the additional pharmacy costs associated with the new intervention are partially offset by savings in other medical costs that result from improved health outcomes. In this case, the predicted budget impact may be acceptable to the budget holder depending on its magnitude.
- *The cost budget is predicted to decrease while health outcomes improve.* Here, the additional pharmacy costs associated with the new intervention are fully offset by savings in other medical costs that result from improved health outcomes. This is an ideal situation, because the budget holder's costs may decrease while the health of the covered population improves.
- *The cost budget is predicted to increase while health outcomes remain unchanged.* This situation may result from an expensive intervention with limited effectiveness *or* from a highly effective intervention with health benefits that are realized after the analysis time horizon (as is often the case for preventives and for chronic diseases). In the latter case, the additional pharmacy costs associated with the new intervention are not offset by savings in other medical costs within the BIA time horizon because the health benefits occur later. In this situation, BIA alone is likely not adequate to support the value story of the new intervention, and developing a cost-effectiveness analysis to complement the BIA may be helpful.

To practice BIA interpretation, consider the results shown in Table 17-3 for the introduction of Drug D for the treatment of asthma. The results show that the introduction of Drug D will increase cost budgets by approximately $90,000 each year, for a total budget impact of $274,112 by year 3 (1.5% increase). The increased pharmacy costs are partially offset by reductions in asthma care costs resulting from reduced use of rescue medications (6.1% reduction) and unscheduled physician visits (14.8% reduction) by year 3. Thus, the introduction of Drug D will increase costs slightly, but patients will be much better managed. These value messages can be presented to a payer, who must then decide whether better asthma management is worth the additional cost.

When assessing BIA results, a common question is, "Are there standard thresholds that budget holders use to accept or reject an intervention?" While there are seldom fixed, publicly available thresholds for BIA like there are for CEA, there are a few jurisdictions that do have general guidelines to consider. These include, but are not limited to, the guidelines summarized in **Table 17-5**. Comparing the BIA results shown in Table 17-3 with the guidance in Table 17-5, we observe that the per-member-per-month budget-impact values associated with adding Drug D to the formulary of a US payer are within manageable/justifiable limits and may be considered affordable.

Reporting

The ISPOR Budget Impact Analysis Good Practice Task Force has provided specific reporting guidance for BIA, and the Consolidated Health

TABLE 17-5. Budget-Impact Threshold Guidelines

Country	Threshold
United States[a]	• No standard threshold; decisions are based on many factors • Per-member-per-month budget-impact values of \$0.014 to \$0.054 may be considered manageable or justifiable[12]
United Kingdom	• NICE/NHS: Budget-impact values more than £40 million in any of the first 3 years prompt commercial discussions[13]
Netherlands	• Decisions are not centered solely around BIA • Full assessment is required when gross expenditure is more than €10 million per year[14] • Full assessment is also required when gross expenditure is between €1 million and €10 million per year and per-patient treatment costs are more than €50,000 per year[14]

BIA = budget-impact analysis; ICER = Institute for Clinical and Economic Review; NHS = National Health Service; NICE = National Institute for Health and Clinical Excellence.

[a] ICER, a research institute that reviews healthcare interventions in the United States but does not make reimbursement decisions, recommended for 2024–2025 an annual prescription drug therapy budget-impact threshold of \$880 million.[15] Note that this threshold applies to the full US population rather than the population of a particular payer.

Economic Evaluation Reporting Standards (CHEERS) offers reporting guidance for economic analyses in general.[2,16] Following these reporting recommendations helps to ensure that the BIA is described in sufficient detail for an interested researcher to reproduce the analysis and replicate the results. To summarize briefly, BIA reports should include several key elements, beginning with background information and a description of the model structure and methods as well as the assumptions, values, and data sources for all input parameters. Appropriately detailed results should be presented in tables or figures, showing costs and health outcomes over the analysis time horizon both for the intervention mix with and without the new intervention as well as for the difference (ie, the budget impact and the health impact). Scenario and sensitivity analyses should be presented to demonstrate the robustness of the model results to changes in modeling assumptions and parameter values. Finally, a discussion section that presents validation, strengths, limitations, and conclusions of the analysis should be included.

While BIA reporting guidelines generally apply regardless of jurisdiction, required or recommended formats may vary. In some countries or regions, the BIA is included in a health technology assessment submission, and in others, separate stand-alone documents may be desired by decision-makers to determine reimbursement. In the United States, the BIA is often included in the Academy of Managed Care Pharmacy (AMCP) dossier that payers may request from the manufacturer of the intervention.[17] Formats and requirements for these reports vary and are updated regularly, so it is important to review the requirements before beginning to write the report. Guidance documents can generally be found on the website of the respective health technology assessment agency.

ARTIFICAL INTELLIGENCE AND BIA

Artificial intelligence (AI) is currently a hot topic with potential to streamline the development of tools used to support decision-making. As such, the use of AI has been assessed, and to date, AI can certainly help with components of BIA development, including both the creation and adaptation of BIA. As with other applications, AI has been found to be useful in facilitating literature reviews, identifying data and data sources, and assisting with updates to equations or programming code. Specific to BIA, a few elements that AI might support include identification of jurisdiction-specific data or creation of code to incorporate additional interventions. Note that AI is not yet ready to take a single prompt and develop an entire BIA, which would include planning an appropriate model structure, identifying the different types of data to include in the analysis, obtaining the data, programming the analysis, reporting results, and compiling a summary of technical content. Rather, because BIA is an organization of a complex set of data and calculations, AI is most useful in supporting the construction of its basic elements.

When using AI, it is important to confirm that any data, data source, or code are correct and appropriately applied, as AI may provide incorrect or fabricated information. Artificial intelligence simply uses efficient algorithms to systematically and mathematically identify patterns and make predictions based on these patterns. Artificial intelligence does not have the critical thinking skills of a human. Furthermore, when using AI, care should be taken with any proprietary information to ensure that the information is safely stored and not fed into public AI sites. As AI is constantly evolving, it is expected to be able to support the development of specific elements of BIA more and more, but at this point, AI should be used as a support tool for the developer rather than a means to produce content or full analyses.

CONCLUSION

Budget-impact analysis is a type of economic assessment that provides short- to mid-term estimates of the financial impact of the introduction of a new healthcare intervention (or changes in the use of an existing intervention) for a specific budget holder. Budget-impact analysis can be used to understand the affordability of a new intervention, inform budget and resource planning, and assess the ability to reach target population health outcomes. Budget-impact analysis estimates are calculated by using data about the population eligible for the intervention, forecasts about use of the new and competing interventions, effects of the interventions on patient health, and the related costs to the budget holder. Results are typically presented over a 3- to 5-year time horizon for two budget scenarios (eg, a world with the new intervention versus a world without) as annual totals or per-member-per-month values.

Because inputs and results will differ for every budget holder, the BIA should be easily customizable. Use of a physical model that is user-friendly and transparent is essential; thus, spreadsheet software is typically a good choice for the programming platform. Quality checking and validation with stakeholders are good practices to ensure credibility of the BIA.

Once the BIA is complete, thoughtful interpretation of results and development of a few clear value messages can help with communication of the value story for the new intervention. Reporting the BIA methods, inputs, results, and value messages following reporting recommendations helps to ensure that the BIA is described in appropriate detail and informs decision-making.

REFERENCES

1. Mauskopf JA, Sullivan SD, Annemans L, et al. Principles of good practice for budget impact analysis: report of the ISPOR Task Force on Good Research Practices—budget impact analysis. *Value Health*. 2007;10(5):336-347. https://doi.org/10.1111/j.1524-4733.2007.00187.x
2. Sullivan SD, Mauskopf JA, Augustovski F, et al. Budget impact analysis—principles of good practice: report of the ISPOR 2012 Budget Impact Analysis Good Practice II Task Force. *Value Health*. 2014;17(1):5-14. https://doi.org/10.1016/j.jval.2013.08.2291
3. Patented Medicine Prices Review Board (PMPRB). Budget impact analysis guidelines for conducting pharmaceutical budget impact analyses for submission to public drug plans in Canada. Updated June 2020. https://www.canada.ca/content/dam/pmprb-cepmb/documents/reports-and-studies/budget-impact-analysis-guidelines/PMPRB-BIA-Guidlines-en.pdf. Accessed February 9, 2026.
4. Australian Government. Department of Health, Disability, and Ageing. Guidelines for preparing a submission to the Pharmaceutical Benefits Advisory Committee (PBAC). Version 5.0, September 2016. https://pbac.pbs.gov.au/. Accessed February 9, 2026.
5. Neyt M, Thiry N, Cleemput I. Belgian guidelines for economic evaluations and budget impact analyses: third edition. Method. Brussels. Belgian Health Care Knowledge Centre (KCE). 2025. KCE Reports 400C. https://kce.fgov.be/sites/default/files/2025-05/KCE400_Method_guidelines_economic_evaluations.pdf. Accessed February 9, 2026.
6. Perelman J, Soares M, Mateus C, et al. Methodological guidelines for economic evaluation studies of health technologies. INFARMED - National Authority of Medicines and Health Products, I.P., Lisbon. Updated December 2019. https://www.infarmed.pt/documents/15786/4001413/Orienta%C3%A7%C3%B5es+metodol%C3%B3gicas+para

+estudos+de+avalia%C3%A7%C3%A3o+econ%C3%B3mica+de+tecnologias+de+sa%C3%BAde+%28EN%29. Accessed February 9, 2026.

7. Mauskopf J, Earnshaw SR, Brogan AJ, et al. *Budget-Impact Analysis of Health Care Interventions: A Practical Guide*. 1st ed. Cham, Switzerland: Springer International Publishing; 2017.

8. U.S. Census Bureau. Annual estimates of the resident population by single year of age and sex for the United States: April 1, 2020, to July 1, 2024 (NC-EST2024-AGESEX-RES). Updated April 2025. https://www.census.gov/data/tables/time-series/demo/popest/2020s-national-detail.html. Accessed February 9, 2026.

9. Centers for Disease Control and Prevention. Diagnoses, deaths, and prevalence of HIV in the United States and 6 territories and freely associated states, 2022. *HIV Surveillance Report*, 2022; vol. 35. Published May 2024. http://www.cdc.gov/hiv-data/nhss/hiv-diagnoses-deaths-prevalence.html Accessed February 9, 2026.

10. Henegar C, Vannappagari V, Viswanathan S, et al. Identifying heavily treatment-experienced patients in a large administrative claims database. Poster presentation at 10th IAS Conference on HIV Science. Mexico City, Mexico. July 21-24, 2019.

11. Hsu R, Fusco J, Henegar C, et al. Clinical outcomes of heavily treatment experienced individuals in the OPERA Cohort. AIDS 2020 e-poster PEB0234. July 6-10, 2020.

12. Liu R, Botteman M. Benchmarking of budget impact results: an updated systematic review of US budget impact analyses. *Value Health*. 2023;26(6):S398-S399. https://doi.org/10.1016/j.jval.2023.03.2226

13. NHS England. Budget impact test threshold consultation—summary of response. Updated January 29, 2025. https://www.england.nhs.uk/long-read/budget-impact-test-threshold-consultation-summary-of-response. Accessed February 9, 2026.

14. Reckers-Droog V, Enzing J, Brouwer W. The role of budget impact and its relationship with cost-effectiveness in reimbursement decisions on health technologies in the Netherlands. *Eur J Health Econ*. 2024;25:1449-1459. https://doi.org/10.1007/s10198-024-01673-3

15. Institute for Clinical and Economic Review (ICER). Value assessment framework—potential budget impact threshold updated for 2024-2025. https://icer.org/our-approach/methods-process/value-assessment-framework/. Accessed February 9, 2026.

16. Husereau D, Drummond M, Augustovski F, et al. Consolidated Health Economic Evaluation Reporting Standards 2022 (CHEERS) 2022 explanation and elaboration: a report of the ISPOR CHEERS II Good Practices Task Force. *Value Health*. 2022;25(1):10-31. https://doi.org/10.1016/j.jval.2021.10.008

17. AMCP format for formulary submissions 5.0: Guidance on submission of pre-approval and post-approval clinical and economic information and evidence. Updated April 2024. https://www.amcp.org/sites/default/files/2024-04/AMCP-Format-5.0-JMCP-web_0.pdf. Accessed February 9, 2026.

Measuring Health-Related Quality of Life, Utility, and Preferences

18

Sorrel Wolowacz, PhD, and Caroline Vass, PhD

As health systems increasingly prioritize patient-centered care and cost-effectiveness, evaluations of medical and policy interventions must extend beyond traditional measures of clinical efficacy. While alleviating disease symptoms and prolonging survival remain essential goals, a central objective of modern healthcare is to enhance patients' overall quality of life and well-being. This broader perspective recognizes that the value of an intervention lies not only in its clinical outcomes but also in how it affects individuals' daily functioning, emotional health, and personal preferences.

This chapter provides a comprehensive overview of the tools and methods used to measure quality of life, utility, and patient preferences—three interrelated concepts that are critical to understanding the full impact of healthcare interventions. By incorporating patients' lived experiences and values, these approaches support more informed, equitable, and patient-centered decision-making in healthcare.

HEALTH-RELATED QUALITY OF LIFE

The field of health economics and outcomes research is widely focused on the measurement of three primary outcomes: clinical, economic, and humanistic, otherwise known as patient-reported outcomes (PROs). Information on quality of life and patient preferences is routinely taken into consideration alongside the safety and efficacy of treatment. In many cases, such as a chronic disease where therapeutic interventions are invasive or a cure is unlikely, quality of life may even be the primary consideration. Outcomes research has increasingly eschewed a narrow focus on clinical indicators of morbidity and mortality, focusing instead on the wider aspects of functioning and well-being.[1]

Quality of life continues to be a loosely defined term, interpreted differently by researchers in different fields.[2] The World Health Organization (WHO) defines health as "not merely the absence of disease or infirmity, but a state of complete physical, mental, and social well-being."[3] This definition of health lends itself to ambiguous interpretations that need to be narrowed down, especially if such information is to be collected in clinical trials where only those aspects of quality of life that are affected by either the disease or the treatment need to be assessed. Hence, the term health-related quality of life (HRQL) is more specific and more appropriate, because it refers to patients' appraisals of their current level of functioning compared with what they perceive to be ideal.[4] Furthermore, it encompasses the domains physical functioning, emotional and cognitive functioning, sexual functioning, general health, and social well-being, all of which are aspects of quality of life that may be impacted by either the disease itself or the treatment. The term PRO refers to a host of outcomes that are provided only by the patient. Examples of these outcomes include symptom severity, perception of daily functioning, feelings of well-being, global impressions of the impact of treatment on daily life, satisfaction with treatment, and

DOI: 10.37573/9781585287666.018

HRQL. Patient-reported outcomes are more representative of the patient's perspective of the impact of the treatment, especially in clinical trials.[5]

The purpose of an HRQL instrument is not merely to measure the presence and severity of symptoms of disease, but also to show how the manifestations of an illness or treatment are experienced by an individual. Because a disease may affect several domains of health, including mental and physical, most researchers tend to use instruments that measure multidimensional traits. There are a range of generic and condition-specific instruments, each with their own advantages and disadvantages that must be evaluated within the context of the needs of any particular study.

EVALUATION OF HRQL INSTRUMENTS

Psychometrics, the science of assessing the measurement characteristics of scales, is used to evaluate HRQL instruments. Psychometric properties for which an instrument should be evaluated include reliability, validity, and responsiveness (ie, sensitivity to clinically significant changes over time). Reliability reflects the extent to which an instrument yields reproducible and consistent results each time it is used under the same condition with the same subjects. The more reliable a measure is, the lower the element of random error. A measure found to be unreliable is not dependable. The reliability of an instrument is normally assessed in two ways: internal reliability/consistency and test–retest reliability.

Internal reliability reflects the homogeneity of items measuring a specific health domain and is normally measured by using Cronbach's alpha coefficient. An alpha value of 0.7 or above is necessary to call a scale internally consistent; however, in general it is optimal to have alpha coefficients greater than 0.85.[6] Cronbach's alpha coefficients closer to a value of 1.0 are indicative of higher levels of homogeneity between the items. This also means that a greater level of confidence can be attributed to the items constituting the domain under investigation. However, in instances where alpha coefficients greater than 0.95 are reported, caution should be exercised, because it could possibly indicate that several of the items are in fact measuring the same thing.

Test–retest reliability is a measure of an instrument's ability to produce data that are consistent or stable over time. It is normally determined by using Cohen's Kappa or Pearson's or Spearman's correlation coefficient. Normally, levels in excess of 0.6 indicate adequate test–retest reliability.[6,7] This test–retest reliability is assessed by applying the measure to the same population at different points in time under the same conditions and looking at the statistical association between the two sets of results.

Validity is defined as the extent to which an instrument measures what it is supposed to measure and does not measure what it is not supposed to measure. The concept refers to nonrandom or systematic measurement error. Of the several different types of validity, construct validity is especially relevant. Because in most cases no absolute criterion (ie, no "gold standard") exists against which to validate an instrument, one becomes involved in collecting empirical evidence to support the inference that a particular measure has meaning. A measure of physical health may be tested against a measure of activities of daily living, with the prediction that the correlation should be positive. If this proves to be the case, it would be evidence of convergent validity. To the extent that it can be demonstrated that the measure does not correlate with variables to which it should not be related, discriminant validity is made evident. For example, a measure of physical function should not be highly correlated with a measure of mental health. Another form of validity, content validity, refers to the adequacy with which a domain has been defined and sampled. While content validity is a more precise expression than face validity (which is defined by its reasonableness in representing a particular HRQL domain), the two terms are often used interchangeably.

Responsiveness is the extent to which an instrument can detect true differences within the construct being measured. It is geared toward measuring changes within patients in terms of their health status over time. To evaluate treatment efficacy, it is essential that an HRQL instrument has demonstrated an ability to detect small but meaningful changes over time. If such information is unavailable, then the study can be designed so that at its conclusion HRQL changes can be compared with changes in clinical status, intervening health events, interventions of known or expected efficacy, or direct reports of change by patients or providers, among other items. Responsiveness in many ways confirms the validity of an instrument by checking to see whether the estimated responses occurred in conjunction with changes in the patient's health status.[8] In the past, responsiveness has not received sufficient attention in the development of HRQL questionnaires; however, investigators are increasingly providing this information as part of an instrument's psychometric properties. In addition, the meaning of responsiveness statistics has become a focus of much needed research.[9-12]

To date, a vast proportion of the HRQL instruments have been developed in English-speaking countries, such as the United States and the United Kingdom. Even though the reliability and validity of these instruments have been established, these psychometric properties might not translate to other countries/cultures. Beliefs and values about health and the interpretation of symptoms may differ significantly among cultures. Culturally adapting an HRQL questionnaire indicates that the language and meaning within the instrument are consistent with that of the target country.[13] The approach that has been used most commonly to translate a measure from one culture to another involves a forward/backward translation process of an original source language document into the target language. Additional guidelines for the adaptation of a measure from one cultural context to another may be found in the literature.[14,15]

HEALTH UTILITY ASSESSMENT

Health utility is a special measure of HRQL, which represents the strength of preference for a given health-related outcome on a cardinal numeric scale, where a value of 1.0 represents full health, 0.0 represents death, and negative values represent health states considered worse than death.[16,17] Health utility estimates are used in cost-utility analyses (CUAs), a special case of cost-effectiveness analysis in which health benefits are usually measured in terms of quality-adjusted life-years (QALYs).[18] Utility weights are used to adjust a patient's time in a given health state to reflect the quality of life typically experienced in that health state. Cost-utility analyses are used for health technology assessment (HTA) and increasingly by pricing and reimbursement authorities in many countries to establish whether the cost of a new intervention can be justified in terms of expected health benefits. The decisions made by these authorities affect patients' access to treatments, physicians' ability to use them, the product's price, and the return that manufacturers realize on their product. Health utility estimates are among the most important data inputs in cost-utility models, because they translate the efficacy observed in clinical trials into the anticipated treatment benefits that are considered by decision-makers. The accuracy and precision of cost-utility model results depend heavily on the quality of the health utility estimates.[19]

The economic evaluation of a new healthcare intervention requires a comparison of the new intervention's costs and benefits with those for existing treatments. Economic evaluations are used to compare both the value of alternative treatments for a single health condition as well as the value of treatments for other health conditions. The latter comparison is especially important when total healthcare expenditures are subject to a budget limit, thus ensuring that the new intervention does not displace more cost-effective interventions for other health conditions.

In order to compare the value of interventions across different health conditions, it is necessary that the measures for costs and benefits are ones that can be used for any health condition and any type of healthcare intervention. Costs are always measured in currency units and are the same for interventions for different conditions. However, the benefits associated with a new treatment may differ for different health conditions and different types of interventions. For one condition, the main benefit from a new intervention could be to reduce mortality (eg, surfactant prophylaxis or rescue therapy for respiratory distress syndrome for very premature infants), whereas for another condition the main benefit could be to reduce pain (eg, a new migraine drug).

Comparing the value of interventions for different conditions requires mapping all of these very different benefits into a single unit of measure, reflecting both improvements in life expectancy and quality of life. Quality-adjusted life-years are computed by adjusting the number of years that a patient lives by a measure of the utility associated with the health state(s) in which the person spends their life. For example, if an intervention confers 2 extra years of life at a utility weight of 0.75, then the intervention would confer an additional 1.5 QALYs (2 × 0.75) to the patient. **Figure 18-1** depicts a hypothetical example of the calculation of QALYs gained for new interventions for both an acute (influenza) and a chronic illness (HIV infection) where health utility declines over time with disease progression.

High-quality utility data are defined as estimates that are aligned with the definitions of the economic model health states and/or events, free from known sources of bias, and measured by using a validated method, appropriate to the condition and population of interest and the perspective of the decision-maker for whom the economic model is being developed.[19]

HEALTH UTILITY ESTIMATION

Health utility is a representation of strength of preference for a given health-related outcome. Therefore, utility measurement requires a preference-based method, and values must be anchored on 1.0 representing full health and 0.0 representing a health state equivalent to dead. Negative values represent health states worse than dead. Time trade-off and standard gamble methods have been used to estimate utility weights, supplemented by other methods, such as discrete choice experiments discussed later in the chapter.

A time trade-off utility estimate can be obtained for either a person's current health status or for hypothetical health state descriptions. In a time trade-off exercise (**Figure 18-2**), participants are asked whether they prefer a relatively short but fixed period of time living in a certain suboptimal health state or a variable amount of time (x) living in full health. The amount of time living in full health is varied until the participant is indifferent between the two options. The utility weight for the health state is then calculated as the value of x (in years) at the point of indifference divided by the fixed period of time. For example, if the participant is found to be indifferent between 10 years in a given health state and 8 years in full health, the utility weight would be 8/10 = 0.8 (Figure 18-2). When applied in an economic model, QALYs for each year lived in the health state will be calculated as 1 × 0.8, reflecting the time trade-off valuation that 1 year in the health state is equivalent to 0.8 years in full health.

For health states worse than dead, adjustments are made to the methods, such as lead-time trade-off. For example, an additional 10 years of full health is added to each life, allowing more time to be traded off for particularly onerous health states. A varying amount of time x living in full health (where x is 0 to 10 years) is compared with 10 years living in full health followed by another 10 years living in an exceptionally bad health state. The amount of time living in full health (x) is varied until indifference is reached. The utility value of the health state worse than death is then calculated as the value of x – 10 at the point of indifference divided by 10.

In standard gamble methods (**Figure 18-3**), participants are asked to choose between (1) a suboptimal health state and (2) a gamble with a chance of full health (p) and a risk of immediate death (1 – p). The probability p is altered until the participant is indifferent. The health state utility value is represented by p (ie, the probability of returning to full health).

Although time trade-off and standard gamble methods are grounded in utility theory, they are seldom used directly to measure health utility. There are several reasons for this, including the following:

- Ethical issues in asking patients to trade off years of life, or gamble with their health status, particularly in vulnerable populations
- Practical difficulties in their application in clinical trials and observational studies
- Most decision-makers (eg, HTA agencies) are interested in the preferences of the general population in their juris-

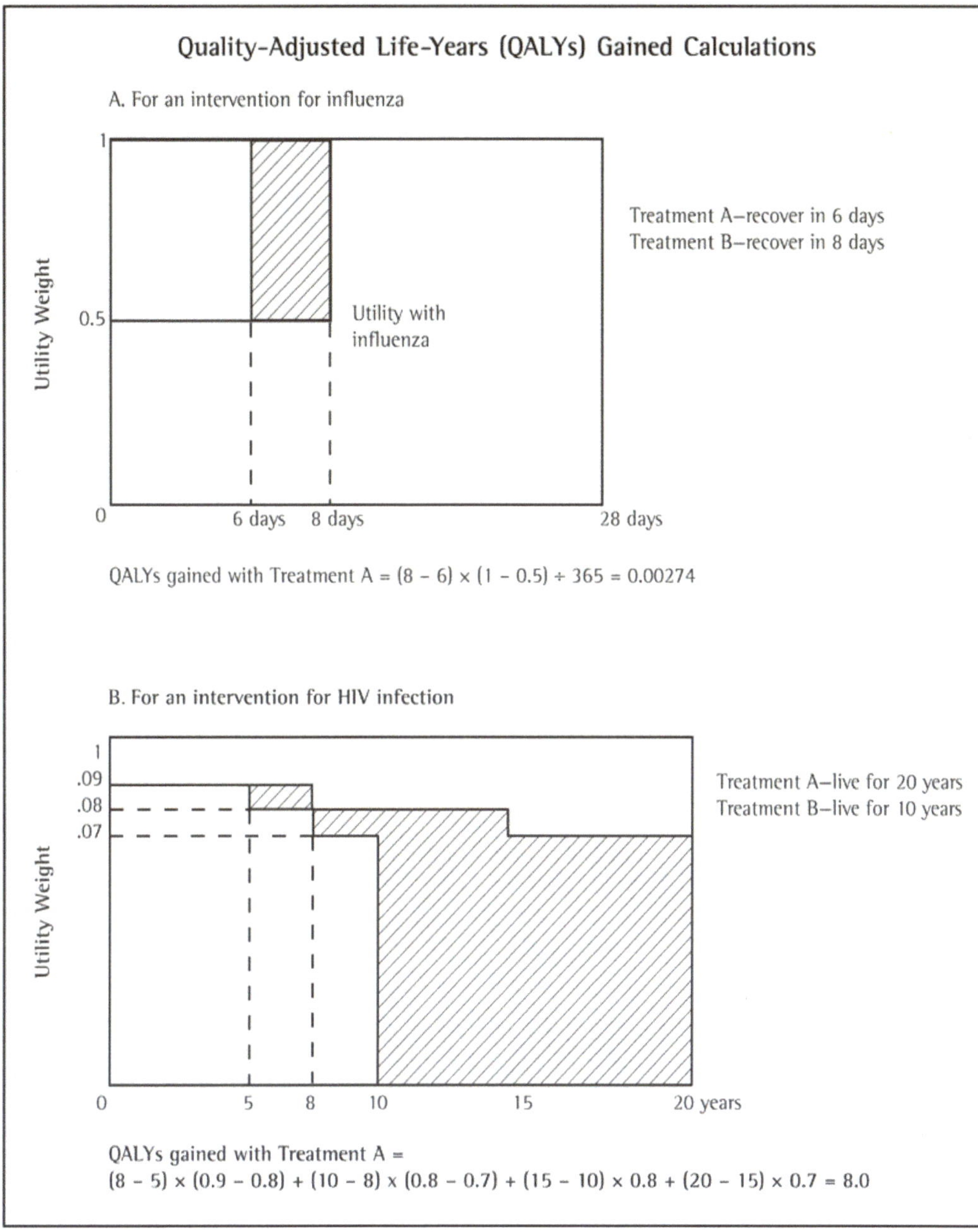

FIGURE 18-1. **Quality-adjusted life-years (QALYs) gained calculation.**

dictions rather than the preferences of the patient population. This is not only because decision-making should be ideally impartial across all health conditions and needs, but also because taxes on the general population often fund the health services.

HEALTH UTILITY INSTRUMENTS

To overcome these issues, utility instruments have been developed that collect health status information from patients via a questionnaire and provide

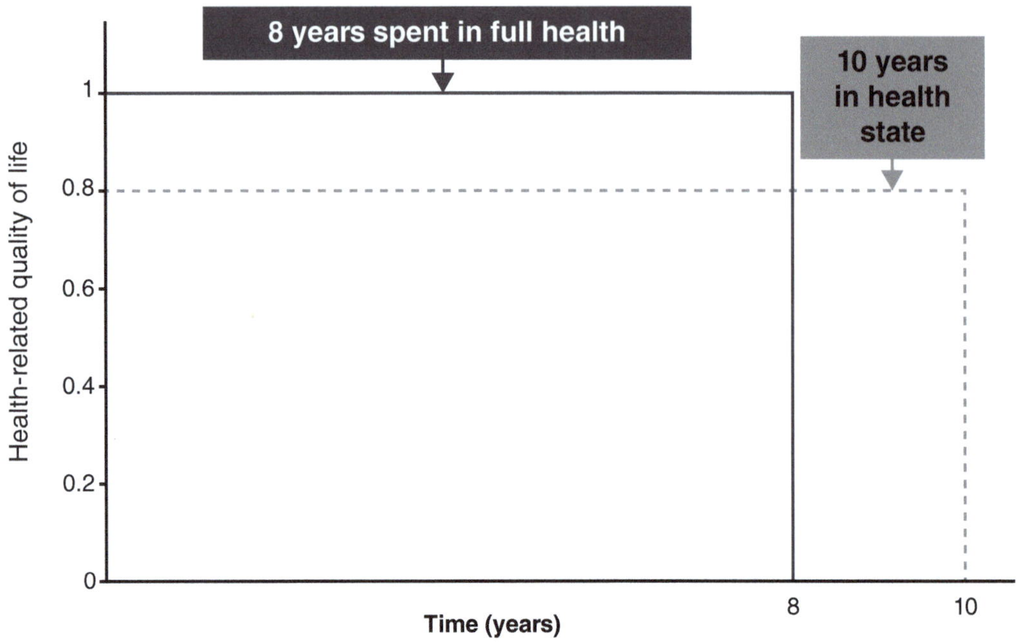

FIGURE 18-2. **Example of a time trade-off point of indifference.**

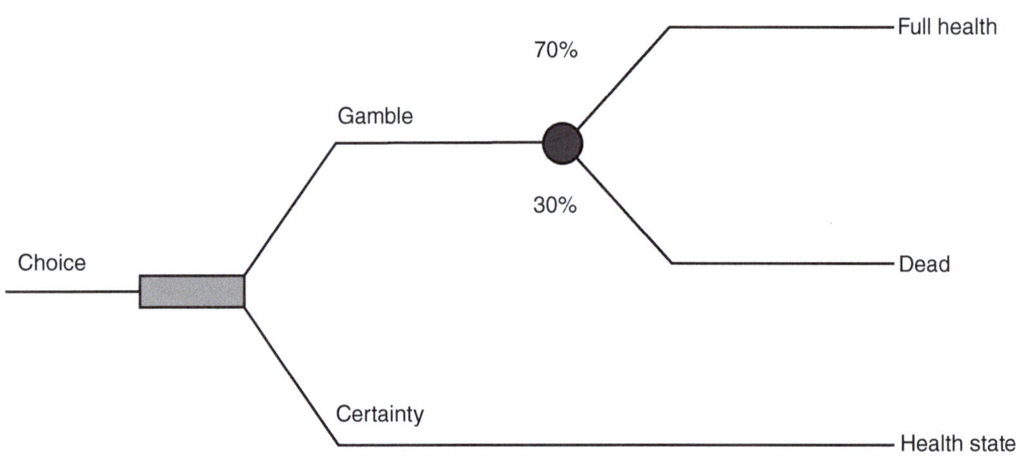

FIGURE 18-3. **Example of a standard gamble point of indifference.**

a preference-based value set (or tariff), which is used to calculate health utility estimates based on patient's responses to the questionnaire. These are often termed "preference-based measures" or "multi-attribute utility measures." A number of utility instruments have been developed; the EQ-5D has been the most widely studied and utilized, and it is described briefly in the next section.[20]

The EQ-5D is a generic utility measure, designed for use in a broad range of health conditions. It encompasses five dimensions of health: mobility, self-care, usual activities, pain/discomfort, and anxiety/depression. Responses in each of the five dimensions of health describe a range of levels of impairment. The EQ-5D is generally self-administered and can be completed in a few minutes. As illustrated by **Figure 18-4**, it consists of two components:

- The descriptive system (or health state classification system), ie, the questionnaire, and the set of health states defined by the possible permutations and

Questionnaire

Under each heading, please choose the ONE answer that best describes your health TODAY.

MOBILITY
- I have no problems in walking about ☐
- I have slight problems in walking about ☑
- I have moderate problems in walking about ☐
- I have severe problems in walking about ☐
- I am unable to walk about ☐

SELF-CARE
- I have no problems washing or dressing myself ☐
- I have slight problems washing or dressing myself ☐
- I have moderate problems washing or dressing myself ☑
- I have severe problems washing or dressing myself ☐
- I am unable to wash or dress myself ☐

USUAL ACTIVITIES *(e.g. work, study, housework, family or leisure activities)*
- I have no problems doing my usual activities ☐
- I have slight problems doing my usual activities ☑
- I have moderate problems doing my usual activities ☐
- I have severe problems doing my usual activities ☐
- I am unable to do my usual activities ☐

PAIN / DISCOMFORT
- I have no pain or discomfort ☐
- I have slight pain or discomfort ☐
- I have moderate pain or discomfort ☐
- I have severe pain or discomfort ☑
- I have extreme pain or discomfort ☐

ANXIETY/DEPRESSION
- I am not anxious or depressed ☐
- I am slightly anxious or depressed ☐
- I am moderately anxious or depressed ☐
- I am severely anxious or depressed ☐
- I am extremely anxious or depressed ☑

2

Value Set

	Central estimate	Health state 23245
Constant	1,000	1,000
Mobility		
slight	0.051	⇒ 0.051
moderate	0.063	
severe	0.212	
unable	0.275	
Self-care		
slight	0.057	
moderate	0.076	⇒ 0.076
severe	0.181	
unable	0.217	
Usual activities		
slight	0.051	⇒ 0.051
moderate	0.067	
severe	0.174	
unable	0.190	
Pain/discomfort		
slight	0.060	
moderate	0.075	
severe	0.276	⇒ 0.276
extreme	0.341	
Anxiety/depression		
slight	0.079	
moderate	0.104	
severe	0.296	
extreme	0.301	⇒ 0.301
Probability (group 1)	0.397	0.397x0.427 +
Probability (group 2)	0.270	0.270x0.939 +
Probability (group 3)	0.333	0.333x1.635 =
Slope (group 1)	0.427	0.9675
Slope (group 2)	0.939	
Slope (group 3)	1.635	
Value for health state 23245	1 -0.9675x(0.051+ 0.076 +0.051+ 0.276 +0.301) =	0.270

FIGURE 18-4. The two components of the EQ-5D.

Reproduction of this EuroQol instrument is not allowed. For use of this EuroQol instrument or any other EuroQol instrument, please submit a request by using the online registration page on www.euroqol.org.

Source: Devlin NJ, Shah KK, Feng Y, et al. Valuing health-related quality of life: an EQ-5D-5L value set for England. *Health Econ.* 2018;27:7–22. https://doi.org/10.1002/hec.3564

combinations of patient responses. The questionnaire has five items and either three or five response levels. The three-level version describes $3^5 = 243$ possible health states and the five-level version describes $5^5 = 3{,}125$ possible health states.

- The value sets (or tariffs), which are used to calculate utility weights for each patient's health state, based on their completed questionnaire. Value sets are available that represent the preferences of the general population in a wide range of countries and have been developed by using time trade-off and other methods to value each of the health states.
- Respondents complete the questionnaire to indicate their current health status (e.g. as shown in **Figure 18-4** left) and the corresponding utility weight for that respondent is calculated using the value set (as shown in **Figure 18-4** right). The average utility weight for a population can then be estimated from the individual patient-level data.

The EQ-5D questionnaire also includes a visual analogue scale (VAS) which records the respondents self-related health. The VAS scores are generally not used to provide utility estimates, because the anchor points of 100 and 0 do not represent full health and death (they are labeled as the best and worst health you can imagine), and the scores do not reflect any preference for health status. The information can be used as a qualitative measure of health outcome as judged by the individual respondent.

The EQ-5D has been the most widely studied and utilized utility instrument. Recognizing that different instruments and methods result in differences in utility estimates, and decision-makers need to ensure consistency of decision-making across health conditions, most decision-makers prefer EQ-5D utility data. However, it is recognized that EQ-5D may not be appropriate for all health conditions or populations: for example, hearing impairments, multiple sclerosis, personality disorders, schizophrenia, and dementia.[21] It is important to consider whether EQ-5D might not capture the important impacts of a given health condition on health status and quality of life and to collect evidence to that effect if needed.

If EQ-5D data are not available or appropriate, a variety of alternative methods can be considered. Most decision-makers recognize a hirearchy of methods as described in **Figure 18-5**. Each of these alternative methods is described below.

Mapping from a patient-reported quality-of-life measure to EQ-5D or another preference-based utility measure involves estimating a relationship between a patient-reported outcome measure and a preference-based measure by analyzing patient-level data for both measures collected in the same population using a statistical model. As a result, the statistical model (or mapping algorithm) theoretically provides utility estimates that are equivalent to EQ-5D estimates and can be used when patient-reported outcome data are available, but utility data are not. It can also be used to map from one preference-based measure to another (eg, to map the SF-6D, a preference-based utility measure derived from SF-36 data, to the EQ-5D). A database of mapping algorithms is maintained by the University of Oxford.[22] It is important to carefully review the quality of mapping algorithms and appropriateness for the population of interest; the original dataset used to develop the algorithm may reflect a different population and/or may have encompassed only a limited range of health states, which would produce poor predictions of utility outside of that range. Mapping is also not useful for improving the sensitivity of

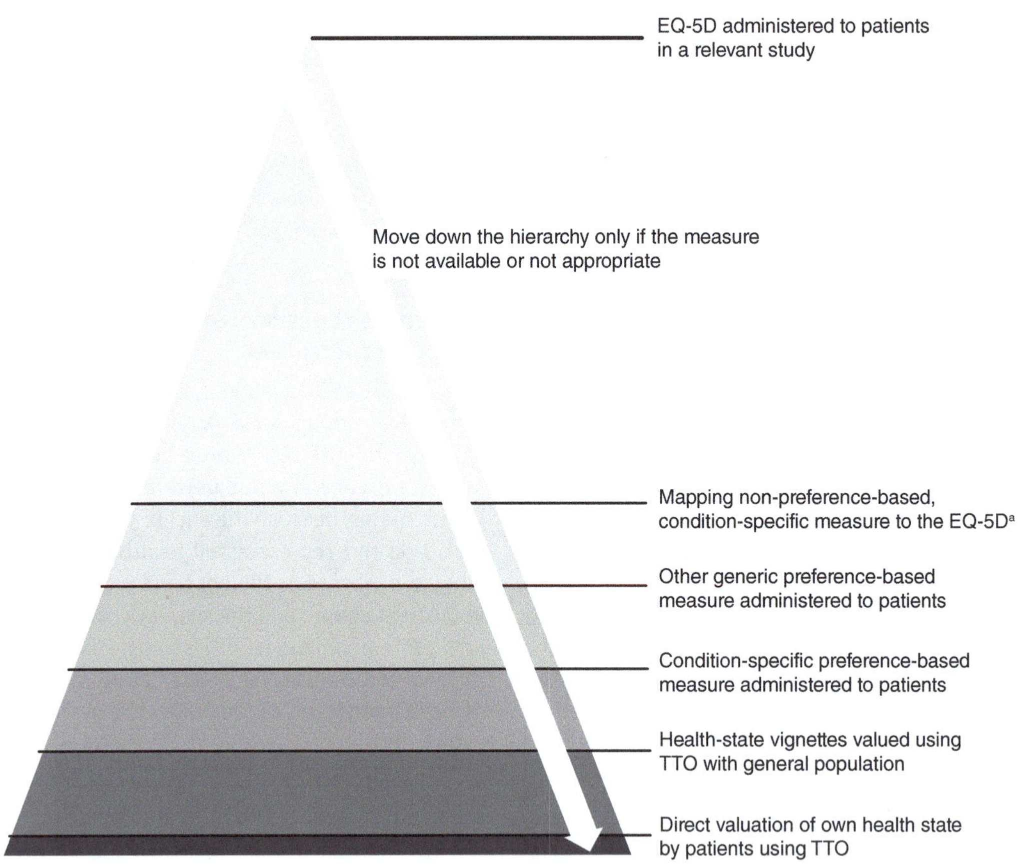

FIGURE 18-5. Utility measure hierarchy (based on a synthesis of HTA agency methods guides).
TTO = Time trade-off
[a] Only if EQ-5D is expected to be an appropriate measure but no EQ-5D data are available

EQ-5D in a given health condition. If EQ-5D is not sensitive, then using its data to develop the mapping algorithm also would not fully reflect health status and quality of life in that condition, and the sensitivity of any condition-specific measure would be lost when mapped to EQ-5D.

Other generic preference-based measures have been designed for use in a broad range of health conditions. Examples include the Health Utilities Index (HUI), 15 dimensions (15D), Assessment of Quality of Life (AQoL), and Medical Outcomes Study Short Form 6 Dimension (SF-6D).[23-28] These differ in content and size of the descriptive system, the method of valuation, and the populations used to value health states. As such, these may be more appropriate than EQ-5D for some health conditions.

Condition-specific preference-based measures may have a useful role when a generic measure is not appropriate, sensitive, or responsive.[29] Examples include the Asthma Quality of Life 5 Dimensions (AQL-5D) and European Organisation for Research and Treatment of Cancer Quality of Life Utility – Core 10 Dimensions (EORTC QLU-C10D).[30,31]

Vignette valuation studies are an altogether different approach in which health state descriptions (vignettes) are valued using a preference-based method (typically time trade-off). These methods are prone to bias, and the validity of their utility estimates depends on the accuracy and level of detail of the health state descriptions. It is not possible for vignettes to include all aspects of the patient experience or the full range of experiences within a health state among patients, but they are useful and generally considered acceptable in cases where patient-completed preference-based measures are not feasible (for example in rare diseases) or no measure is appropriate for the health condition or population.[32]

There are now a variety of generic preference-based measures designed for children and young people.[33] Also, the importance of considering caregivers in economic evaluations is increasingly being recognized.[34] Although preference-based measures were not designed for caregivers, EQ-5D has been used, and a new measure is in development, which aims to be appropriate for caregivers as well as patients.[35,36]

UTILITY STUDY DESIGN CONSIDERATIONS

A review of existing estimates available in the published literature is an important starting point to determine whether high-quality utility estimates relevant to the economic model are available and whether new research is needed. In any new research, as important to data quality as the selection of the utility measure, is the design of the study in which utility data are collected.[19] Prospective data collection in clinical trials and open label extension studies represent an important opportunity and an efficient way to collect utility data. However, careful design is critical to the quality and usefulness of the data. Because the primary use of utility data is for economic evaluation, most commonly performed via an economic model, the design should optimize the collection of utility estimates for model health states and/or events. Particular care may be needed in selection of the timing of assessments, respondents (eg, whether a proxy respondent may be needed for patients too ill to complete a measure, or young children), and mode of administration. In some cases, it may not be possible to collect all data needed for a model within the registration trial, and additional work may be needed to provide a complete set of estimates for all the modeled health states. Prospective longitudinal or cross-sectional observational studies or surveys may be able to capture a fuller range of health states, also reflecting the real-world patient population rather than patients selected for trials. Early-access or compassionate-use–type programs, Phase IV studies, registries, and other post-licensing commitments can be an efficient way to capture data. Although such studies may be performed too late in the product development program to provide estimates for HTA submissions of new technologies, the data may be useful for reassessments and ongoing cost-utility research for products.[19]

SUMMARY AND CONTEXT

As mentioned previously, health utility estimates are among the most important data inputs in CUAs, which are increasingly used to guide decisions about access to healthcare interventions. High-quality utility estimates are required that are aligned with the definitions of the economic model health states and/or events, free from known sources of bias, and measured by using a validated method, appropriate to the condition and population of interest and the perspective of decision-maker for whom the economic model is being developed. The EQ-5D is the most widely used and researched utility measure, and it is preferred or accepted by most decision-makers. However, it is recognized that it may not be appropriate for all health conditions and populations, and a range of other methods are available. Careful selection of the measure and study design is important to optimize the quality and relevance of utility estimates, which inform important decisions governing patients access to new treatments.

Utility estimates alone do not capture the full spectrum of patient and public values. They are typically derived from a limited set of health state descriptions and may not reflect the nuanced trade-offs that individuals are willing to make between different treatment attributes, such as side effects, convenience, and cost. Moreover, utility instruments often rely on general population preferences, which may differ from those of patients or caregivers directly affected by a condition or intervention. To address these limitations and to enable a fuller understanding of value in healthcare, researchers increasingly turn to preference assessment methods.

PREFERENCE ASSESSMENT

Preference assessment methods are designed to quantify preferences by eliciting how individuals prioritize and make trade-offs based on the different attributes of healthcare interventions. Many of these methods are grounded on Lancaster's theory that utility (or value) is derived from the attributes of treatments (or goods or services).[37] The rest of this chapter focuses on the primary preference-based methods, highlighting their methodologic considerations and practical applications in health outcomes research.

DISCRETE CHOICE EXPERIMENTS AND BEST-WORST SCALING CASE 3

Attribute trade-off–based stated preference methods include discrete choice experiments (DCEs), conjoint analysis, and best-worst scaling (BWS) case 3. In each, respondents are presented with a series of hypothetical scenarios comprising two or more alternatives (eg, treatments, tests, screening programs, vaccines) where they state (through choosing, rating or ranking) the option that they prefer. The alternatives in each scenario are described in terms of their attributes and levels. Choices made over a series of scenarios indicate the relative value of the attributes and levels and allows estimation of the trade-offs between different attributes (ie, how they balance the attributes to maximize their utility). In a DCE, respondents make a choice among a discrete set of two or more options. Conjoint analysis refers to rating or ranking of the options. Best-worst scaling case 3 is when the choice is for most preferred and least preferred, and a less common variant asks respondents to select the best and second-best options from three or more.

The generation of alternatives and choice sets from a selection of attributes and levels is called the experimental design. It is rarely possible to present all combinations of attribute levels to respondents, so a fraction is presented instead. Designs are sometimes chosen from the full factorial at random, but most often the fraction is created with various statistical properties in mind. Orthogonal designs have level balance (ie, all attribute levels occur with equal frequency) and ensure each level appears equally often in combination with every other attribute level.[38] This eliminates covariance between attributes, isolating the independent effect of each level on choice and allowing for causal interpretation of the results (ie, how a change in an attribute affects the probability of choosing an option). Another option is a D-efficient design, which involves minimizing the inverse of the variance-covariance matrix in a maximum likelihood estimation.[39] A software algorithm generally searches for a design that maximizes this efficiency. Researchers used to assume that parameters equal zero when generating D-efficient designs, but more recent advances use a Bayesian approach and incorporate prior assumptions (expected values) to improve statistical efficiency.[40] Blocking the fractional factorial design can reduce the number of choice sets a respondent sees even further to minimize response fatigue, as long as the sample size is sufficient.

Discrete choice experiments generate cross-sectional data and are typically analyzed by using discrete choice models.[40,41] These models (ie, not chosen = 0 and chosen = 1) use probability regressions, which typically assume either a logistic (logit) or normal (probit) distribution. Popular models include latent class analysis and either conditional logit, mixed logit, or random parameters logit.[42] These assume that respondents choose the option that maximizes their utility, but there is also a random element to their choice.

Sample size calculations for DCEs often need *a priori* estimation of the effect size, the specification of the likely utility function, and assumptions about the choice design. More attributes and more levels mean more parameters to estimate, which in turn requires more observations and a larger sample size. Likewise, more complex models estimating more parameters will require more respondents. A typical DCE requires a sample between 100 and 300 respondents.[40]

Figure 18-6 shows an example of a choice set from a breast-screening DCE used to elicit preferences from 1,000 women of screening age in the United Kingdom. The choice set required women to balance the effectiveness of the screening at detecting cancers (true positives), the chance that it would detect something that was not actually cancer (false positives), and the cost incurred to participate. In addition to the two options shown, women were given a third option of no screening to reflect their real-world choice.

Analyses revealed distinct groups of women (classes) with similar preference patterns (**Figure 18-7**). The largest group was designated as Pc-1 and accounted for almost a third of the sample (32.3%). Women in this class treated the detection attribute as most important and had a large negative coefficient on the "No Screening" parameter, suggesting tremendous disutility in the absence of a breast-screening program.

	Programme A	Programme B	No Screening
Women who will have cancers detected by screening	7% 	10% 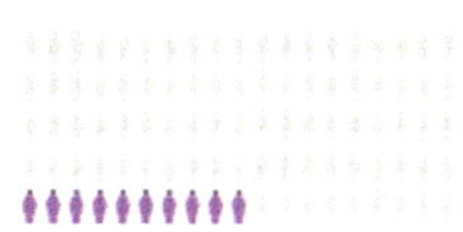	None: no cancers detected
Women who will have an unnecessary follow-up	1% 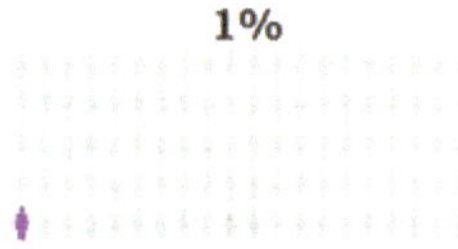	10% 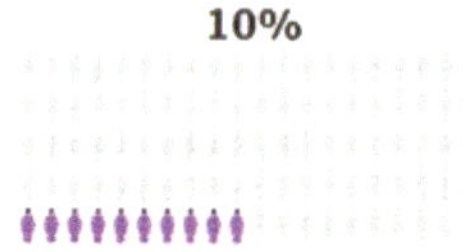	None: no unnecessary follow-up
Out-of-pocket cost to you of screening programme per screen	£150 per screen (£750 over your lifetime) 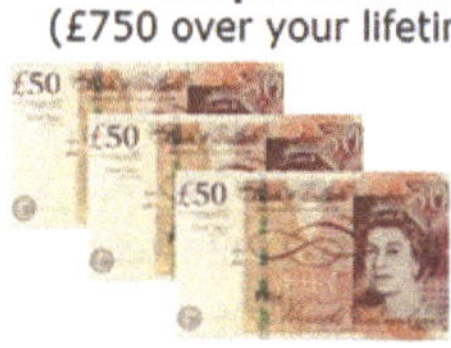	£200 per screen (£1,000 over your lifetime) 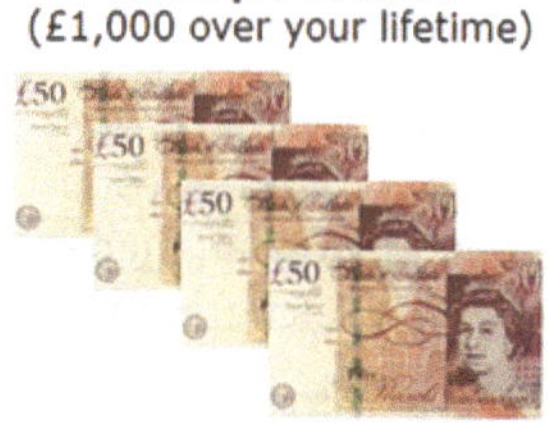	None: no cost to you
	○	○	○

FIGURE 18-6. **Example DCE choice question.**

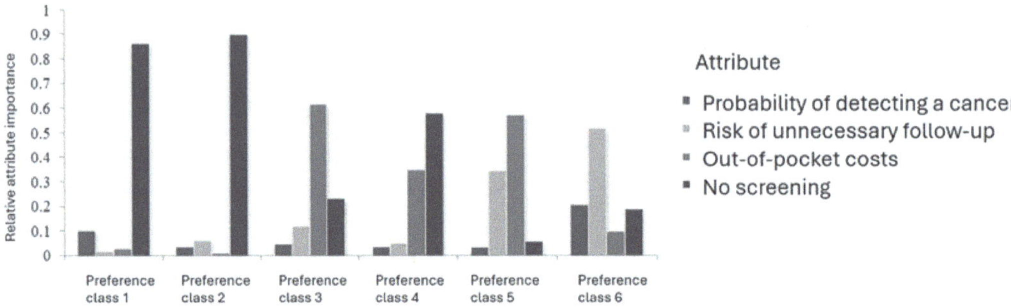

FIGURE 18-7. Example DCE results using latent class analysis to quantify preference heterogeneity.

Note: Preference classes were selected through an iterative process involving comparisons of the Akaike information criterion (AIC), the Bayesian information criterion (BIC), and consistent Akaike information criterion (CAIC).

Women in the Pc-4 group (18.7% of the sample) also had a large negative coefficient on the "No Screening" parameter but were distinguished for considering cost to be the most important attribute. The Pc-5 group agreed that cost was most important and felt it was closely followed by the risk of unnecessary follow-up. But their coefficient for "No Screening" was positive (although statistically insignificant), indicating that they would rather not participate in a screening program.[43]

Trade-off analysis revealed a marginal willingness to pay of ~£79 (2013 prices) for a 1% point increase in the probability of detecting a cancer and that women were, on average, willing to accept nearly two additional unnecessary follow-ups (1.72) for an additional cancer detected per 100 women screened. Assuming a 10% probability of detecting a cancer, a 10% risk of unnecessary follow-up, and a lifetime screening cost of £100, the probability of a woman choosing screening over no screening was estimated to be ~85%.[43]

Discrete choice experiments have become a cornerstone of preference elicitation, earning widespread recognition from pivotal decision-making bodies, such as the Food and Drug Administration and European Medicines Agency.[44-46] Although DCEs can answer many research questions, including the relative importance of various attributes, the trade-offs individuals are willing to make, and the potential uptake of different options, they are also complex and require a large sample size. Consequently, the successful implementation of DCEs requires a robust foundation of experimental design and analysis and a suitable sample size (ideally, at least 250 respondents answering 8–12 questions) to ensure that the results are reliable.

BEST-WORST SCALING CASE 1

Best-worst scaling case 1, also known as object case, is supported by the psychological premise that individuals can better identify extremes (eg, the best and the worst) when presented with a list of objects. These objects, sometimes referred to as items, criteria, and/or attributes, may be aspects of a treatment, outcomes in a trial, or domains of a measure. In BWS, a list of objects is created, and each respondent is presented with a series of choice sets containing a subset of these objects.

Typically, respondents are asked to select which is "best" and which is "worst" or a variation of this, such as their most and least preferred, which is most and least important, or which they most agree with and least agree with from the subset. The framing will be determined by the research question, and different frames and phrasing will reveal different information about respondents' preferences. Repeated choices over a series of questions reveal the ranking of the objects on an underlying latent scale. For this reason, BWS case 1 is often seen as an alternative to rating scales, such as Likert questions, with the added advantage that it eliminates scale-interpretation issues (ie, is one person's "good" equivalent to another person's "very good" or does 5 of 10 really reflect the midpoint?) and bunching (ie, every aspect of health is "very important"). Although the design of BWS exercises may be more challenging and individual questions may take longer for respondents to complete, BWS often requires respondents to answer fewer questions and can provide more robust and reliable data than simple ordinal response categories or scale responses.[47]

The subset of objects presented in the choice tasks are created by using an experimental design to encourage desirable statistical properties. One design property often considered is balance, which entails giving each object equal opportunity to be selected by showing it an equal number of times and an equal number of times with each object. Approaches for analyzing BWS data vary in complexity. The simplest analytical approach is a "count analysis," which involves counting the number of times an item was selected best or worst and sometimes weighting this by the number of times it appeared depending on the properties of the experimental design. A count analysis can provide individual-level ranking and rating of all objects. As respondents provide answers over multiple choice sets, there are opportunities to analyze these cross-sectional data with logit- or probit-based discrete choice models. Alternatively, maximum-difference models, which assume that an individual makes a choice by simultaneously selecting the option with the biggest difference in utility, also can be estimated; however, these are less often implemented in practice.[48]

Figures 18-8 and **18-9** give examples of a BWS case 1 choice question and study results.[49] The study sought to better understand trial decision-making by considering how caregivers and patients prioritize 13 factors when considering participation in a gene therapy trial. The BWS choice questions (Figure 18-8) asked respondents to choose the item they would care most and least about when deciding whether to join a trial. Respondents completed 11 of these choice questions with a subset of five trial attributes. Analysis of the BWS case 1 data revealed that respondents prioritized improved muscle function and cared relatively less about the need for muscle biopsies or potential for randomization to placebo (Figure 18-9).

Relative to other preference methods, BWS case 1 can be relatively simple and easy to design and analyze. It is often chosen over other preference methods when the anticipated sample size is limited (eg, rare diseases), there is a need to understand individual-level

First choose the item that you would care about the most if you were deciding whether to join the gene therapy trial. Then choose the item that you would care about the least. You have to answer both to move on.

Which would you care about the most when deciding whether to join the trial? Which would you care about the least?

I care about this the most		I care about this the least
○	Two muscle biopsies required	○
●	Limits later use of gene therapies or CRISPR	○
○	Chance of improved muscle function	○
○	Risk of death (low risk)	○
○	Any benefits last 10 years	●

FIGURE 18-8. Example BWS case 1 choice question.

Source: Paquin RS, Fischer R, Mansfield C, et al. Priorities when deciding on participation in early-phase gene therapy trials for Duchenne muscular dystrophy: a best-worst scaling experiment in caregivers and adult patients. *Orphanet J Rare Dis.* 2019;14(1):102. https://doi.org/10.1186/s13023-019-1069-6

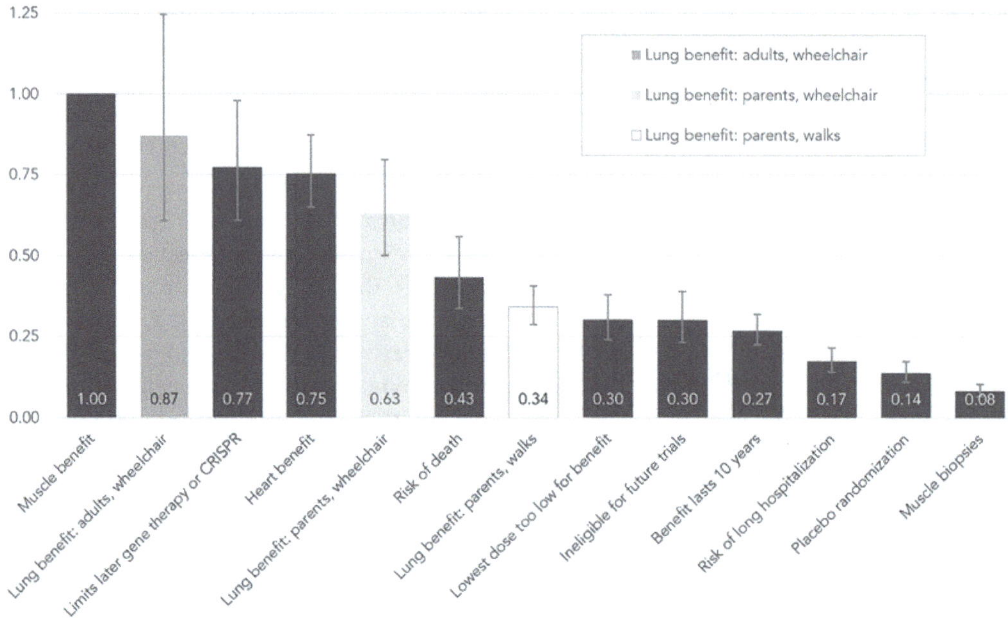

FIGURE 18-9. Example BWS case 1 results.

Source: Paquin RS, Fischer R, Mansfield C, et al. Priorities when deciding on participation in early-phase gene therapy trials for Duchenne muscular dystrophy: a best-worst scaling experiment in caregivers and adult patients. *Orphanet J Rare Dis.* 2019;14(1):102. https://doi.org/10.1186/s13023-019-1069-6

preferences (eg, for a decision aid), there is an especially long list of attributes, or the analysis requires simplicity (eg, because of computing- or time-constraints). However, this simplicity comes at the expense of being able to answer complex research questions. BWS case 1 does not provide trade-off information, so it is unable to provide evidence on marginal rates of substitution between objects or on thresholds, such as maximum acceptable risk or willingness to pay.

BEST-WORST SCALING CASE 2

Best-worst scaling case 2, also known as profile case, is similar to BWS case 1 in that it has respondents select a variant of the best or worst, but differs in that respondents also select the attribute level. It is similar to DCE in that it describes alternatives in terms of both attributes and levels, only this time individuals are presented with a single profile at a time rather than comparing across multiple alternatives. The resulting profiles must be informed by an experimental design, and these designs tend to be more like a DCE.[50] Although a simple count analysis can be conducted, many studies employ discrete choice–type models.

Best-worst scaling case 2 is often used in studies eliciting preferences for health states, and the method informed weighting for measures, such as the Investigating Choice Experiments for the Preferences of Older People–Capability (ICECAP) and the Child Health Utility (CHU-9D, EQ-5D Youth version [EQ-5D-Y]) literatures.[51-53] **Figure 18-10** provides an example of a BWS case 2 choice question from a study where young patients aged 11 to 16 years were presented with questions related to teeth quality (eg, tooth pain, ability to eat) and a level related to the attribute (eg, a bit, a lot).[54] Patients were asked to indicate which attribute level would be the best part and worst part. **Table 18-1** shows the results, which were used as weights in a dental cavities–specific measure of oral health-related quality of life (after combining with adult-generated DCE weights). The reference level was the

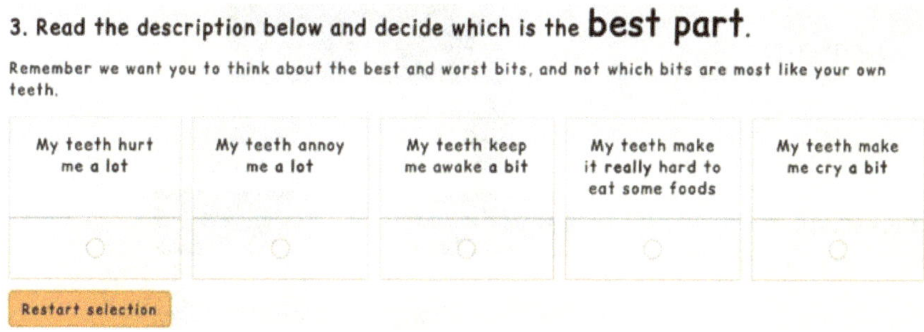

FIGURE 18-10. Example BWS case 2 choice question.

Source: Rogers HJ, Sagabiel J, Marshman Z, et al. Adolescent valuation of CARIES-QC-U: a child-centred preference-based measure of dental caries. *Health Qual Life Outcomes.* 2022;20(1):18. https://doi.org/10.1186/s12955-022-01918-w

TABLE 18-1. Example BWS Case 2 Results

Variables	Standard Model
Hurt1	*Reference*
Hurt2	−2.235***
Hurt3	−3.406***
Annoy1	−0.959***
Annoy2	−1.989***
Annoy3	−2.72***
Awake1	−0.866***
Awake2	−2.322***
Awake3	−2.827***
Eat1	−0.949***
Eat2	−1.874***
Eat3	−2.543***
Cry1	-0.266***
Cry2	−2.039***
Cry3	−3.097***

Source: Rogers HJ, Sagabiel J, Marshman Z, et al. Adolescent valuation of CARIES-QC-U: a child-centred preference-based measure of dental caries. *Health Qual Life Outcomes.* 2022;20(1):18. https://doi.org/10.1186/s12955-022-01918-w

"best" level (chosen best with the highest frequency), which was no hurting at all. The other levels for all other attributes were negative and consistently exhibit logical soundness (increasingly inferior levels are perceived as worse). The largest decrements in utility were between Cry1 and Cry3 and Hurt1 and Hurt 3, showing moving from *my teeth do not make me cry* to *my teeth make me cry a lot* and from *my teeth do not hurt me at all* to *my teeth hurt me a lot* have the biggest impact on child patients and are the most important attributes.

Best-worst scaling case 2 can yield more insights than the ranking of objects offered BWS case 1 and may arguably be easier to implement than DCEs with the option for simple designs and analysis. The method may therefore be useful when the research question is evolving. It may also be useful when the questions need to be simple, as considering one profile at a time and selecting best or worst levels is arguably easier than a DCE. This is perhaps why the study design seems to have been used more often with children and older adults.

THRESHOLDING METHODS

Threshold-based approaches to preference elicitation seek to find combinations of attributes (eg, benefits and risks, benefits and

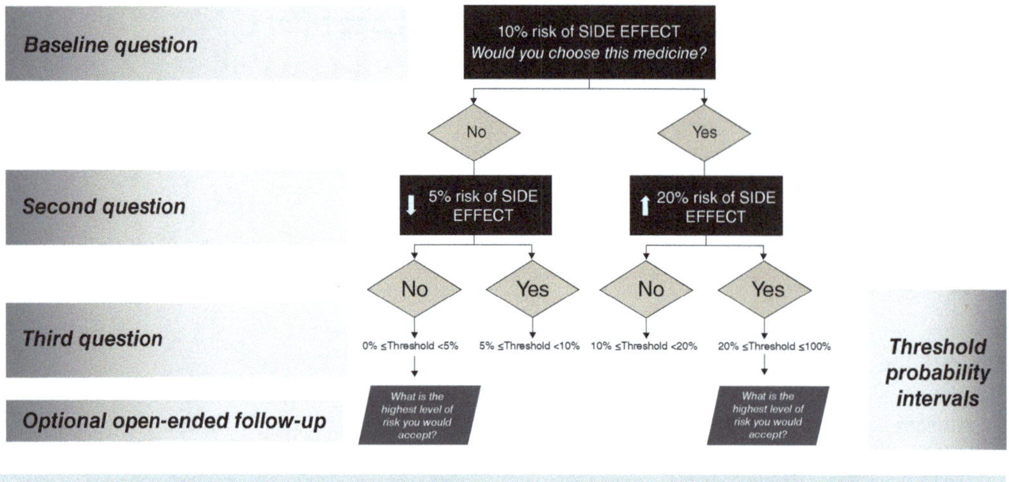

FIGURE 18-11. **Example probabilistic thresholding question series.**

costs, benefits and length of life) that offer the same level of utility. These methods typically vary the value of one attribute in an option until the participant is indifferent between the alternatives. In a thresholding study, a respondent is presented with a choice between two healthcare options: the "reference option" is usually current health or standard of care, and the "target option" presents an increase in both the benefit and burden so that respondents are required to make a trade-off when choosing their preferred alternative.

Thresholding methods can include either standard gambles or time trade-offs, as described previously, or contingent valuation where willingness to pay is the metric, revealing a monetary valuation. Studies are also increasingly implementing the "probabilistic threshold technique" where probabilistic attributes (typically a risk of harm) are used to quantify preferences.[55]

In a thresholding series, the initial question usually presents the same attributes in the reference and target options. **Figure 18-11** shows how the series is implemented: if the reference option is chosen first, the key attribute of the target is made better, and the question is repeated. If the target is chosen first, the key attribute of the target is made worse, and the question is repeated. The procedure is repeated until the researcher can identify the threshold level where the respondent is indifferent between the reference and target options shown by the intervals in Figure 18-11. If the respondents' preference lies outside the ranges presented in the series, an open-ended follow-up question can be asked to understand exactly where their threshold lies.

The results of a thresholding exercise can be presented as a histogram, or an interval regression can be used to model the upper and lower limits of the range in which the threshold value is known to lie. Threshold techniques offer researchers a relatively simple approach to preference quantification with no need for experimental design. Their results are easier to interpret, and studies can be conducted with relatively small sample sizes as they yield preference information at the individual level. However, eliciting preferences can be challenging, because multiple series are required, which can be burdensome for respondents.

CONCLUSION

A wide range of methods are available for quantifying preferences in health and healthcare, including BWS, DCE, and thresholding techniques. These methods vary in complexity, data requirements, and the types of insights provided. Simple methods, such as a BWS case 1, can be implemented relatively quickly in smaller samples but cannot provide trade-off information. In contrast, DCEs are more resource-intensive but offer rich data on the relative importance of attributes and the trade-offs individuals are willing to make. Selecting the appropriate preference assessment method depends on the research question, the characteristics of the target population, and practical considerations, such as sample size.

While preference methods help us to understand how individuals value different features of healthcare interventions, utility assessment translates those preferences into a standardized metric—typically on a scale from 0 (death) to 1 (full health)—that can be used in economic evaluations. Health utility estimates translate clinical outcomes into QALYs, enabling comparisons across diverse health conditions and treatments. While the EQ-5D remains the most widely used and accepted utility instrument, it is not universally appropriate and there are a range of viable alternatives.

Understanding how to measure quality of life, preferences, and patient utilities is essential for conducting rigorous health outcomes research and informing evidence-based decision-making in healthcare. By integrating these approaches, researchers and decision-makers can better align healthcare interventions with the needs, values, and priorities of the populations they serve.

REFERENCES

1. Berzon RA, Mauskopf JA, Simeon GP. Choosing a health profile (descriptive) and/or a patient-preference (utility) measure for a clinical trial. In: Spilker B, ed. *Quality of Life and Pharmacoeconomics in Clinical Trials*. 2nd ed. Marietta, GA: Lippincott-Raven; 1995.
2. Chumney ECG, Delinokov S, Fuldeore M, et al. What exactly do you mean by that? A summary of discrepancies in the definitions of key pharmacoeconomic and outcomes research terms: a white paper. *ISPOR Connections*. 2004;9(1):6.
3. World Health Organization. *The First Ten Years of the World Health Organization*. Geneva, Switzerland. WHO; 1958.
4. Cella DF, Tulsky DS. Measuring quality of life today: methodological aspects. *Oncology (Williston Park)*. 1990;4(5):29-38; discussion 69. PMID: 2143408
5. Wiklund I. Assessment of patient-reported outcomes in clinical trials: the example of health-related quality of life. *Fundam Clin Pharmacol*. 2004;18(3):351-363. https://doi.org/10.1111/j.1472-8206.2004.00234.x
6. Nunnally JC. *Psychometric Theory*. 2nd ed. New York: Basic Books; 1978.
7. McDowell I, Newell C. *Measuring Health: A Guide to Rating Scales and Questionnaires*. 2nd ed. Oxford: Oxford University Press; 1996.
8. Jenkinson C, McGee H. *Health Status Measurement: A Brief but Critical Introduction*. London: Radcliffe Medical Press; 1998.
9. Hays RD, Anderson R, Revicki DA. Psychometric evaluation and interpretation of health-related quality of life data. In: Shumaker SA, Berzon RA, eds. *The International Assessment of Health-related Quality of Life: Theory, Translation, Measurement and Analysis*. Morrison, CO: Rapid Communications; 1995:103-114.
10. Lydick EG, Epstein RS. Clinical significance of quality of life data. In: Spilker B, ed. *Quality of Life and Pharmacoeconomics in Clinical Trials*. 2nd ed. Lippincott-Raven; 1995:461-465.
11. Juniper EF, Guyatt GH, Willan A, Griffith LE. Determining a minimal important change in a disease-specific quality of life questionnaire. *J Clin Epidemiol*. 1994;47(1):81-87. https://doi.org/10.1016/0895-4356(94)90036-1
12. Jaeschke R, Singer J, Guyatt GH. Measurement of health status: ascertaining the minimal clinically important difference. *Control Clin Trials*. 1989;10(4):407-415. https://doi.org/10.1016/0197-2456(89)90005-6
13. Hunt SM, McKenna S. Cross-cultural comparability of quality of life measures. *Br J Med Econ*. 1992;4:17-23. https://doi.org/10.1177/009286159302700223
14. Bullinger M, Anderson R, Cella D, Aaronson N. Developing and evaluating cross-cultural instruments from minimum requirements to optimal models. *Qual Life Res*. 1993;2(6):451-459. https://doi.org/10.1007/bf00422219
15. Hui C, Triandis HC. Measurement in cross-cultural psychology: a review and comparison of strategies. *Cross Cultural Psychol*. 1985;16:131-152. https://doi.org/10.1177/0022002185016002001
16. Lenert L, Kaplan RM. Validity and interpretation of preference-based measures of health-related quality of life. *Med Care*. 2000;38(9 Suppl):II 138-150. https://doi.org/10.1097/00005650-200009002-00021

17. Feeny D. A utility approach to the assessment of health-related quality of life. *Med Care*. 2000;38(9 Suppl):II 51-54. https://doi.org/10.1097/00005650-200009002-00022
18. Robinson R. Cost-utility analysis. *BMJ*. 1993;307(6908):859-862. https://doi.org/10.1136/bmj.307.6908.859
19. Wolowacz SE, Briggs A, Belozeroff V, et al. Estimating health-state utility for economic models in clinical studies: an ISPOR Good Research Practices Task Force Report. *Value Health*. 2016;19(6):704-719. https://doi.org/10.1016/j.jval.2016.06.001
20. The EuroQoL Group. EuroQol: a new facility for the measurement of health-related quality of life. *Health Policy*. 1990;16(3):199-208. https://doi.org/10.1016/0168-8510(90)90421-9
21. Finch AP, Brazier JE, Mukuria C. What is the evidence for the performance of generic preference-based measures? A systematic overview of reviews. *Eur J Health Econ*. 2018;19(4):557-570. https://doi.org/10.1007/s10198-017-0902-x
22. Dakin H, Abel L, Burns R, et al. HERC database of mapping studies. Version 9.0. Updated December 1, 2023. http://www.herc.ox.ac.uk/downloads/herc-database-of-mapping-studies. Accessed March 25, 2026.
23. Feeny D, Furlong W, Boyle M, Torrance GW. Multi-attribute health status classification systems. Health Utilities Index. *Pharmacoeconomics*. 1995;7(6):490-502. https://doi.org/10.2165/00019053-199507060-00004
24. Horsman J, Furlong W, Feeny D, Torrance G. The Health Utilities Index (HUI): concepts, measurement properties and applications. *Health Qual Life Outcomes*. 2003 Oct 16;1:54. https://doi.org/10.1186/1477-7525-1-54
25. Sintonen H, Pekurinen M. A generic 15 dimensional measure of health-related quality of life (15D). *J Soc Med*. 1998;26:85-96.
26. Maxwell A, Özmen M, Iezzi A, Richardson J. Deriving population norms for the AQoL-6D and AQoL-8D multi-attribute utility instruments from web-based data. *Qual Life Res*. 2016;25(12):3209-3219. https://doi.org/10.1007/s11136-016-1337-z
27. Brazier J, Roberts J, Deverill M. The estimation of a preference-based measure of health from the SF-36. *J Health Econ*. 2002;21(2):271-292. https://doi.org/10.1016/s0167-6296(01)00130-8
28. Brazier J, Roberts J, Tsuchiya A, Busschbach J. A comparison of the EQ-5D and SF-6D across seven patient groups. *Health Econ*. 2004;13(9):873-884. https://doi.org/10.1002/hec.866
29. Rowen D, Brazier J, Ara R, Azzabi Zouraq I. The role of condition-specific preference-based measures in health technology assessment. *Pharmacoeconomics*. 2017;35(Suppl 1):33-41. https://doi.org/10.1007/s40273-017-0546-9
30. Yang Y, Brazier JE, Tsuchiya A, Young TA. Estimating a preference-based index for a 5-dimensional health state classification for asthma derived from the asthma quality of life questionnaire. *Med Decis Making*. 2011;31(2):281-291. https://doi.org/10.1177/0272989x10379646
31. King MT, Costa DS, Aaronson NK, et al. QLU-C10D: a health state classification system for a multi-attribute utility measure based on the EORTC QLQ-C30. *Qual Life Res*. 2016;25(3):625-636. https://doi.org/10.1007/s11136-015-1217-y
32. Matza LS, Stewart KD, Lloyd AJ, et al. Vignette-based utilities: usefulness, limitations, and methodological recommendations. *Value Health*. 2021;24(6):812-821. https://doi.org/10.1016/j.jval.2020.12.017
33. Bégo-Le Bagousse G, Jia X, Wolowacz S, et al. Health utility estimation in children and adolescents: a review of health technology assessments. *Curr Med Res Opin*. 2020;36(7):1209-1224. https://doi.org/10.1080/03007995.2020.1762553
34. Basarir H, Brockbank J, Knight C, Wolowacz S. The inclusion of the utility values for carers and family members in HTAs: a case study of recent NICE appraisals in the UK. Poster presented at the 2019 ISPOR 24th annual international meeting, May 22, 2019, New Orleans, LA [abstract]. *Value Health Reg Issues*. 2019;22(Suppl 2):S330.
35. Wittenberg E, James LP, Prosser LA. Spillover effects on caregivers' and family members' utility: a systematic review of the literature. *Pharmacoeconomics*. 2019;37(4):475-499. https://doi.org/10.1007/s40273-019-00768-7
36. Mukuria C, Peasgood T, McDool E, et al. Valuing the EQ health and wellbeing short using time trade-off and a discrete choice experiment: a feasibility study. *Value Health*. 2023;26(7):1073-1084. https://doi.org/10.1016/j.jval.2023.02.008
37. Lancaster KJ. A new approach to consumer theory. *J Polit Econ*. 1966;74(2):132-157. https://doi.org/10.1086/259131

38. Street DJ, Burgess L. *The Construction of Optimal Stated Choice Experiments: Theory and Methods*. 1st ed. Hoboken, NJ: Wiley Interscience; 2007.
39. Reed Johnson F, Lancsar E, Marshall D, et al. Constructing experimental designs for discrete-choice experiments: report of the ISPOR Conjoint Analysis Experimental Design Good Research Practices Task Force. *Value Health*. 2013;16(1):3-13. https://doi.org/10.1016/j.jval.2012.08.2223
40. Soekhai V, de Bekker-Grob EW, Ellis AR, Vass CM. Discrete choice experiments in health economics: past, present and future. *Pharmacoeconomics*. 2019;37(2):201-226. https://doi.org/10.1007/s40273-018-0734-2
41. Hauber AB, González JM, Groothuis-Oudshoorn CG, et al. Statistical methods for the analysis of discrete choice experiments: a report of the ISPOR Conjoint Analysis Good Research Practices Task Force. *Value Health*. 2016;19(4):300-315. https://doi.org/10.1016/j.jval.2016.04.004
42. Vass C, Boeri M, Karim S, et al. Accounting for preference heterogeneity in discrete-choice experiments: an ISPOR Special Interest Group Report. *Value Health*. 2022;25(5):685-694. https://doi.org/10.1016/j.jval.2022.01.012
43. Vass CM, Rigby D, Payne K. Investigating the heterogeneity in women's preferences for breast screening: does the communication of risk matter? *Value Health*. 2018;21(2):219-228. https://doi.org/10.1016/j.jval.2017.07.010
44. FDA. Patient preference information – voluntary submission, review in premarket approval applications, humanitarian device exemption applications, and de novo requests, and inclusion in decision summaries and device labeling. 2016. https://www.fda.gov/regulatory-information/search-fda-guidance-documents/patient-preference-information-voluntary-submission-review-premarket-approval-applications. Accessed February 5, 2026.
45. The PREFER Consortium. PREFER recommendations: why, when and how to assess and use patient preferences in medical product decision-making. 2022. https://doi.org/10.5281/zenodo.6470922
46. Bouvy JC, Cowie L, Lovett R, et al. Use of patient preference studies in HTA decision making: a NICE perspective. *Patient*. 2020;13(2):145-149. https://doi.org/10.1007/s40271-019-00408-4
47. Burton N, Burton M, Rigby D, et al. Best-worst scaling improves measurement of first impressions. *Cogn Res Princ Implic*. 2019;4(1):36. https://doi.org/10.1186/s41235-019-0183-2
48. Schuster ALR, Crossnohere NL, Campoamor NB, et al. The rise of best-worst scaling for prioritization: a transdisciplinary literature review. *J Choice Model*. 2024;50. https://doi.org/10.1016/j.jocm.2023.100466
49. Paquin RS, Fischer R, Mansfield C, et al. Priorities when deciding on participation in early-phase gene therapy trials for Duchenne muscular dystrophy: a best-worst scaling experiment in caregivers and adult patients. *Orphanet J Rare Dis*. 2019;14(1):102. https://doi.org/10.1186/s13023-019-1069-6
50. Cheung KL, Wijnen BF, Hollin IL, et al. Using best-worst scaling to investigate preferences in health care. *Pharmacoeconomics*. 2016;34(12):1195-1209. https://doi.org/10.1007/s40273-016-0429-5
51. Coast J, Flynn TN, Natarajan L, et al. Valuing the ICECAP capability index for older people. *Soc Sci Med*. 2008;67(5):874-882. https://doi.org/10.1016/j.socscimed.2008.05.015
52. Ratcliffe J, Flynn T, Terlich F, et al. Developing adolescent-specific health state values for economic evaluation: an application of profile case best-worst scaling to the Child Health Utility 9D. *Pharmacoeconomics*. 2012;30(8):713-727. https://doi.org/10.2165/11597900-000000000-00000
53. Dalziel K, Catchpool M, García-Lorenzo B, et al. Feasibility, validity and differences in adolescent and adult EQ-5D-Y health state valuation in Australia and Spain: an application of best-worst scaling. *Pharmacoeconomics*. 2020;38(5):499-513. https://doi.org/10.1007/s40273-020-00884-9
54. Rogers HJ, Sagabiel J, Marshman Z, et al. Adolescent valuation of CARIES-QC-U: a child-centred preference-based measure of dental caries. *Health Qual Life Outcomes*. 2022;20(1):18. https://doi.org/10.1186/s12955-022-01918-w
55. Hauber B, Coulter J. Using the threshold technique to elicit patient preferences: an introduction to the method and an overview of existing empirical applications. *Appl Health Econ Health Policy*. 2020;18(1):31-46. https://doi.org/10.1007/s40258-019-00521-3

Cost-Utility Analysis 19

Elinor G. Borgert, PhD, MSc, and
Kevin Wiley, PhD, MPH

Recall from Chapter 16 that in a cost-effectiveness analysis (CEA), the incremental cost of a program is compared with the incremental health effects of that program, and the health effects are measured in natural units such as life-years gained. Although widely used and important, there are two main drawbacks with this form of analysis. The first is that a CEA focuses on a single outcome of effect even though given medical intervention may have a spectrum of outcomes to consider. These could include life-years gained, physiologic improvements or compromises, treatment side effects, and other quality-of-life issues. A second issue is that comparisons with the resulting incremental cost-effectiveness ratios (ICERs) are limited to those using the same outcome measures, and precludes comparisons with those of other programs when different units of health effects have been used for different programs.

To overcome these problems with a traditional CEA, researchers often turn to a cost-utility analysis (CUA). It is frequently treated as simply a special form of CEA in which the denominator is standardized to measure outcomes in quality-adjusted life-years (QALYs).[1,2] The construction of QALYs recognizes that the output of a particular healthcare intervention cannot be considered merely in terms of extra years of life; it adjusts or weights these years of life by the quality of those years.

This adjustment accounts for the fact that there are two important aspects of any health-related intervention: (1) the resulting quantity of life (life expectancy or mortality) gained and (2) the resulting quality of life (morbidity, which is more difficult to measure) gained. As a uniform measure of health outcomes, QALYs are designed to reflect simultaneous improvements in morbidity and mortality resulting from a given intervention.[1]

The results of a CUA are presented in an ICER measured as cost per QALY ($/QALY), which indicates the cost required to generate the equivalent of 1 additional year of perfect health (1 QALY) using the formula:

$$\frac{\text{Cost of intervention A} - \text{Cost of intervention B}}{\text{QALYs of intervention A} - \text{QALYs of intervention B}}$$

By providing a method through which these various outcomes can be combined into a single composite outcome (the QALY), CUAs allow researchers to compare their results with those of other CUA studies. Doing so greatly facilitates interdisease as well as intradisease comparisons; investments in magnetic resonance imaging scans can then be compared with both Doppler screening and aspirin therapy to determine which program generates the greatest utility for a given monetary outlay.

Cost-utility analysis is most appropriately used in the following situations:[1]

1. *When health-related quality of life is the important outcome.* Researchers comparing alternative treatments for arthritis evaluate the programs based on how well they improve the patients' physical, social, and psychological functioning; arthritis treatments are not expected to influence patient mortality.
2. *When health-related quality of life is one of the important outcomes (ie, when the program affects both morbidity and mortality).* Many cancer treatments improve both longevity and long-term

DOI: 10.37573/9781585287666.019

quality of life but can significantly decrease the patients' quality of life in the short term (during the treatment process itself).

3. *When the programs being compared have a wide range of different outcomes.* Decision-makers wanting to maximize the health benefits with a limited budget must have a common tool to evaluate the expected health benefits derived from a uniform investment of resources in competing programs.
4. *When researchers wish to compare a program to others that have already been evaluated using a CUA.* A formulary committee deciding whether or not to expand its list to include the latest drugs for several different conditions must have a common tool to evaluate the expected health benefits.

Healthcare policymakers around the world are increasingly using cost-utility data to determine which procedures to provide and which pharmaceuticals to include in drug formularies. The United Kingdom has its National Institute for Health and Care Excellence (NICE), Canada has its Canadian Agency for Drugs and Technologies in Health (CADTH), and Australia has its Pharmaceutical Benefits Advisory Committee (PBAC), all of which have long since added cost-utility data to their criteria for healthcare coverage.[3] New treatments must compete with each other and existing treatments and demonstrate greater cost-effectiveness before being included on formularies in these countries.

Decision-makers could potentially even list interventions in a league table, which ranks them according to the magnitude of their ICERs (**Table 19-1**). Although theoretically useful, league tables have largely fallen out of favor in recent decades. For one, it is difficult to compare the results of a number of independent CUAs unless key methodological features are standardized to ensure a level playing field. Many of these, such as the choice of discount rate, the range of costs and consequences considered, and the choice of comparison treatments, are the same choices that need to be made when conducting a CEA or cost-benefit analysis (CBA).[2,12] But for CUAs, the method of estimating utility values for health states is an important additional consideration and not an easy one. Furthermore, the rise of real-world data and adaptive reimbursement models makes static league tables less useful.

In theory, once comparable CUA study results are ranked, decision-makers would have three options. They could (1) begin with a limited budget and purchase the most cost-effective interventions for a population first, working their way down the league table until the budget is exhausted; (2) determine a cost-effectiveness threshold and then provide all cost-effective interventions to a population; or (3) use the cost-effectiveness data available in a league table as one of many factors to consider in deciding which interventions to provide. Until CUAs are fully standardized, the latter is the only feasible option open to healthcare decision-makers. However, the second also garners a great deal of attention as researchers and decision-makers attempt to determine the cost-effectiveness threshold.

The $50,000 threshold has long been the most cited $/QALY threshold in CUAs, but there is a great deal of disagreement about this subjective benchmark. The original use of this threshold seems to be Medicare's decision in the 1980s to cover dialysis in patients with chronic renal failure at an ICER within this range.[2,13] Its real appeal appears to lie in the convenience of a round number. Many believe that the actual cost-effectiveness threshold is significantly higher, and ICERs ranging from $50,000 to $200,000 per QALY are commonly described as cost effective today.[14-17]

For example, several CUAs have evaluated the Oregon State Medicaid program after individuals were randomly selected to receive medical services through Medicaid or to continue with uninsured medical care. In one such analysis, providing routine depression screenings through Medicaid resulted in better/earlier treatments and an ICER of $62,000 per QALY gained. The authors compared this with a cost-effective threshold of $130,000 per QALY to argue that the program intervention was cost effective.[18,19]

The statistical value-of-life literature, which uses willingness to pay surveys and revealed-preference approaches to infer the value of life from actual behavior, supports the assertion that interventions with ICERs of

TABLE 19-1. League Table of CUAs with Ratios Converted to 1998 US Dollars

Intervention	Comparator	Target Population	Reference	$/QALY
Warfarin	Aspirin	65-year-old with nonvalvular atrial fibrillation and high risk for stroke	Gage et al. (1995)[4]	Cost-saving
Warfarin	Aspirin	65-year-old with nonvalvular atrial fibrillation and medium risk for stroke	Gage et al. (1995)[4]	Cost-saving
Fortification with folic acid at 0.7 mg/100 g of cereal grain product	No fortification program to prevent congenital abnormalities	All women in United States capable of becoming pregnant	Neumann et al. (2016)[2]	Cost-saving
Pneumococcal pneumonia vaccination	No vaccination	People > 64 years	Sisk et al. (1997)[5]	Cost-saving
Nefazodone	Step approach (nefazodone if imipramine fails)	30-year-old women with one previous episode of major depression	Revicki et al. (1997)[6]	$2,800
Captopril	No captopril	80-year-old patients surviving myocardial infarction	Tsevat et al. (1995)[7]	$4,300
Nefazodone	Imipramine	30-year-old women with one previous episode of major depression	Revicki et al. (1997)[6]	$4,500
Captopril	No captopril	70-year-old patients surviving myocardial infarction	Tsevat et al. (1995)[7]	$5,900
Fluoxetine	Imipramine	30-year-old women with one previous episode of major depression	Revicki et al. (1997)[6]	$7,000
Warfarin	Aspirin	65-year-old with nonvalvular atrial fibrillation and medium risk for stroke	Gage et al. (1995)[4]	$8,800
Warfarin	No therapy	65-year-old with nonvalvular atrial fibrillation and low risk for stroke	Gage et al. (1995)[4]	$15,000
Interferon-α2b with melphalan and prednisone	Conventional treatment	Patients with multiple myeloma	Nord et al. (1997)[8]	$19,000
Driver-side air bag	No air bags	Driving population and passengers	Graham et al. (1997)[9]	$27,000
One-time Doppler ultrasound screening	No screening	Asymptomatic 60-year-old men with a low prevalence of > 59% carotid stenosis	Derdeyn et al. (1996)[10]	$56,000
Continuing care from a community psychiatric nurse	Continuing care from a general practitioner	Patients with a range of nonpsychotic problems	Revicki et al. (1997)[6]	$69,000
Dual air bags	Driver-side air bag only	Driving population and passengers	Graham et al. (1997)[9]	$69,000
MRI scan of head	CT scan of head	35-year-old women presenting with single episode of asymmetric neurological symptom suggesting possible neurological disorder	Mushlin et al. (1997)[11]	$110,000
Annual Doppler ultrasound screening	One-time Doppler ultrasound screening	Asymptomatic 60-year-old men with a low prevalence of > 59% carotid stenosis	Derdeyn et al. (1996)[10]	Dominated

CT = computed tomography; CUAs = cost-utility analysis; MRI = magnetic resonance imaging; QALY = quality-adjusted life-year.

Source: Adapted from Mushlin AI, Mooney C, Holloway RG. The cost effectiveness of magnetic resonance imaging for patients with equivocal neurological symptoms. *Int J Technol Assess Health Care.* 1997;13:21-34.

$200,000/QALY or higher could be considered cost-effective.[14] However, the general recommendation remains that cost-effectiveness information should be used alongside other considerations, such as budget-impact analyses and feasibility considerations, in a transparent decision-making process, rather than in isolation based on a single threshold value.[16] For more on these considerations, refer to Chapters 17 and 20.

However, several measurement issues must be considered in constructing both utility weights and quality-of-life measures, as explored in Chapter 18. Furthermore, the difficulties in measuring utility values and incorporating them into QALYs are inherently subjective and may lack the precision of clinical endpoints.[20] Generic health-related quality-of-life instruments may fail to detect subtle, treatment-specific health effects.[21] Conversely, disease-specific instruments may fail to detect unanticipated health effects, particularly in domains such as mental health.[20,22,23] Although an improvement over purely clinical measures in this regard, they still may not fully capture the effects of nonhealth events, such as economic or social factors.[24,25] Also, QALYs may undervalue interventions for individuals with disabilities or chronic conditions, which may raise ethical issues about fairness in resource allocation.[26-28]

While CUAs remain essential tools in determining value, their limitations must be addressed through robust statistical techniques, sensitivity analyses, and careful interpretation to ensure accurate and meaningful evaluations of healthcare interventions.

No discussion of CUAs would be complete without mentioning distributional CEAs (DCEAs). Distributional CEAs are relatively new to the literature and offer novel methodologies that build on a CUA's use of QALYs and adds a distributional lens to explicitly assess equity.[29] A recent publication estimated that Medicare funding for inpatient COVID-19 treatments yielded 735,569 net QALYs and reduced the population-level burden of health inequality by 0.23%. Despite data limitations and modeling assumptions, the study demonstrated that equitable investment in COVID-19 care can simultaneously improve overall health and reduce disparities in the US healthcare system.[30]

In rural areas with limited access to specialty care, DCEAs could provide a valuable framework for evaluating not just the efficiency but also the equity of healthcare interventions. For example, Medicare coverage of quarterly telehealth endocrinology visits for adults with type 2 diabetes may yield modest improvements in clinical outcomes at a population level but substantial gains for those living in underserved rural communities. Traditional cost-effectiveness models may overlook how access barriers disproportionately affect rural patients, who often face long travel distances, lost wages, and delayed treatment. By explicitly considering social variables and applying equity weights, DCEAs can highlight how redistributing healthcare resources to historically underserved populations might improve not only individual outcomes but also overall societal health equity. When analyzed through a distributional lens, interventions such as telehealth may emerge as preferable policy options owing to their potential to narrow health disparities and to improve fairness in outcome distribution.

However, DCEAs are limited by the difficulty of obtaining reliable, subgroup-specific data, such as differential telehealth adoption rates or diabetes-related outcomes among rural populations, which can affect the accuracy of modeled equity impacts. Additionally, assumptions about equity weights and social preferences may vary by context and are not always standardized, making it challenging for policymakers to accurately interpret distributional trade-offs.[31,32]

In conclusion, CUA offers a powerful framework for evaluating healthcare interventions by integrating both morbidity and mortality into a single, standardized metric: the QALY. This allows for more comprehensive comparisons across diverse treatments and conditions, especially when health-related quality of life is a significant outcome. Cost-utility analyses enable decision-makers to assess value in a consistent manner, facilitating resource allocation in environments with constrained budgets.

However, while CUAs provide a valuable tool for health economics, they are not without limitations. The subjectivity involved in measuring utility values, challenges of capturing nuanced health effects, and ethical concerns about equity—particularly for populations with chronic conditions or disabilities—highlight the need for cautious interpretation. Moreover, the reliance on cost-effectiveness thresholds, such as the oft cited $50,000 per QALY, remains contentious and should not be the sole determinant in policy decisions.

Ultimately, CUAs should be viewed as one component of a broader decision-making process. When combined with other considerations—such as budget impact, feasibility, and societal values—they can support more transparent, equitable, and effective healthcare policies. As methodologies continue to evolve and real-world data becomes more integrated, CUAs will remain a cornerstone of health economic evaluations.

REFERENCES

1. Drummond MF, Obrien BJ, Stoddart GL, Torrance GW. *Methods Economic Evaluation Health Care Programmes*. Oxford: Oxford University Press; 1997.
2. Neumann PJ, Russell LB, Siegel JE, et al. Using cost-effectiveness analysis in health and medicine. In: *Cost-Effectiveness in Health and Medicine*. Oxford: Oxford University Press; 2016:1-38. https://doi.org/10.1093/acprof:oso/9780190492939.003.0001
3. George B, Harris A, Mitchell A. Cost-effectiveness analysis and the consistency of decision making: evidence from pharmaceutical reimbursement in Australia (1991 to 1996). *Pharmacoeconomics*. 2001;19(11):1103-1109. https://doi.org/10.2165/00019053-200119110-00004
4. Gage BF, Cardinalli AB, Albers GW. Cost-effectiveness of warfarin and aspirin for prophylaxis of stroke in patients with non-valvular atrial fibrillation. *JAMA*. 1995;274:1839-1845. PMID: 7500532
5. Sisk JE, Moskowitz AJ, Whang W, et al. Cost-effectiveness of vaccination against pneumococcal bacteremia among elderly people. *JAMA*. 1997;278(16):1333-1339. https://doi.org/10.1001/jama.1997.03550160053038
6. Revicki DA, Brown RE, Keller MB, et al. Cost-effectiveness of newer antidepressants compared with tricyclic antidepressants in managed care settings. *J Clin Psychiatry*. 1997;58(2):47-58. https://doi.org/10.4088/jcp.v58n0201
7. Tsevat J, Duke D, Goldman L, et al. Cost-effectiveness of captopril therapy after myocardial infarction. *J Am Coll Cardiol*. 1995;26(4):914-919. https://doi.org/10.1016/0735-1097(95)00284-1
8. Nord E, Wisløff F, Hjorth M, Westin J. Cost-utility analysis of melphalan plus prednisone with or without interferon-α2b in newly diagnosed multiple myeloma. *Pharmacoeconomics*. 1997;12(1):89-103. https://doi.org/10.2165/00019053-199712010-00009
9. Graham JD, Thompson KM, Goldie SJ, et al. The cost-effectiveness of air bags by seating position. *JAMA*. 1997;278(17):1418-1425. PMID: 9356000
10. Derdeyn CP, Powers WJ. Cost-effectiveness of screening for asymptomatic carotid atherosclerotic disease. *Stroke*. 1996;27(11):1944-1950. https://doi.org/10.1161/01.str.27.11.1944
11. Mushlin AI, Mooney C, Holloway RG. The cost-effectiveness of magnetic resonance imaging for patients with equivocal neurological symptoms. *Int J Technol Assess Health Care*. 1997;13:21-34. https://doi.org/10.1017/s0266462300010205
12. Drummond M, Torrance G, Mason J. Cost-effectiveness league tables: more harm than good? *Soc Sci Med*. 1993;37:33-40. https://doi.org/10.1016/0277-9536(93)90315-u
13. Grosse SD. Assessing cost-effectiveness in healthcare: history of the $50,000 per QALY threshold. *Expert Rev Pharmacoecon Outcomes Res*. 2008;8(2):165-178. https://doi.org/10.1586/14737167.8.2.165
14. Hirth RA, Chernew ME, Miller E, et al. Willingness to pay for a quality-adjusted life year: in search of a standard. *Med Decis Mak*. 2000;20(3):332-342. https://doi.org/10.1177/0272989X0002000310
15. Ryen L, Svensson M. The willingness to pay for a quality adjusted life year: a review of the empirical literature. *Health Econ*. 2014;24(10):1289-1301. https://doi.org/10.1002/hec.3085
16. Bertram MY, Lauer JA, De Joncheere K, et al. Cost-effectiveness thresholds: pros and cons. *Bull World Health Organ*. 2016;94(12):925-930. https://doi.org/10.2471/BLT.15.164418
17. Neumann PJ, Cohen JT, Weinstein MC. Updating cost-effectiveness: curious resilience $50,000-per-QALY threshold. *N Engl J Med*. 2014;371(9):796-797. https://doi.org/10.1056/NEJMp1405158

18. Muening PA, Quan R, Chiuzan C, Glied S. Considering whether Medicaid is worth the cost: revisiting the Oregon health study. *Am L Pub Health*. 2015;105:866-871. https://doi.org/10.2105/AJPH.2014.302485
19. Baicker K, Taubman SL, Allen HL. The Oregon experiment—effects of Medicaid on clinical outcomes. *N Engl J Med*. 2013;368(18):1713-1722. https://doi.org/10.1056/NEJMsa1212321
20. Tengs TO. Cost-effectiveness versus cost-utility analysis of interventions for cancer: does adjusting for health-related quality of life really matter? *Value Health*. 2004;7(1):70-78. https://doi.org/10.1111/j.1524-4733.2004.71246.x
21. Claxton K. Exploring uncertainty in cost-effectiveness analysis. *Pharmacoeconomics*. 2008;26(9):781-798. https://doi.org/10.2165/00019053-200826090-00008
22. Pyne JM, Fortney JC, Tripathi SP, et al. Cost-effectiveness analysis of a rural telemedicine collaborative care intervention for depression. *Arch Gen Psychiatry*. 2010;67(8):812-821. https://doi.org/10.1001/archgenpsychiatry.2010.82
23. Diamond GA, Kaul S. Cost, effectiveness, and cost-effectiveness. *Circ Cardiovasc Qual Outcomes*. 2009;2(1):49-54. https://doi.org/10.1161/CIRCOUTCOMES.108.793406
24. Shields GE, Elvidge J. Challenges in synthesising cost-effectiveness estimates. *Syst Rev*. 2020;9(1):289. https://doi.org/10.1186/s13643-020-01536-x
25. Prosser LA, Stinnett AA, Goldman PA, et al. Cost-effectiveness of cholesterol-lowering therapies according to selected patient characteristics. *Ann Intern Med*. 2000;132(10):769-779. https://doi.org/10.7326/0003-4819-132-10-200005160-00002
26. Nord E, Daniels N, Kamlet M. QALYs: some challenges. *Value Health*. 2009;12 Suppl 1:S10-S15. https://doi.org/10.1111/j.1524-4733.2009.00516.x
27. Rubin JL, Lopez A, Booth J, et al. Limitations of standard cost-effectiveness methods for health technology assessment of treatments for rare, chronic diseases: a case study of treatment for cystic fibrosis. *J Med Econ*. 2022;25(1):783-791. https://doi.org/10.1080/13696998.2022.2077550
28. Weintraub WS, Cohen DJ. The limits of cost-effectiveness analysis. *Circ Cardiovasc Qual Outcomes*. 2009;2(1):55-58. https://doi.org/10.1161/CIRCOUTCOMES.108.812321
29. Cookson R, Griffin S, Norheim OF, Culyer AJ, eds. *Distributional Cost-Effectiveness Analysis: Quantifying Health Equity Impacts and Trade-Offs*. Oxford: Oxford University Press; 2020.
30. Kowal S, Ng CD, Schuldt R, et al. The impact of funding inpatient treatments for COVID-19 on health equity in the United States: a distributional cost-effectiveness analysis. *Value Health*. 2023;26(2):216-225. https://doi.org/10.1016/j.jval.2022.08.010
31. Steijger D, Chatterjee C, Groot W, Pavlova M. Challenges and limitations in distributional cost-effectiveness analysis: a systematic literature review. *Int J Environ Res Public Health*. 2022;20(1):505. https://doi.org/10.3390/ijerph20010505
32. Yang F, Angus C, Duarte A, et al. Impact of socioeconomic differences on distributional cost-effectiveness analysis. *Med Decis Mak*. 2020;40(5):606-618. https://doi.org/10.1177/0272989X20935883

Cost-Benefit Analysis 20

Elinor G. Borgert, PhD, MSc

INTRODUCTION

Healthcare systems around the world are challenged with allocating limited resources in an attempt to maximize societal well-being. Unlike other sectors of the economy, the healthcare market is handicapped by complex market failures, information asymmetries, and third-party payers, all of which complicate the efficient distribution of services. As a result, traditional market mechanisms often fall short in guiding optimal investment decisions in health technologies, treatments, and services. This chapter explores how cost-benefit analysis (CBA), a tool grounded in welfare economics, can help to fill this gap by providing a structured framework for evaluating whether health interventions generate more value than they consume.

While perfect competition rarely exists in any sector, many markets still manage to allocate resources efficiently through the decentralized decisions of individuals and firms. For example, no formal analysis is typically required to determine whether a new hamburger restaurant should open; market forces will reward efficient ventures and eliminate inefficient ones. This self-regulating mechanism works, because consumers understand what they are buying, production costs are predictable, and—crucially—people pay directly for what they consume. In contrast, healthcare decisions frequently lack these conditions, particularly the alignment of costs and consumption at the individual level. As a result, choices about adopting new technologies, pharmaceuticals, or services often fail to reflect true societal efficiency. Because we cannot reliably assume that each healthcare resource allocation decision is efficient on average, researchers must do the work of the market and evaluate the efficiency of decisions in a research setting.

It is important to acknowledge at the outset that the use of CBA for questions regarding healthcare and policy has been largely eschewed in favor of cost-effectiveness analysis (CEA) or cost-utility analysis (CUA). This is not owing to any inherent advantage of the more common methods. In fact, the framework used within CBAs is much more consistent with how other (nonhealth-related) interventions and policies are evaluated before implementation. These evaluations are based on how much individuals are willing to pay for a product and where they can get the "most bang for their buck." A common approach is to convert all the benefits of competing programs into monetary terms so that the net economic benefit of each can be compared, facilitating a more efficient allocation of resources across different sectors of society.

In contrast, a CUA's focus on quality-adjusted life-years (QALYs) means that it is limited to informing only the allocative efficiency of resources within the healthcare sector (see Chapter 19). A CEA is even more narrowly focused on a single disease-specific outcome measure (see Chapter 16). For example, when considering the cost-effectiveness of beta-blockers compared with aspirin therapy following a myocardial infarction (MI), a typical CEA will consider the difference in the costs of each therapy alongside the difference in their intended benefit, the number of recurrent MI episodes that could be prevented over

DOI: 10.37573/9781585287666.020

1 year of treatment. This points to a number of limitations:

1. A CEA ignores the many other potential benefits that might result from either of these two treatments, such as reduced incidents of angina, reduced severity of the MIs that do occur, and reduced mortality.
2. It similarly fails to account for any differences in side effects or other negative outcomes with the two treatments.
3. A CEA cannot compare the resource allocation for post-MI treatment to alternative uses of those same resources (eg, applied to prenatal care or very low birthweight deliveries), because the relevant outcomes of interest can be very different.

There are also some healthcare issues for which CEAs and CUAs are wholly unsuited. For instance, their use to assess fertility treatments would raise considerable methodological challenges, because the object is to create new life rather than extend, save, or improve the health-related quality of life.

This chapter reviews the economic principles that support CBA, discusses the general methods, and briefly reviews traditional barriers to its use. It concludes with a discussion of more recent advances in the field of health services research as it relates to CBAs.

EFFICIENCY AS AN ECONOMIC GOAL

Welfare economics is the study of how the allocation of resources and goods affects the welfare or well-being of society as a whole. These fundamental concepts are embodied in CBAs and can be easily illustrated by using a simple model that would be familiar to most students of economics. **Figure 20-1** presents a graph of a simple (and heavily stylized) market for hamburgers. The downward sloping line represents the demand for hamburgers in this hypothetical market—where the demand (the maximum amount that consumers are willing and able to pay for each additional hamburger produced) also represents the marginal

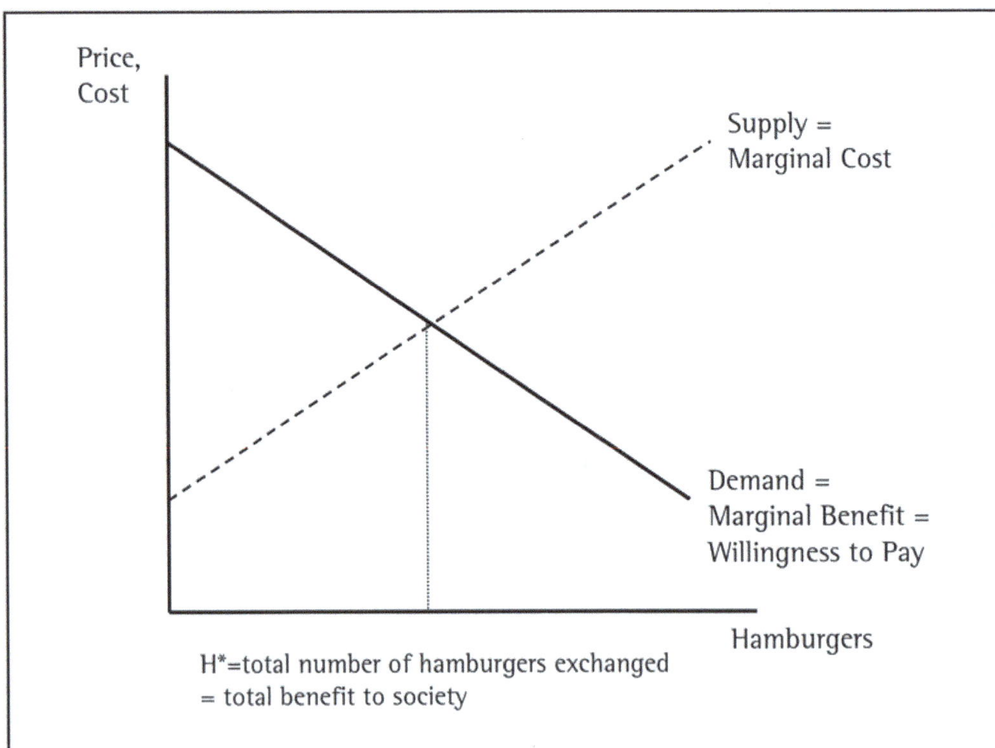

FIGURE 20-1. **Hypothetical market for hamburgers.**

benefit to society from consuming hamburgers. This identity must hold true, because rational agents would only be willing to pay (out of pocket) as much for the last unit they consume as that unit brings them in value. Thus, the area underneath the demand curve for each unit represents the additional benefit that society receives from consuming that unit. The sum of these, up to the total number of hamburgers exchanged (H*), is the total benefit society receives from consuming hamburgers. Similarly, the upward sloping curve represents the supply or marginal cost curve and reflects the fact that because inputs (such as capital and labor) are not perfect substitutes, the opportunity cost of producing each additional hamburger will tend to rise as production increases. The area under the supply curve represents the additional opportunity cost in terms of resources that society must use up in order to produce each additional unit. The sum of these additional costs, up to the total number of hamburgers exchanged, is equal to the total opportunity cost to society from the production of hamburgers.

In standard economic markets, such as those for hamburgers, supply and demand interact to ensure that H* is actually produced, such that society retains as large an excess of total benefit over total opportunity costs. This excess benefit is known as surplus, and maximizing surplus is assured in competitive markets with no intervention. A CBA would simply amount to measuring the total benefit, measuring the total opportunity costs, and subtracting the two from each other to get a measure of surplus. Thus, one can see that a CBA is, in principle, quite simple. The objective is just to measure the surplus represented in Figure 20-1 to ensure that it is positive and to verify that any proposed increases in hamburger production would add to that surplus.

The theoretical foundation of this welfarist approach is based on the idea that each individual is the best judge of their own welfare or well-being. This welfare can be measured by the perceived value of goods and services in terms of the maximum amount they would be willing to pay for them. In the example of the hamburger market, a person will purchase one if they value the hamburger at a rate equal to or more than the price. The simplicity of this transaction negates the need for any sort of formal CBA.

Decisions about healthcare are much more complicated. With widespread health insurance (such that very few people pay for care completely out of pocket), the market demand curve fails to represent the true marginal benefit curve to society. As a result, the area under the demand curve will grossly overstate the true benefits from consumption, and healthcare markets will tend to misallocate resources. This is why economists must step in to attempt to independently measure marginal benefits (in dollar terms), marginal costs, and the difference between the two: the surplus.

MEASURING BENEFITS FROM HEALTH INTERVENTIONS

There has been something of a rebirth in CBA since the early 1990s.[1-4] This rebirth is partly due to the increased attention that economists have paid to educating their clinical brethren about the superior theoretical and conceptual foundations of CBA compared with CEA/CUA. It is clear, for example, that if the perspective of the analysis is society, and if society is seeking to maximize welfare (social surplus), then CBA is the best (if not only) tool.[5]

However, the growth of CBAs has also been spurred by the introduction of contingent valuation methods (primarily from the environmental economics literature), which seek to assign willingness to pay (WTP) for nonmarket goods through the use of survey methods. A number of studies have demonstrated the generality of converting multidimensional preferences into a monetary index of WTP by using "yes/no" or other dichotomous questions.[6] An increasingly popular method for estimating WTP is the discrete choice experiment (DCE). As discussed in Chapter 18, DCEs present individuals with a series of hypothetical scenarios in which they must choose between alternatives that vary in attributes such as effectiveness, side effects, and cost. By analyzing these choices, researchers can infer the relative importance of each attribute and estimate the monetary value that individuals place on specific health outcomes. Discrete choice experiments are particularly useful when valuing complex interventions with multiple dimensions of benefit, and they are gaining traction in both regulatory and health technology assessment settings as a robust tool for preference elicitation. This method asks survey respondents whether they would be willing to pay a specific amount of money out of pocket for access to some treatment, technology, or health outcome. The dollar amount may be fixed, vary across a small number of values, or have unique values for each respondent.[7] Regression techniques are used to relate the "yes/no" answers to the dollar values asked and other characteristics of the respondents. The regression parameters can be used to predict WTP for the intervention in question.

The applications of this technique are broad and growing. For example, WTP methods have been applied to health outcomes, such as the value of reductions in the severity of angina pectoris attacks, avoiding migraine headaches, and avoiding postoperative nausea.[1,5,8,9] Willingness to pay has also been applied to healthcare services, such as preventive medicine, treatment for depression, chemotherapy, and in vitro fertilization.[10-13] It has only been in the past couple of decades that clinical researchers have appeared to fully embrace the method of contingent valuation assessment of WTP as a measure of the dollar value of benefits in health. Cost-benefit analysis may be well on its way to achieving the position of acceptance and even preference that it warrants, given its firm foundation in welfare theory.

HOW TO CONDUCT A CBA

The general approach for a CBA is relatively straightforward, as outlined in Gold et al.[14] Fundamentally, it involves identifying all opportunity costs associated with the intervention in question and comparing them to the dollar value of all benefits that accrue from the intervention. If the dollar values of the benefits exceed the opportunity costs, then the intervention improves social welfare and should be adopted. Conversely, if the opportunity costs exceed the benefits, then social surpluses will be reduced, and the intervention should not be adopted. The process involves five steps:

Step One: Identify All Opportunity Costs

- Identify the direct costs of potential treatment (eg, costs of the intervention, costs of clinical personnel required to provide treatment, costs of supplies associated with treatment).
- Identify indirect costs associated with potential treatment and recovery (eg, value of time lost from work or other activities associated with treatment, costs of ancillary healthcare that must be increased because of treatment).
- Identify expected costs associated with adverse outcomes from treatment (eg, the dollar cost of treatment for some adverse event × the probability of the adverse event occurring during treatment).

Step Two: Identify Clinical Benefits

- Identify changes in the level of morbidity.
  - ◊ Identify changes in primary health indicators (eg, reduction in heart attacks associated with treatment for hypertension).
  - ◊ Identify changes in secondary health indicators (eg, reduction in blood pressure associated with treatment for hypertension).
- Identify changes in life expectancy/mortality.

Step Three: Identify Ancillary Benefits

- Consider whether the treatment will require fewer resources than current practice.
- Consider whether the treatment might save on nonhealth resources compared with current practice.

Step Four: Value All Benefits

- Assign dollar values to all clinical and ancillary benefits, which may involve conducting a WTP study for these benefits.

Step Five: Decision Rule

- As much as possible within existing budget constraints, implement an intervention if the net benefit is positive or its benefit/cost ratio is > 1.

EXAMPLES

This process is illustrated nicely in a study of the costs and benefits of hormone replacement therapy (HRT).[15] In this paper, the author sought to determine whether HRT yields greater benefits to women than the costs of providing the therapy. One interesting aspect of the analysis is that HRT has a wide range of benefits, in that it alleviates a range of menopausal symptoms. The author avoided the need to capture and value each benefit of the therapy individually by implementing a WTP methodology. They simply asked the women who were undergoing HRT to consider all of the benefits they had received and incorporate them into a single WTP measure.

The researchers administered a questionnaire to 104 women in a department of gynecology of a Swedish hospital. The questionnaire contained a contingent valuation question where they were asked whether they would be willing to pay one of eight possible prices. The responses were used in a logit regression to calculate the mean WTP for HRT among the women in the sample. The author found the mean WTP for HRT was approximately SEK 42,000 (roughly $5,314). The actual costs of the therapy were then calculated by summing up the costs of the medication and the office visits required to monitor the therapy. These costs ranged between SEK 1,600 to 2,200 (approximately $202 to $278). Thus, the perceived value of the benefits was significantly more than the cost, implying that social welfare in Sweden was enhanced with the use of HRT.

A second example of a pharmacological CBA focused on intranasal steroids for allergic rhinitis.[16] As in the previous example, given the range of benefits that are derived from alleviating the symptoms of allergic rhinitis, independently assessing clinical benefits and assigning distinct values to these benefits would be a daunting task. Consequently, a WTP method was employed. The authors administered their instrument to 242 patients with an allergic rhinitis diagnosis who had been randomized into one of two treatment arms. Each patient was administered a WTP instrument prior to the trial (where the hypothetical benefits were described). In this case, the patients were asked an open-ended question ("How much would you be willing to pay realistically each week to get rid of your ragweed hay fever and all the problems it brings?"). Patients were asked the same set of questions after completing the clinical trial. Mean WTP was $12.95 per week. Opportunity costs of the therapy were tracked in the study and included the dollar cost of the therapy, the number of unscheduled visits to the study physician and any other physician or clinic, and time off of work due to hay fever symptoms. Average per week opportunity costs were approximately $7.15. Again, because the dollar value of benefits exceeded the dollar value of costs, the therapy in question enhanced social welfare.

BARRIERS TO BENEFIT MEASUREMENT

Measuring benefits satisfactorily has always been the Achilles' heel of CBAs. The main issue is that it is empirically difficult and even conceptually problematic to assign dollar values to the types of benefits (such as improvements in health, avoided deaths, or gains in years of life) that are important in clinical research.[5,17] It is certainly the case that early attempts to assign dollar values to a year of life were weak, often resorting to measuring labor market productivity.

There is now a large literature on revealed preference methods, which infer the value of a health outcome from observed behaviors. These typically value a year of life by examining real-life choices people make in response to incremental changes in the risk of death. They can also value changes in mortality from investments in social programs such as seat belt or airline safety regulation.[18] The use of surveys in contingent valuations has also gained traction. However, WTP measurements, such as those described, may still be susceptible to framing bias. Responses may be sensitive to survey methodology, descriptions of hypothetical/offered scenarios, the ways questions are phrased, and the reference case.

Willingness to pay estimates may also be correlated with ability to pay, leading to results that intrinsically favor the more well-off.

In addition, a growing body of work utilizes contingent valuation methods to assess the value of improvements in health, such as reductions in the severity of angina pectoris or osteoarthritis. These recent advances in the economics literature have somewhat ameliorated the empirical concerns about CBA.

However, a conceptual problem remains. Many clinicians are unwilling to accept the ethical implications of assigning finite, measurable values to human life. To this complaint, one needs only conduct a simple thought experiment. Consider the spectacular wrecks that occasionally occur in auto racing. After the wreckage has come to a stop, it is not unusual to see the driver walking away from the accident unharmed. This raises the question of why we have so many deaths on US highways (where the highest observed speeds are much below that of the average auto race). The answer, of course, is that it simply costs too much to build cars, such as those used in racing for daily use; while it is feasible, there is not a demand for such expensive cars. This means, of course, that individuals regularly trade off an increased risk of death for money (in the form of less expensive cars), implying that nearly no one in the US driving public sets an infinite value on his or her own life. Recognizing that the value each of us places on our own life is not infinite, the conceptual objection collapses, leaving only the empirical problems addressed above.

As mentioned previously, CBAs have been greeted with skepticism largely, because many clinicians and clinical researchers are uncomfortable settling a dollar value on a year of human life.[14] Faced with this insurmountable obstacle to CBAs, clinical researchers have most often resorted to CUAs. However, frequently these CUAs are conducted where there is no comparison option; that is, a single average cost-effectiveness ratio is calculated at something like $75,000 per QALY gained. In the absence of any other information, health services researchers are at a loss. Is $75,000 to save a year of one life in perfect health considered good/reasonable or bad/too expensive? When faced with this position and as mentioned previously in Chapter 19, researchers resort to threshold values, such as asserting that $50,000 per life year saved is definitively "good," that any gain between $50,000 and $100,000 per QALY gained may be good, and that anything greater than $200,000 per life year saved is "bad."[19,20] The astute reader will notice that such analyses are simply poorly conducted CBAs, where the dollar value of a year of life in perfect health is arbitrarily set at $50,000 with certainty and $100,000 with some uncertainty. It is ironic that clinical researchers who would decry the economists' practice of setting a dollar value on life as cold-hearted would resort to this tack, because health economists have long tended to value a year of life somewhere north of $400,000.[20]

CONCLUSION

The healthcare sector is characterized by many barriers to entry which prevent normal market forces from ensuring that resource allocations are efficient and maximize welfare. Consequently, it falls to economists and other health services researchers to calculate the net benefits of treatment and other resource allocation decisions. Because social welfare is theoretically based on the difference between the dollar value of total benefits and the dollar value of total opportunity costs, CBA is considered by many to be the "gold standard" method for health economic evaluations. Cost-benefit analysis involves measuring the value of benefits and subtracting from that the measured value of all costs (direct and indirect) of the decision in question. Since the 1990s, the most widely applied tool for assigning dollar values to benefits has been to estimate patient or social WTP for the therapy in question. Such WTP methods typically involve asking contingent valuation questions (either open ended "how much would you pay" questions, or dichotomous "would you pay a given amount" questions). The value of this approach is that it allows the respondent to incorporate all dimensions of perceived benefit into a single dollar amount. Additionally, the tools of contingent valuation estimation have become increasingly sophisticated. Given the growing acceptance of WTP studies in recent years, the future of CBA in health economic and health services research remains promising.

REFERENCES

1. Johannesson M, Jonsson B, Borgquist L. Willingness to pay for antihypertensive therapy–results of a Swedish pilot study. *J Health Econ*. 1991;10:461-473. https://doi.org/10.1016/0167-6296(91)90025-i
2. Robinson A. No prescription for despair. *Can Med Assoc J*. 1993;149:639-643. PMID: 8364820
3. O'Brien B, Gafni A. When do the "dollars" make sense? Toward a conceptual framework for contingent valuation studies in health care. *Med Decis Making* 1996;16:288-299. https://doi.org/10.1177/0272989X9601600314
4. Diener A, O'Brien B, Gafni A. Health care contingent valuation studies: a review and classification of the literature. *Health Econ*. 1998;7:313-326. https://doi.org/10.1002/(sici)1099-1050(199806)7:4<313::aid-hec350>3.0.co;2-b
5. Kenkel D. On valuing morbidity, CEA, and being rude. *J Health Econ*. 1997;16:749-757. https://doi.org/10.1016/s0167-6296(97)00027-1
6. van der Pol M, Ryan M, Donaldson C. Valuing food safety improvements using willingness to pay. *Appl Health Econ Health Policy*. 2003;2:99-107. PMID: 14619281
7. Bradford W, Kleit AN, Krousel-Wood MA, Re RM. Willingness to pay for telemedicine assessed by the double-bounded dichotomous choice method. *J Telemed Telecare*. 2004;10(6):325-330. https://doi.org/10.1258/1357633042601991
8. Chestnut L, Keller LR, Lambert LE, Rowe RD. Measuring heart patients' willingness to pay for changes in angina symptoms. *Med Decis Making*. 1996;16:65-77. https://doi.org/10.1177/0272989X9601600115
9. Tong A. Clinical guidelines: can they be effective? *Nurs Times*. 2001;97:3-4. PMID: 11954337
10. Corso P, Hammitt JK, Graham JD, et al. Assessing preferences for prevention versus treatment using willingness to pay. *Med Decis Making*. 2002;22:S92-S101. https://doi.org/10.1177/027298902237713
11. O'Brien W, VanEgeren L, Mumby P. Predicting health behaviors using measures of optimism and perceived risk. *Health Values: J Health Behav Ed Promotion*. 1995;19:21-28. https://psycnet.apa.org/record/1995-30557-001
12. Ortega A, Dranitsaris G, Puodziunas A. A clinical and economic evaluation of red blood cell transfusions in patients receiving cancer chemotherapy. *Int J Technol Assess Health Care*. 1998;14:788-798. https://doi.org/10.1017/s0266462300012083
13. Keller E, Botha W, Chambers GM. Does *in vitro* fertilization (IVF) treatment provide good value for money? A cost-benefit analysis. *Front Glob Womens Health*. 2023;4:971553. https://doi.org/10.3389/fgwh.2023.971553
14. Gold M, Siegel JE, Russell LB, Weinstein MC, eds. *Cost-Effectiveness in Health and Medicine*. Oxford: Oxford University Press; 1996.
15. Zethraeus N. Willingness to pay for hormone replacement therapy. *Health Econ*. 1998;7:31-38. https://doi.org/10.1002/(sici)1099-1050(199802)7:1<31::aid-hec316>3.0.co;2-7
16. Keith P, Haddon J, Birch S. A cost-benefit analysis using a willingness-to-pay questionnaire of intranasal budesonide for seasonal allergic rhinitis. *Ann Allergy Asthma Immunol*. 2000;84:55-62. https://doi.org/10.1016/s1081-1206(10)62741-x
17. Vass CM, Payne K. Using discrete choice experiments to inform the benefit-risk assessment of medicines: are we ready yet? *Pharmacoeconomics*. 2017;35(9):859-866. https://doi.org/10.1007/s40273-017-0518-0
18. Viscusi W, Magat W, Scharff R. Asymmetric assessments in valuing pharmaceutical risks. *Med Care*. 1996;34:DS34-47. PMID: 8969313
19. Ubel P, Hirth RA, Chernew ME, Fendrick AM. What is the price of life and why doesn't it increase at the rate of inflation? *Arch Intern Med*. 2003;163:1637-1647. https://doi.org/10.1001/archinte.163.14.1637
20. Hirth R, Chernew ME, Miller E, et al. Willingness to pay for a quality-adjusted life year: in search of a standard. *Med Decis Making*. 2000;20:332-342. https://doi.org/10.1177/0272989X0002000310

GLOSSARY

Accrual accounting: Approach that records revenue when it is earned and expenses when they are incurred, regardless of when cash changes hands.

Alternative hypothesis: The statement for which evidence is sought in a statistical test; if the null hypothesis is rejected, the alternative hypothesis is the conclusion that is supported.

Analysis of variance (ANOVA): A statistical test used to examine differences in means among three or more groups.

Appointment no-show rate: The percentage of scheduled outpatient appointments that patients fail to attend without prior notification.

Artificial intelligence (AI): The field of computer science focused on creating systems that can perform tasks that typically require human intelligence, such as learning, reasoning, problem-solving, and decision-making.

Association: A relationship between two variables where changes in one tend to be related to changes in the other.

Attributable risk (AR): The difference in disease incidence between the exposed and unexposed groups, indicating the excess risk due to the exposure.

Attribute: A feature or characteristic of a medical product—such as efficacy or effectiveness, safety, means of administration, duration of effect, duration of use, or burden on patients or caregivers—that may affect benefit-risk considerations.

Average length of stay (ALOS): The duration of a patient's hospital stay, from admission to discharge.

Bed occupancy rate: The percentage of occupied beds in a hospital over a specific time period.

Bias: A systematic error that leads to an incorrect parameter estimate or an inaccurate prediction.

Bias assessment: Evaluation of the extent to which systematic errors may affect the validity of study results.

Binary variables: A variable that has two possible values, such as "yes or no" or "true or false."

Boolean operators: Logical operators (and, or, not) used to combine search terms in database queries.

Brand reputation: The collective assessment of a healthcare organization's credibility, reliability, and quality, as perceived by patients, staff, stakeholders, and the broader community.

Budget: An estimate of income and expenditures for a fixed period of time.

Budget holder: The audience for or the perspective of the budget, typically a payer, such as a health plan or government body that is responsible for payment.

Case-control study: An observational study where subjects are selected based on the presence (cases) or absence (controls) of a disease, and past exposure to a potential risk factor is compared between the two groups.

Case fatality rate: A measure used to assess the severity of a disease by calculating the proportion of individuals diagnosed with a disease who die from it within a specified time period.

Case report: A detailed report of the symptoms, diagnosis, treatment, and follow-up of an individual patient, often used to highlight novel or unusual occurrences.

Case series: A collection of case reports involving patients who were given similar treatment or have similar characteristics, used to identify patterns and generate hypotheses.

Cash accounting: Records revenue and expenses at the time cash changes hands, regardless of when services were provided.

DOI: 10.37573/9781585287666.BM

Categorical (nominal) variables: Variables that have at least two categories without any intrinsic ordering.

Causal diagram: A graphic representation of causal relationships between factors.

Charge (list price): The amount a healthcare provider sets/bills for services rendered before any discounts or adjustments.

Charity care: A type of discount to charges that the provider billed for services provided to a patient later deemed not able to pay.

Chi-square test: A statistical test used to examine associations between two variables when the data are nominal categories (ie, smoker/nonsmoker and hypertension [yes/no]).

Clinical outcomes: Measurable changes in health, function, or quality of life that result from a patient's medical care or treatment.

Cohort study: An observational study where a group of disease-free individuals is followed over time to assess the incidence of disease based on their exposure status.

Collinearity: A situation in which independent or predictor variables are highly linearly related.

Complete case analysis: A method for handling missing data by including only those observations (cases) that have no missing values for any of the variables required in the analysis.

Confidence intervals: Defines boundaries within which the true population parameter is likely to fall, most often calculated at the 95% confidence interval.

Confounder: A third variable that distorts the apparent relationship between an exposure (independent variable) and an outcome (dependent variable), because it is associated with both but is not on the causal pathway between the two.

Confounding: A situation in which the observed association between an exposure and an outcome is distorted by the presence of another variable related to both.

Contingent valuation method: A method to assign willingness to pay values for nonmarket goods using survey methods.

Continuous variables: Variables with numerical values that can assume any value in a specified range.

Contractual adjustments: A type of discount to charges that is negotiated with a payer.

Control group: A group of subjects in a study who do not have the disease or outcome of interest and are used as a comparison to the case group.

Correlation analysis: Measurement of the strength and direction of the relationship between two or more variables without implying causation.

Cost: The total dollar value assigned to resources used to sell a product or provide a resource.

Cost-benefit analysis (CBA): A decision-making framework that compares the monetary value of benefits to the monetary value of costs of an intervention.

Cost-effectiveness analysis (CEA): Technique used to compare the cost and consequences of treatment alternatives that have a common nonmonetary outcome.

Cost-effectiveness ratio: A measure of economic efficiency calculated by dividing the cost of treatment by a nonmonetary outcome, such as years of life saved or cases prevented.

Cost-effectiveness threshold: A benchmark value (often expressed in cost per QALY) used to determine whether a health intervention provides good value for money.

Cost per patient visit: The average cost incurred by the healthcare organization for each outpatient visit.

Cost-utility analysis (CUA): A type of economic evaluation that compares the costs and health outcomes of different interventions, with outcomes measured in terms of utility, typically using QALYs.

Critical success factors (CSFs): Essential areas of activity that must be performed well for an organization to achieve its mission.

Cross-sectional study: A study that analyzes data from a population at a specific point in time to determine the prevalence of an outcome or condition, without establishing causality or temporal sequence.

Daily census: The number of hospital inpatients present at a specific time of the day.

Data extraction: The process of systematically collecting information from included studies for analysis.

Data interoperability: The ability of different IT systems to communicate, exchange, and use data effectively.

Days at home: A metric tracking the number of days that patients spend at home as opposed to in healthcare facilities.

Days not in hospital: The total number of days patients remain out of the hospital during a specified period.

Days of therapy avoided: The total number of days a patient would have received a specific medication (often antibiotics or high-cost drugs) but did not owing to appropriate discontinuation, dose adjustment, or substitution based on clinical judgment.

Decision tree model: A sequence of treatment decisions and probabilistic health outcomes over time in a series of chance and decision nodes.

Demand (marginal benefit curve): The maximum amount that consumers are willing and able to pay for each additional unit of product produced.

Dependent variable: Outcome variable, or the one that is to be predicted or explained.

Descriptive statistics: The act of summarizing data into a useful form for understanding the study sample, including measures of central tendency (mean, median, and mode) and measures of variability (standard deviation, standard error of the mean, and range).

Difference-in-differences: A design that measures trends in outcomes over time and subtracts the differences between treatment groups to estimate the causal effect of a treatment.

Direct cost: The immediate, out-of-pocket expenses directly associated with a health intervention, such as medical supplies, clinical personnel, medications, and facility use required to deliver the treatment.

Discounting: Technique used to adjust future costs and consequences to current dollars; used to account for the time value of money.

Discrete choice experiment (DCE): A survey-based method used to elicit preferences by asking individuals to choose between hypothetical alternatives that differ in attributes, such as effectiveness, side effects, and cost.

Discrete variables: Variables that can take on only a finite number of distinct values.

Distributional CEA: Analysis that combines the objectives of maximizing health and minimizing unfair variation in health when evaluating population health interventions.

Ecologic fallacy: The incorrect assumption that relationships observed for groups necessarily hold for individuals within those groups.

Ecologic study: The relationship between exposure and disease at the group or population level rather than the individual level.

Effectiveness: Effects of treatment under real-world, everyday practice conditions.

Efficacy: Effects of a treatment under the controlled conditions of a clinical trial.

Efficiency: Output or outcome achieved at the lowest possible cost.

Electronic health record (EHR): A collection of electronically stored patient medical information that can be accessed and communicated digitally.

Eligible population: The population of individuals who are eligible to receive the intervention of interest within the jurisdiction of the healthcare budget holder.

Emergency department (ED) utilization rate: Measurement of how frequently a population uses ED services over a specific period, typically expressed per 1,000 individuals per year.

Endpoints: The specific outcomes measured in a study to assess the effect of an intervention, which may be qualitative or quantitative.

Expense: The cost attributed to service provision for a particular period of time (the reporting period).

External validity: The extent to which the results of a study can be generalized to other people, settings, and situations.

Fisher's exact test: A statistical test used instead of a chi-square test when any cell in the matrix has an expected frequency of less than 5 and the sample is between 20 and 40.

Fixed cost: A cost that occurs no matter how often it is used to generate revenue (eg, a building payment).

Flowchart: A diagram representing the systematic review process used to illustrate the study selection pathway.

Forest plot: A method of visualizing the results of a meta-analysis that includes the effects from individual studies and the pooled effects.

Generalized estimating equation (GEE) model: Method used for analyzing correlated data—such as repeated measures, clustered data, or longitudinal data—where observations within the same group or subject are not independent.

Generalized linear models (GLMs): A broad class of statistical models that extend linear models to nonlinear relationships, accommodating a wide variety of outcome distributions.

Governance and strategy: The system of leadership, policies, structures, and oversight used by boards and senior management to ensure accountability, transparency, ethical conduct, and effective performance.

Gross charge: The total amount billed (not collected) for services before any contractual allowances or discounts.

Health technology assessment (HTA): Evaluations of the clinical effectiveness, cost-effectiveness, and broader social and ethical implications of health interventions to inform decision-making.

Hospital-acquired infection (HAI) rate: The rate of infections acquired during hospital stays, often measured per 1,000 patient days.

Hypothesis testing: The statistical act of comparing the null and alternative hypotheses to determine whether there is a significant effect on the outcome.

Incidence: The rate at which new cases of a disease occur in a population at risk over a specified time period.

Incident population: The population newly eligible for the intervention of interest in a specific time period.

Incremental cost-effectiveness ratio (ICER): A metric used to assess the additional cost per additional unit of health benefit (usually per QALY) when comparing two interventions.

Independent variable: The predictor variable that might influence or be associated with the outcome (dependent) variable.

Indirect cost: A cost that supports multiple products or services and is not directly attributable to a single product or service (eg, the cost of the electricity used for a surgery).

Inference: A conclusion reached on the basis of evidence and reasoning.

Inferential statistics: Statistics used to make inferences about a population from a sample.

Instrumental variable: A predictor for getting the treatment that has no effect on outcomes and is used to mimic random assignment with observational data.

Integrating advanced technology: The adoption and implementation of innovative digital tools and systems to enhance clinical care, operational efficiency, patient safety, and health outcomes.

Interaction: A situation where the effect of one variable on the dependent variable differs based on the level of another variable.

Internal validity: Confidence that an observed effect is truly due to the intervention and not other factors.

Interquartile range: The interval between the 25th and 75th percentile values, so a measure of variability directly related to the median.

Interrupted time series: A longitudinal design used to measure differences in outcomes before and after an intervention.

Intervention: A new or existing pharmaceutical, vaccine, medical device, diagnostic, surgical approach, digital application, or anything else that may be used to support the medical treatment of a patient.

Intervention mix: A group of interventions that are being used by the population of interest.

Inverse probability weighting: Use of patient demographics and other nontreatment variables in a logistic regression to estimate the probability for both treated and untreated patients being in the treated group; these probabilities are then used as weights in the outcome analyses.

Key performance indicators (KPIs): Quantifiable measures used to evaluate organizational success.

Lead time: The period between early detection of disease and the time of its usual clinical presentation.

League table: A ranked list of health interventions based on their ICERs used to compare the relative cost-effectiveness of multiple options.

Length of stay (LOS): The duration of a patient's hospital stay from admission to discharge.

Linear model: A linear (straight line) relationship between one or more independent variables and a dependent variable.

Linkage variable: Variable that predicts critical outcomes or specific levels of resource use in modeling.

Logistic regression: Statistical method used for modeling the relationship between a set of independent variables and a binary dependent variable with two possible outcomes, usually coded as 0 and 1.

Longitudinal study: A research design that involves repeated observations or measurements of the same individuals or groups over an extended period of time.

Machine learning: A type of artificial intelligence that enables systems to learn from data and make predictions or decisions without being explicitly programmed.

Mann-Whitney *U* test (or Wilcoxon rank-sum test): A nonparametric test used to compare differences between two independent groups when the data are ordinal or continuous but not normally distributed.

Mantel-Haenszel chi-square test: A variant of the chi-square test that is used to compare nominal data from independent samples, while controlling for the effect of a confounder.

Markov model: The natural history of disease as a sequence of mutually exclusive health states, defined to capture important clinical traits, such as acute event history.

Maximum acceptable risk (MAR): The greatest increase in probability or magnitude of a harm that a patient would accept to achieve or realize a given benefit.

Mean: The arithmetic average of individual data points; the sum of all data points divided by the number of data points.

Measures of variability: The variability or spread of the data, including standard deviation, standard error of the mean, range, and interquartile range.

Median: Value above (or below) which half of the data points fall, the 50th percentile value of a distribution.

Mediator: A variable that helps to explain how an independent variable (predictor) influences a dependent variable (outcome) as an intermediate step in the causal chain between the two.

Medication reconciliation rate: The percentage of patients who receive medication reconciliation during outpatient visits.

Meta-analysis: A quantitative method that combines results from studies included in a systematic review to assess the pooled effect.

Missing at random (MAR): A missing data mechanism in which the probability of a value being missing depends on observed data but not on the missing data itself.

Missing completely at random (MCAR): Missingness is not related to any observed or unobserved data, so a complete case analysis will produce unbiased estimates.

Missing not at random (MNAR): The probability of missingness that depends on the value of the missing data itself.

Mixed-effects model (or mixed model): A regression model that includes both fixed effects (parameters that apply to the entire population) and random effects (parameters that vary by subject or other units, such as hospitals).

Mode: The most commonly reported value in the dataset.

Moderator: A variable that influences the strength or direction of the relationship between the intervention and the outcome measure.

Mortality rate: A measure of the frequency of occurrence of death in a defined population during a specified time period.

Multivariable model: A model that simultaneously analyzes the relationship between multiple independent variables and a dependent variable.

Multivariate analysis: A specialized model that involves analyzing more than one dependent variable simultaneously to understand relationships among multiple outcomes.

Narrative synthesis: A method of summarizing the findings of included studies without conducting statistical analyses (ie, not a meta-analysis).

Net patient revenue (NPR): The amount recognized as revenue collected for services rendered, equal to gross charges minus all contractual allowances and discounts.

90-day risk-standardized home time: The number of days patients spend at home the first 90 days postdischarge.

Nonlinear model: A type of model where the relationship between the independent variables (predictors) and the dependent variable (outcome) is not linear.

Nonparametric tests: Statistical tests used when the data do not meet conditions for a parametric test, such as when the data are not normally distributed, contain ordinal data, have small sample sizes, or contain outliers.

Normal distribution: A probability distribution where data are symmetric and bell-shaped about the mean.

Null hypothesis: The idea that there is no relationship, difference, or effect between the independent and dependent variables being studied.

Number needed to treat (NNT): The number of patients who need to be treated to prevent one additional adverse outcome, calculated as the inverse of the absolute risk reduction.

Odds ratio (OR): A measure of association in case-control studies that compares the odds of exposure among cases to the odds of exposure among controls.

Operational excellence: The systematic execution of processes and continuous improvement efforts to achieve sustainable, high-quality performance in cost, efficiency, safety, and patient satisfaction.

Ordinal variables: Variables that are measured with a natural order.

Ordinary least squares regression: A fundamental statistical method used to estimate the linear relationship between one dependent variable and one or more independent (predictor) variables.

***P*-value:** The probability of obtaining the observed difference between treatments in a study if there is no "real" difference between treatments in the larger population of interest.

Parameters: Measurements that describe a population.

Parametric tests: Generally more powerful than nonparametric tests and used when data meet several conditions: (1) they follow or nearly follow a normal distribution, (2) variability of the data are approximately equal between groups, (3) measures of patient response are independent and unrelated, and (4) data are continuous.

Patient satisfaction: Measurement of the degree to which patients are content with the healthcare they received, including their interactions with providers, the quality of care, and the overall experience within the healthcare system.

Patient satisfaction score: Metrics derived from patient surveys assessing patient experiences and patient care satisfaction.

Penalized regression: Set of regression techniques that add a penalty term to the linear regression loss function to discourage overly complex models.

Pooling: Combination of the results of many studies into one dataset.

Population: The entire group of individuals, events, or elements that share a common characteristic and from which data may be collected to answer a specific research question.

Power: The probability that a statistical test will detect a true effect or difference when one actually exists—the probability of avoiding a Type II error (false negative).

Preferences: Qualitative or quantitative expressions of how individuals value or prioritize different health outcomes, interventions, or attributes when faced with alternative options.

Prevalent population: The population eligible for the intervention of interest at a particular point in time.

Profit: The excess of revenue over expenses in a reporting period.

Propensity score matching: A technique that relies on patient demographics and other non-treatment variables in a logistic regression to estimate the probability for treatment as a way to mimic randomization between groups.

Proportionate mortality: The percentage of total deaths in a population that are attributable to a particular cause.

Prospective cohort study: A cohort study in which participants are followed into the future from the point of exposure to observe outcomes.

Quality-adjusted life-year (QALY): A measure that combines life expectancy with quality of life.

Quasi-experimental design (QED): A study design that aims to measure causation without the random assignment of participants to treatments.

Random error: A term used in linear regression to account for random variations in the data.

Range: The difference between the largest and the smallest values in the distribution.

Readmission rate: The proportion of patients who return to a hospital for unplanned inpatient care within a defined period (commonly 30 days) of their previous hospital discharge.

Real-world data (RWD): Data relating to patient health status and/or the delivery of healthcare routinely collected from a variety of sources.

Real-world evidence (RWE): The clinical evidence regarding a medical product's use and potential benefits or risks derived from analysis of real-world data (RWD).

Regression: Method used to model and analyze the relationship between a dependent variable (outcome) and one or more independent variables (predictors or explanatory variables).

Regression discontinuity design: A cutoff value for a continuous variable whose measurement cannot be manipulated to estimate causal effect size based on the difference between patients just below and above the cutoff.

Relative risk (RR): A measure of association in cohort studies that compares the risk of disease in the exposed group to the risk in the unexposed group.

Retrospective cohort study: A cohort study that uses existing records to identify exposure and outcome status, with both having occurred before the study begins.

Revenue: The amount of money collected for services.

Sample: A subset of members drawn from a defined population under study.

Selection bias: Differences in baseline characteristics between treated and untreated groups—unrelated to the treatment itself—that affect the likelihood of the outcome, leading to distorted or misleading results.

Semivariable (mixed) cost: A cost that typically begins with a base, fixed amount and then has a variable cost component for each use (eg, base subscription cost to access a resource that is accompanied by a per use variable cost).

Sensitivity analysis: A model's response to variations in the levels of parameters of variables included by answering the "what if" questions.

Standard deviation (SD): The spread of individual measurements about the sample mean to quantify variability.

Standard error of the mean (SEM): Statistic computed from the standard deviation as a measure of precision, quantifying the uncertainty in the estimate of the mean.

Statistical model: A mathematical framework that represents the relationships between variables using probability.

Statistics: The science of collecting, analyzing, interpreting, and presenting data to support decision-making and draw conclusions.

Step cost: A cost that is fixed within a range of some volume of services provided but then steps up to a new level of fixed costs within the next range of volume of services provided or units sold.

Survival analysis: Statistical procedure used when investigators are interested in evaluating the time to the event of interest in study subjects, adjusting for the fact that subjects are followed for differing lengths of time.

Systematic literature review: A structured, comprehensive approach to synthesizing research on a specific question.

Time-driven activity-based costing (TDABC): A micro-costing methodology that assigns a cost to products and services based on the amount of time the resource is used to perform an activity for a specific patient.

Time-to-event analysis: Also called survival analysis, a branch of statistics involving outcomes that involve both an event's occurrence and the time needed to reach that event.

Time to first appointment: The average time a patient receives the first outpatient appointment after a referral or request.

30-day readmission rate: The percentage of patients readmitted to the hospital within 30 days.

Type I error: An error that occurs when one falsely rejects the null hypothesis when it is true, concluding that a significant difference exists between groups when it does not.

Type II error: An error that occurs when one fails to reject the null hypothesis when the alternative hypothesis is true, falsely concluding that no significant difference exists between groups when a true difference does exist.

Univariate analysis: The analysis of a single variable to summarize and find patterns in its distribution, such as central tendency or variability.

Utility: A numerical value (typically between 0 and 1) representing the preference or value individuals place on a specific health state, where 0 is equivalent to death and 1 is perfect health.

Value-based metrics: Tools focusing on patient outcomes relative to healthcare costs.

Variable: A characteristic that is being observed or measured.

Variance: The spread of the data, measuring how far each value in the dataset is from the mean on average.

Willingness to pay (WTP): The maximum amount an individual is willing to pay for a good or service, used to assign monetary value to benefits in a CBA.

Zero-inflated data analysis: Statistical methods designed to handle datasets with an excessive number of zero values.

INDEX

A

B

C

DOI: 10.37573/9781585287666.INDEX

D

E

F

G

H

I

J

K

L

M

N

O

P

Q

R

S

T

U

FSC
www.fsc.org
MIX
Papier | Fördert gute Waldnutzung
FSC® C083411

Kolibri 360 GmbH
Ferdinand-Jühlke-Straße 7
99095 Erfurt, Deutschland
produktsicherheit@kolibri360.de